Health & Fitness
in
Plain English™

Jolie Bookspan, Ph.D.

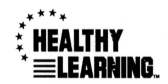

Including

• *Exercise* (everything that works and doesn't—in and out of the gym)

• *Health* (heart, bones, cholesterol, body fat, and weight loss)

• *Vitamins, Health Foods, Nutrition, and Diets*

• *Back Pain, Knee Pain, Headaches, Leg Cramps, Ankle Sprains, and Foot Pain*

• *Fun Facts,* plus an *A-Z Glossary*

ISBN: 1-58518-642-2
Library of Congress Control Number: 2002104557

Book design: Jeanne Hamilton
Cover design: Karen McGuire
Illustrations: Todd Sargood

Healthy Learning
P.O. Box 1828
Monterey, CA 93942
www.healthylearning.com
Fax: (831) 372-6075
Tel: (831) 372-6077

Dedication

To Grandmom, who got her college degree at age 81.

To her, the highest things in life were education and Jack LaLane.

To my wonderful husband and hero, Paul, who listens to me and tries all my ideas.

The Surgeon General

Has Determined

That Lack of Physical Activity

Is Detrimental

to Your Health

— Surgeon General's Report on
Physical Activity and Health, July 1996

Table of Contents

DEDICATION 3

REVIEWERS 6

PREFACE 7

PART I – EXERCISE 9

1. Why Should You Get in Shape?.. 10
2. The Different Aspects of Fitness 18
3. Improving Your Fitness 24
4. What Does "Aerobic" Really Mean? 36
5. What Does "Warm-Up" Really Mean? 49
6. Stretching and the Eight Great Stretching Mistakes 54
7. Abdominal Muscles—Why You Need Good Ones,
   and How to Get Them 68
8. What Exercises Do You Need to Be Fit? 83
9. Good and Bad Exercises 106
10. Just Overdo It and What to Do When You Do Too Much 127
11. Getting Out of Shape and How to Avoid It 136
12. Exercise Gimmicks 141
13. How to Get Started Getting in Shape 144

PART II – NUTRITION 149

14. Nutrition Myths... 150
15. Calculating Food Fat 159
16. Sport Drinks 169
17. Ergogenic Aids—Does Physical Enhancement Await on Your Plate?............... 175
18. Healthy Eating 189
19. How to Lose Weight Without Dieting 203

PART III – HEALTH 215

20. Back and Neck Pain—Why?.. 216
21. Back and Neck Pain—Prevention and Treatment 234
22. Calcium, Protein, Space Flight, Exercise,
    and Your Bones—A Detective Story 264
23. Body Fat—It's Not All Bad 281
24. Problems of Being Overweight... 284
25. Body Fat—How to Tell How Much You've Got.................... 287
26. What to Do About the Shape You're In 293
27. Cardiovascular Disease... 300
28. Good and Bad Cholesterol Explained 310
29. Headaches... 316
30. Leg Cramps and What to Do About Them 326
31. Funny Physical Facts and Foibles... 333

GLOSSARY 341

ABOUT THE AUTHOR 363

Reviewers

Sincere thanks to the following individuals who reviewed this book:

Alan Berg, Ph.D., M.D., *Housecall Doctor. Philadelphia, Pennsylvania*

Russ Gazzara, Ph.D., *Developmental Neurotoxicologist, National Center for Toxicological Research, FDA. Little Rock, Arkansas*

Green Beret Lt. Col. R. Kelly Hill, M.D., *Our Lady of the Lake Regional Medical Center. Baton Rouge, Louisiana.*

David Hsu, Ph.D., M.D., *Department of Neurology, Stanford University Hospital. Stanford, California*

David Josephson, *Josephson Engineering. San Jose, California*

David Koeppel, *Writer, Film Editor, Paramount Pictures. Hollywood, California*

Larry "Scoots" Miller, Ph.D., *Microbiologist. Seattle, Washington*

Alan Moore, M.D., *Board Certified, Obstetrics Gynecology, and Family Medicine. The Woodlands, Texas (osteoporosis chapter)*

Rich Ruoti, Ph.D., P.T., P.C., *BuxMont Physical Therapy. Warminster, Pennsylvania (back pain chapters)*

Audrey Tannenbaum, M.Ed., A.T.C., C.S.C.S., *Athletic Trainer and Maccabean Games Triathlon Gold Medalist. Horsham, Pennsylvania*

Marla Tonseth, M.B.A., P.T., *Physical Therapist, Private Practice. Warrington, Pennsylvania (back pain chapters)*

William B. Young, M.D., *Jefferson Headache Center, Thomas Jefferson University Hospital. Philadelphia, Pennsylvania (headache chapter)*

Preface

Finally. A book on health, nutrition, and fitness, all together, and written in plain English. This book is for everyone, regardless of physical condition or academic background.

Topics in each chapter were selected from questions people ask most frequently. In nontechnical language, this book puts solid information in the place of myths; details hundreds of fun, upbeat ideas for exercise, health, and nutrition; explains the mysterious terminology of fitness; and gives practical, step-by-step suggestions for healthier living. It's all here, from how to lose weight; to what to do about back pain, neck pain, knee pain, headaches, osteoporosis, and leg cramps; to what do good and bad cholesterol mean, and how you can control your own levels. There are answers to those fun little questions about our bodies that everyone wonders about, like why does your foot fall asleep? Why do your joints crackle and pop? Why does it hurt so much to ding your funny bone? At the end of the book, there is a large, annotated glossary. More than a handy reference of definitions, it includes word derivations, key concepts, and fun stories behind the people and information.

With the information in this book, you will be better equipped to make sense of the many claims and counterclaims in exercise, health, and nutrition. You will learn how to get more active and healthy as part of your real life, not just in a gym. You will be able to make informed decisions about your health. You'll even have fun!

Part I

EXERCISE

*A vigorous five-mile walk will do more good for an unhappy
but otherwise healthy adult than all the medicine and
psychology in the world.*

– Paul Dudley White

1. Why Should You Get in Shape?
2. The Different Aspects of Fitness
3. Improving Your Fitness
4. What Does "Aerobic" Really Mean?
5. What Does "Warm-Up" Really Mean?
6. Stretching and the Eight Great Stretching Mistakes
7. Abdominal Muscles—Why You Need Good Ones,
    and How to Get Them
8. What Exercises Do You Need to Be Fit?
9. Good and Bad Exercises
10. Just Overdo It and What to Do
    When You Do Too Much
11. Getting Out of Shape and How to Avoid It
12. Exercise Gimmicks
13. How to Get Started Getting in Shape

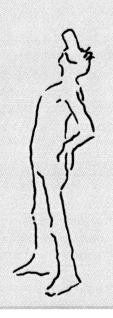

1

Why Should You Get in Shape?

*I don't exercise. What's in it for me? You've got to offer me
more than my life to get me on a StairMaster grunting for two
hours. I view my body as a way of getting my head from one
place to another.*

— Dave Thomas

Good physical condition is important for everyone. This is true even if you are
not an athlete. Good fitness reduces your risk of many serious diseases, delays
several common effects of aging, increases your tolerance to heat and cold, increases
muscle, and reduces fat. Regular exercise, and the wellness it brings, helps you
cope with stress and feel better in general. Good physical fitness can improve your
safety and comfort during your daily life and recreational activities, and preserve
your mobility and independence. How is this all so?

Better Health

An active lifestyle makes major positive changes in your health and well-being.
Common Western ills, such as heart and blood vessel disease, obesity, some types
of diabetes, and many musculoskeletal problems, are known as *hypokinetic* diseases
(*hypo-* means "less than" or "not enough," and *kinetic* means "activity"). Hypokinetic
disease is a fancy term for illness related to, or even caused by, being sedentary and
out of shape.

- Epidemiologic studies suggest that regular exercise lowers incidence of breast cancer in women, and colon and reproductive tract cancer risk in both men and women.

- Resistance exercise thickens bones, important in osteoporosis prevention (Chapter 22).

- Cardiovascular fitness through aerobic exercise reduces your risk of early death from vascular disease, heart disease, and high blood pressure, all major killers of both men and women (Chapter 27).

- Sudden death from heart attack is more common in an out-of-shape person who exerts past capacity than in those who regularly exercise.

Delayed Aging

Although your chronological years increase, you can become functionally younger with exercise. It's difficult to separate the toll of aging from just sitting around too much. Still, getting slower and weaker as years pass is not solely an inescapable aging process. To varying degrees, it comes from not enough activity.

Your body functions decline predictably, both with aging and without enough physical activity.

- As years pass without exercise, your muscular strength, speed, and power all drop off sharply.

- After about age 30, the deterioration would run about 0.75% to 1% per year if you didn't exercise regularly.

- The maximum amount of oxygen your body can use to make energy, an important indicator of fitness, would drop about 10% each decade from ages 20 to 60.

- Without flexibility exercises, joints tighten with passing years until ordinary reaching and bending can become difficult and, in many cases, impossible.

- Being inactive or injured diminishes your sense of balance. Fear of falling, or the real falls that result, often keep a person from further outings or activity. A vicious cycle of inactivity, deconditioning, and ever-decreasing balance can leave you housebound, even chairbound.

Regular exercise, stretching, and balance practice considerably slow, even reverse, all this loss, meaning gains equivalent to stopping or reversing years of aging. Older people who exercise, move, balance, and stretch have many of the functional characteristics of a chronologically younger person. They can reach, bend, and move easily. They can negotiate uneven sidewalks and other terrain. They can carry their own packages, go out, and have fun. The anti-aging effect of exercise is possible for all age groups. Geriatric populations on exercise programs considerably improve strength and mobility. Often, physical gains are enough to remove their need for walkers, wheelchairs, and canes. They improve self-sufficiency so much that, once again, they can carry out their own activities of daily living. All from regular exercise.

Fewer, Less Serious Injuries

Better physical fitness may lower your risk of joint injury during regular physical activity. Pushing beyond capacity, which is easy to do when you don't have much capacity to begin with, can easily lead to pain and overuse injuries. Lt. Col. Bruce H. Jones, M.D., Chief of the Occupational Medicine Division of the U.S. Army Research Institute of Environmental Medicine, reported on data from army recruits. He found that those of lower physical fitness had consistently higher injury rate than those of higher fitness.

Good flexibility seems to be important to reduce injuries. A tight-jointed exerciser may have a higher incidence of muscle pulls and strains. Tight shoulders strain when reaching overhead. To facilitate reaching with tight shoulders, people often arch their backs, throwing their body weight plus what they lift right onto their low backs. Someone with tight back muscles is back pain waiting to happen. Tight hips and backs can make you unable to sit up straight. The resulting rounded back pressures discs to degenerate and move outward. Muscle tightness pulls you into round-shouldered poor posture and makes standing up properly feel unnatural. Although men usually have less natural flexibility than women, particularly of the lower extremities where injury rates are high, they can attain healthful flexibility with regular stretching. It is not the case that having big muscles or lifting weights reduces flexibility; lack of stretching reduces flexibility. More on flexibility in Chapter 6.

Good balance skills decrease risk of falls, near-falls, slips, and all the injuries that come with them. Instead of training balance, people often stop activity, which further decreases balance and other physical abilities. Practicing balance restores independence, improves fitness and mobility, and allows more activity with less chance of injury from falling or dropping things during a slip.

Everyone needs physical exercise for general health and injury prevention. Without it, a vicious cycle of inactivity and injury grows. If you are sedentary, begin to become more active, working within your safety and comfort zone to make activity a lifetime habit, rather than a chore to endure and avoid.

Positive Mood

Regular exercise is thought to affect your mood positively in several ways.

- In the short term, a vigorously exercising body is thought to manufacture a class of hormones called endorphins, although specifics are not established. The word *endorphin* is a contraction of "endogenous (made from within) morphine-like substance." It's not definitely known, but feasible, that endorphins improve mood after hard workouts by releasing chemicals that stimulate your brain's pleasure center.

- In the long term, exercise increases your overall fitness so that you can do things you enjoy more often and more comfortably.

- Regular exercise is established to reduce premenstrual symptoms and cramping during menses.

- Regular exercise helps decrease moodiness and sugar cravings that often strike in the late afternoons, by increasing insulin sensitivity. That means less insulin mobilizes to process a given load of carbohydrate. This seems to be the case no matter what time of day you exercise, as long as you exercise regularly. Your blood sugar maintains a steadier level, reducing the swings that produce food cravings and moodiness.

- Regular exercise seems to be associated with reduced symptoms of depression and anxiety.

- Greater physical ability, body awareness, and improved body shape and health with exercise might also make you happy. Overall, the specifics of how exercise improves your emotional state are not clearly mapped. Still, there is evidence for a relationship between long-term exercising and increased feeling of well-being and ability to face emotional stress.

Reduced Fatigue

It may seem backward that exercising makes you less tired, while not exercising leaves you tired, but exercise works to reduce your overall levels of fatigue.

- The out-of-shape body doesn't use oxygen efficiently. When your body can't supply the oxygen your muscles demand, you tire easily doing ordinary activities.

- Out-of-shape muscles find simple tasks tiring, while strong muscles can easily accomplish them.

- Weak, out-of-shape muscles can't do the work to hold your posture all day. They give up, leaving you slumped, achy, and "out of gas."

- Regular exercise raises your body's level of physical "readiness," making you feel energetic.

- Regular exercise makes many physical changes in your body, including more blood volume and oxygen-carrying blood cells; more blood vessels to carry the blood; blood vessels that are less clogged with fatty deposits; better strength and tone of your various body parts; and other changes that make you feel vital and energetic.

A vicious cycle occurs when you are too out-of-shape to exercise enough to get much exercise benefit. Sitting around makes you tired and weak, which reduces your ability and inclination to exercise.

A positive cycle comes when you stick with an exercise program until you become accustomed to regular exercise, and can exercise hard enough to make gains, which, in turn, allows you to do more and feel better and more energetic.

> A brisk walk or other short exercise can
> "pick you up" more than a candy bar.

Better Tolerance to Heat

Exercise in the heat has been described as probably the single greatest stress on the human cardiovascular system. When you improve your physical fitness, your body makes changes that improve your ability to tolerate heat and do activity in the heat.

Blood supply to your heart and limb muscles is crucial for you to move around. You also need to shunt blood to your skin to take heat away from your body to cool you. Because there is only a finite amount of blood to go around, competition develops.

- A fitter person has more total body fluid volume, including blood volume, and can pump more blood with each heartbeat.

- The fitter person can supply blood to muscles for movement and skin for cooling, without running short for either one.

- Fitter people increase how much they can sweat for cooling.

- With increased fluids to go around for cooling, body core temperature will not rise as high at the same exercise intensity as in an out-of-shape person.

- The out-of-shape person has less cooling capacity and decreased ability to do activities safely in the heat.

More than any other factor, physical fitness reduces your susceptibility to overheating. If you get out of shape again, you lose your adaptations. Improved fitness, and the improved heat tolerance that comes with it, is not only for athletes who exercise in the heat, but for everyone who spends any time in the heat.

Better Tolerance to Cold

Physical fitness improves tolerance to exercise in cold environments, although to a lesser extent than in heat. Even so, the structural and metabolic changes that occur with regular exercise appear to keep you warmer in the cold.

- Increased muscle mass, which you get through resistance exercise, increases heat production and storage.

- A fit person can do more exercise to keep warm in the cold.

- A fit person tolerates a lower body temperature than an unfit person before shivering starts.

Exercise in the cold improves your cold tolerance much more than exercise alone.

Recreational Fun and Safety

A high degree of muscular strength, cardiovascular endurance, and muscular endurance positively affects your capacity for exertion, common to many activities you enjoy for sport and health. You need your exercise reserves for extended efforts like long runs, roller blading, biking, and swimming; and for shorter, more intense efforts, like a few hard matches of tennis, moving furniture, doing home repair, the changing demands of a weekend hike, carrying groceries and kids, or doing household chores.

- Someone with high cardiovascular capacity can more easily run, hike, bike, skate, dance, or swim a distance that is difficult for someone with less cardiovascular adaptation.

- Better fitness makes daily chores around the house and yard easier.

- Fitter people perceive less exertion at the same exercise intensity so they can do more before pooping out. They carry more, lift more, and move more, all without feeling tired.

- Fitter people are less likely to have heart trouble during activities.

Being in good condition may make the difference between a difficult situation and an easy jaunt.

Fat Loss

Exercise burns calories so you can lose weight, or even eat more without gaining weight. Regular exercise burns fat and shifts your body to a mode where it burns more fat for fuel in general and during exercise. When your body preferentially burns fat, it extends the supply of the carbohydrates stored in your muscles and liver, thereby extending your exercise capacity.

Getting "In Shape" vs. Getting Healthy

You hear all the confusing recommendations—some sources say you need five days a week of hard exercise, others claim you need only three days a week of moderate exercise. The answer is simple. Different levels of exercise will give you different levels of results. Mild to moderate exercise three days a week will begin to improve your health. Your disease risks will begin to go down, and you will start feeling and looking better. Exercising more vigorously and more often makes bigger changes. This does not mean you have to kill yourself. Overdoing exercise will not get you much more gain than regular, vigorous exercise, but it increases your risk of injury.

> The Surgeon General's Report on Physical Activity and Health, released in 1996, defines moderate exercise as using about 150 calories per day, or 1,000 calories a week. This is about a half hour of medium-intensity exercise per day.

You don't need to go to a gym. Be active as a way of daily life, in a variety of ways, and you need never see the inside of a gym. This book will show you how to be fit from an active daily "real" life, not just gym exercises.

What Is "Fitness as a Lifestyle"?

Exercising to be healthy doesn't sound like fun to many people. For them, "fitness" means stopping their "real life," putting on clothes they feel self-conscious in, driving to some gym they don't feel comfortable in, with strangers they don't relate to, and doing uncomfortable, arbitrary motions that have no similarity to their "real life." But they do it because they "should" or because they "have to." Or maybe they just don't do it. What's healthy about being so stressed? Unfortunately, "fitness as a lifestyle" to many means going to a gym every day or two, then stopping and going back to their "real life"—slouching, sitting around, bending wrong all day, using poor posture, walking heavily, sitting round-shouldered, taking elevators, driving everywhere while sitting slouched, and avoiding all movement.

Fitness should relate to what you do all day every day. It doesn't mean "doing" exercises. It's like how math is often taught. You could learn to balance a checkbook and figure what 18% interest and "minimum payment" really add up to every month. But instead, it's "How many apples and oranges Johnny has." Then people call math "irrelevant." You need math for your real life, and fitness is the same. You need to stand, sit, and walk with good posture; use your legs, not your back, for lifting and bending all day; use shock absorption when you walk; and use your body all day, not just sit. People do squats with a trainer for an hour (paying to learn proper form and straight back), then bend right over at the waist to put the weight down when they are finished. People do lunges for their legs in exercise classes, then bend right over at the waist to pick up their things when they leave. This book will give you hundreds of ways to use your body properly and get fit in your real life, and have true fitness as your real lifestyle.

> Fitness is for your "real life," not just in a gym.
> Why do leg exercises in a gym, then bend wrong all day, not using your legs, to pick things up?

It Pays

Being in good physical condition is important to your life, even if you never want to play sports or climb mountains. The many health and well-being payoffs contribute to safe, healthful, and fun living every day.

2

The Different Aspects of Fitness

You've got to be very careful if you don't know where you are going, because you might not get there.

—Yogi Berra

There are different ways you can be in shape. You need to know the different aspects of fitness so that you can know where you're going with your fitness program. Each different fitness aspect needs different types of exercise. Without exercising each in its own way, you "might not get there."

Why Different Aspects of Fitness?

Swimming, walking, and jogging increase your cardiovascular (aerobic) endurance, but not your strength. Dashing for a bus or playing baseball doesn't improve your ability to go long distances. Taking long daily walks or runs will not build big muscles. Neither will sit-ups take fat off your stomach; for that, you need aerobic work. Weightlifting for strength is usually not aerobic exercise, despite what health clubs tell you. Stretching makes you more flexible, not stronger. Why?

Cardiovascular endurance, anaerobic capacity, muscular strength, power, and muscular endurance are different body systems, both structurally and chemically. Different activities make different adaptations in your different systems, giving you different kinds of fitness. To walk or run long distances, you need to train for distance. Being fit in only one way won't be much help to the other things you need to do. For lifting grocery bags, strong biceps (among other muscles) separate those people struggling from those lifting easily. Big biceps won't help your swimming, because swimming doesn't use the biceps much. To get the effect you want, you need to do the right training. This chapter tells the interesting story behind each specific adaptation to different exercise. Then Chapter 3 tells specifically how to improve each aspect of your fitness.

Cardiovascular Endurance (Aerobic Capacity)

Cardiovascular endurance is also called cardiorespiratory endurance or aerobic capacity. It's the ability of your heart and lungs and their interconnected system of blood vessels to supply oxygen and nutrients to the parts that move you around. Your body uses this oxygen to make energy, so the process is called *aerobic*, which means "with oxygen."

Your cardiovascular endurance determines how long you can walk, run, bike, dance, skate, ski, jog, hike, shop, or swim at your chosen pace. It contributes to how tired you will be at the end of doing things you need to do all day. It affects your general health. Improving your aerobic condition makes getting where you want to go easier, and means you can get through your day more easily and with less fatigue. See Chapter 4, "What Does 'Aerobic' Really Mean?" for the details on what it means to be aerobic.

Anaerobic Capacity

Not all activities are aerobic. With fast activity, your body doesn't have a chance to activate its aerobic system. Your body has to use quick and ready-stored fuel, not oxygen, so it is called *anaerobic. Anaerobic* means "without oxygen." You have only enough of this special stored "quick" energy for a few minutes of anaerobic activity. If you continue activity at a pace that is too fast for you, your body can't switch over to its oxygen-using aerobic system to any great extent. Your body continues trying to use your stored fuel, but your demand exceeds the supply, and you run out of fuel. If you don't slow down so that your body can switch to the aerobic system that can make more energy, your body will stop you, gasping in your tracks—anaerobic.

You use your anaerobic system to run for a bus, get out of your chair, lift packages and children, throw things, hold your breath, go up a flight of stairs, get out of a burning building, and do any short, hard activity. Developing your anaerobic system will make all these activities easier and safer. If your body is not prepared for short, quick activities, you can wind up hurting yourself and missing the bus besides. Your anaerobic system is explained more in Chapter 4, "What Does 'Aerobic' Really Mean?"

Strength

Muscular strength is usually measured by the maximum force your muscles can generate in a single effort. You need strength to lift and carry weights, packages, children, groceries, and yourself easily, and without struggle. By increasing your strength through weightlifting, you can move around more easily, and reduce your chance of musculoskeletal injury while doing it.

Elderly and debilitated people who could not previously even lift themselves out of their chairs become more mobile after strengthening programs, allowing them to walk unaided once again. Many people won't kneel down or sit on the floor because they are too weak to get back up. That is not aging, that is the need to regain the strength to do it.

Some people believe that women should not do weightlifting (for any number of reasons, including the fear of getting large muscles). Weightlifting is important for health. Even women who don't do activities commonly regarded as strength activities need strength to do daily activities like carrying several 20-pound grocery bags and a 40-pound child. Weightlifting to increase muscular strength also strengthens bones. The pull of muscle against bone thickens the bone. The stronger a muscle, the more it can pull on the bones it attaches to. Weightlifting is a key part of osteoporosis prevention.

> Weightlifting to strengthen muscles
> also thickens bones, helping prevent osteoporosis.
>
> If you are afraid to kneel or sit on the floor because you can't
> get back up, you need to regain the strength
> (and balance skills) to do it.

Extra muscle helps you stay warm in winter and is your chief calorie burner. Building more muscle through strength training means that you burn more calories every day.

> Every pound of muscle you gain through strength training
> increases your metabolic rate by about 50 calories per day.
>
> If you gain five pounds of muscle, you burn about 250 more
> calories every day, even when just sitting around.

Power

In exercise physiology, power is measured by how fast you can be strong. It's a product of speed and strength together. You call on power to lift things, throw things, move things, hit things, dash out of the way of cars, or catch a falling child or package.

Different activities need different amounts of strength compared to speed. To throw the discus and lob a tennis ball, you take a light weight and hurl it fast and far away. Offensive linemen try to do the same to heavy defensive backs and tackles. A higher strength component compared to how fast you move, for example in bench pressing or lifting any weight, is called strength-dominated power. Swimming, running, jumping, baseball, and tennis use primarily speed-dominated power.

Power is not just for athletes. When you increase your power, you can move things and yourself around more quickly and easily, with less chance of injury while doing so. It may save your life in an emergency, or help you save someone else's life.

Muscular Endurance

Walking, jogging, biking, skating, and swimming involve many, many leg or arm repetitions against the relatively light resistance of the ground, the bicycle pedal, or the water. High repetitions against low resistance call on muscular endurance.

Muscular endurance is different from cardiovascular endurance. It is just endurance of the specific muscles you are working, not your heart and aerobic system. Untrained muscles do not have muscular endurance. They will get tired before you are out of breath. Trained muscles have specific changes in their cells and how they function that increase endurance capacity. These adaptations don't change muscle size.

Improved muscular endurance makes long walks, runs, rides, and swims easier, and reduces your chance of leg cramps. For carrying things around, and just getting through the day, muscular endurance of your back muscles can make the difference between an uneventful day and a tired, achy back that night.

Flexibility

Flexibility is the ability to move easily and safely through a range of motion. You need good flexibility to reach shelves and cabinets without straining and arching, bend to tie your shoes and pick things up, paint or cut your own toenails, scratch your own back, and safely do recreational activities.

Several body areas appear susceptible to injury from poor flexibility. The range of motion required to strain tight low-back muscles is quite small, accounting for many painful backs. Tight hips and shoulders prevent healthy posture. With good flexibility, you may suffer fewer injuries to your muscles and the tough fibrous structures called tendons that attach your muscles to your bones.

Regular stretching reduces many problems of poor posture and tight, achy joints. See the next chapter on "Improving Your Fitness" for a section on flexibility, and Chapter 6, "Stretching and the Eight Great Stretching Mistakes."

Balance

Balance is an often forgotten aspect of fitness. Good balance is essential to preventing falls and the injuries that result from them. A vicious cycle develops when you get out of shape and decrease your balance skills along with all your other "use-it-or-lose-it" abilities. You become more afraid to fall and more afraid to bend down or do activities. You do less, further lose balance skills, and so on, losing more and more independence. Many people become housebound or even chairbound—terrified of falls. Walking heavily is often a sign of poor balance. Walking heavily is hard on the joints and can contribute to a lot of aches and pains. A slip or misstep while walking with packages, for example, can either be easily rebalanced with good equilibrium skills, or result in a cascade of shoulder, neck, or back strain from sudden repositioning; a sprained ankle; and various impact injuries from the fall.

Balance is highly trainable. Ways to improve balance are described in Chapter 8, "What Exercises Do You Need to Be Fit?" and Chapter 9, "Good and Bad Exercises," in the section on good foot exercises.

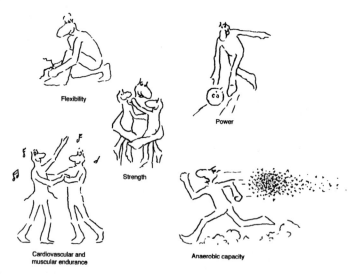

Figure 2.1. There are several components to fitness. You need them all, not just for sports, but for your everyday life and health.

Aspects of Fitness

Cardiovascular Endurance, also called aerobic fitness — Ability of your heart and lungs, and their system of blood vessels, to supply oxygen and nutrients to the parts that move you around. Enables you to run, swim, bike, skate, walk, ski, and dance farther and longer, with less effort.

Anaerobic Capacity — Stored fuel system for short, intense activity. Enables you to run or swim short distances quickly, exert against resistances like pushing open a stuck door, and do strenuous exercise.

Strength — Ability to move a heavy weight once, or a few times. Increasing your strength makes it easier to lift weights and move yourself around.

Power — Ability to move weight quickly. You call on power to push, pull, punch, throw, and lift things and yourself quickly.

Muscular Endurance — Ability to move a light weight repeatedly. You need muscular endurance of your legs to walk, jog, and cycle long distances, and go dancing all night. You need muscular endurance of your arms to swim.

Flexibility — Ability to move easily and safely through a range of motion, and to even just stand and walk without hunching. Healthy flexibility—not too much, not too little—can reduce pulls and strains.

Balance — Ability to keep your body stable and in position without swaying, slipping, or falling. Crucial to preventing falls and near-falls, and the injuries that come with them, and to avoiding the slips that make you drop things on your foot. Injury and disuse diminish balance.

Not Just One

You need all the different aspects of fitness for a healthy, comfortable life. Doing only one sport or exercise that develops only one aspect of fitness is robbing you, and possibly setting the stage for health problems. The next chapter explains how to develop each different aspect of fitness.

3

Improving Your Fitness

Speaking generally, all parts of the whole body which have a function, if used in moderation and exercised in labours to which each is accustomed, become thereby healthy and well-developed, and age slowly; but if unused and left idle, they become liable to disease, defective in growth, and age quickly.

– Hippocrates

A little over 2,500 years ago, the Greek athlete Milo realized he could increase strength by using workloads above those normally encountered. He began lifting a young calf every day. The calf's maturing weight provided progressive resistance until, it was said, he carried the grown bull around the Olympic arena. He became a military hero, and was undefeated as an Olympic wrestler.

Whether Milo lifted an increasingly heavy calf in legend or in fact, it is well-established that fitness improves by progressively increasing the load, a process called overload. Routinely carrying increasingly heavy loads, for example, increases strength. Progressively raising the number of times you lift a light weight improves muscular endurance. Progressively swimming farther extends your cardiovascular endurance. Increasing your joint range of motion improves your flexibility.

Thin people can be out of shape. Average weight people can be out of shape. Fat people can be in or out of shape but still want to drop some fat. Even athletic people can be out of shape. Understanding differences among aspects of fitness was covered in the previous chapter. This chapter covers how to train each of your different aspects of fitness, so you can get in the shape you want.

Cardiovascular Endurance

You can improve your cardiovascular status through continuous low-intensity large-muscle activity, like walking, running, skating, dancing, biking, cross-country skiing, and swimming.

If your activity is too hard for your fitness level, you will get out of breath and need to stop, cutting the aerobic benefits short. If your intensity is too low, as in slow walking or exercise class "floor work" of leg lifts and abdominal crunches, you will not gain aerobic exercise benefit (or burn as many calories). Keep an easy, moderate pace to make easy, moderate progress.

Exercise studies find a close match between how hard your body actually works and how hard you consider the activity. That means you can easily monitor your work load. A pace you find to be medium effort usually is a medium load on your system, and is about right for exercising for general cardiovascular fitness. A good rule of thumb is to be able to carry on a conversation. If you are too out of breath to talk, you are working at an intensity that is too high to be mostly aerobic. That's not bad; it means you're working hard. See the next chapter, "What Does 'Aerobic' Really Mean?" for more on this interesting subject.

> Recommendations call for regular moderate exercise to improve your health. But what is moderate?
> Luckily, your body is smart. Exercise that feels moderate is moderate. Exercise that feels too easy really is too easy.

Anaerobic Capacity

You need good anaerobic capacity to get you through short, hard exertions—dashing to catch a bus, going up a flight of stairs, throwing a ball, sliding home in baseball, moving things, carrying someone to safety. Improve your anaerobic capacity through high-intensity, short-duration activity like sprint runs, swims, and going up stairs. Alternate sprints with rests.

Gradually work up to 30 seconds of hard anaerobic work, then one minute of aerobic "rest," which is easy, mild activity, until your heart rate returns to normal. Then increase the times and the repetitions, keeping the 1:2 ratio of anaerobic work to active rest.

As with aerobic activity, you can tell your intensity by how it feels. You are anaerobic when you are working hard and fast enough to be out of breath, and the workload feels taxing, even uncomfortable. Train for this, and what was previously uncomfortable becomes possible, and eventually easy.

Strength

Strength training is good for you. Some people reject lifting for fear of hurting themselves or becoming bulky. Done properly, strength training will make you look trimmer and reduce your chance of injury from other activities. Strength training increases your ability to do the physical work of any of your favorite activities, firms your muscles, strengthens your joints, and increases your amount of muscle, which burns calories and keeps you warm. Lifting weights is an important part of osteoporosis prevention because the stress of muscle pulling against bone increases bone density.

> Weightlifting increases bone density, important to prevent thinning bones.

How Do You Get Stronger?

Your body makes several adaptations to increase your strength when you start a weightlifting program. Usually, the first adaptation is a learning effect, which immediately increases the amount you can lift, even before any physical changes occur in your muscles. Then, three physical changes begin. The firing rate of nerves serving your muscles increases; the number of nerve-muscle units, called motor units, that can fire together increases; and you increase the size (cross-sectional area) of your muscle.

For the first three to four weeks, it is the neural factors that predominate to increase your strength. After that, strength increases in young males primarily by increasing size of the muscle. Women and older men increase strength more through neural mechanisms than size, even when they make the same strength increases as young men. Obviously, women and older men can increase muscle size through training, but size is not the only predictor of strength. Strong things may come in small packages.

How Do Your Muscles Get Stronger?

- The firing rate of nerves serving your muscles increases.

- More nerve-muscle units can fire together.

- Your muscle cells themselves get bigger.

Because maximum strength contributes to winning specific Olympic events and, even more crucial, football games, studies have subjected strength training methods to microscopic scrutiny. It has been found that to get stronger you need to contract muscles at close to the maximum they are able to contract. That takes heavy weight, and that is why most exercise class "floor work" does not strengthen. Your leg is not heavy enough. You need a weight that is so heavy that after 8 to 10 lifts you are just about unable to lift it again. It's almost heretical to say swimming won't make you strong. But like floor work without weights in exercise classes, water is not heavy enough to make your muscles work maximally after only 8 to 10 strokes. That doesn't mean swimming and water exercises are not good for you in other ways. It means they are not major strength builders, unless you are debilitated from sickness or injury or do large numbers of laps at high speeds, which increase your intensity and total work.

Most studies agree the maximum number of times to lift a heavy weight consecutively to maximize strength gain is between 4 and 10 repetitions, or "reps." These same studies find less gain with more or fewer reps. Why? If you can do more reps with the same amount of weight, you are not using a weight heavy enough for maximum strength gain. Fewer reps don't sufficiently overload a muscle to gain strength. Strength work will "tone," or firm you up, more than leg lifts or arm circles, for example, which are high repetitions using light weights.

What about recommendations for weightlifting that say to do 8 to 12 repetitions? That also works. It will not maximize strength building quite so much, but it uses a slightly lighter weight, making the activity safer. For the recreational lifter, the 8 to 12 repetition recommendation is probably preferable. For the serious strength builder, who has good training and supervision, the heavier weight, fewer repetition recommendation better applies.

One group of repetitions is called a set. Slowly and safely work up to three sets of repetitions. But start easy. Try one set to start. After a week or so, if this easy start produces no pain or other problems, increase gradually until you can comfortably do two to three sets. Lift the weight through as complete a range of motion as is comfortable. Control the weight to avoid risk of injury.

How to Train to Get Stronger

- Carefully experiment to find the heaviest weight that you can comfortably and safely lift 4 to 8 times (repetitions) for serious, supervised strength building, or 8 to 12 repetitions for a general strengthening program.

- The "heaviest weight you can lift 4 to 8 times" may be your own body—getting up from a chair or the floor, doing push-ups, pull-ups, lunges, or squats, and especially, bending properly all day.

- Work up to three sets of repetitions.

- Rest one to four minutes between each set.

Between each set, you need rest. Rest allows you to recover enough to maximize muscular tension for the next set. One to four minutes of rest between each set is usually enough. Allow a minimum of a full day between weight training sessions for muscle repair and strength building processes to proceed without interference. When you have progressed to where you can easily lift the weight for three sets, increase the weight.

Balance is important. That means strengthening muscles opposite each other. For example, strengthening your abdominal muscles without strengthening your back muscles opposite them often causes your "abs" to chronically pull your torso with more tension than your back muscles. The result is back pain and poor posture. Chapter 7 details abdominal muscles, and Chapters 20 and 21 cover back pain and back exercises.

> Many people exercise their abdominal muscles, then never contract their back muscles to strengthen them, too.
> Poor posture and back pain can result.
> It is a shame that gyms and "health" clubs
> have "abs only" classes.

What about eating more protein to get stronger? Many popular fitness magazines sell protein supplements, stating you need extra protein to build muscle. This is rarely true. The Western diet usually provides much more protein than you need, even with heavy activity. You ordinarily do not need to eat additional protein to increase strength or musculature. Making sure you eat enough carbohydrate to fuel your exercise has been found to help. Not getting enough carbohydrate is fatiguing. For more on healthy eating, see Chapter 18.

Lifting is important to everyone's fitness plan. It's a myth that being strong reduces your coordination or flexibility. You can be strong with poor coordination, but not too strong.

> It is not true that if you stop exercising, your muscles will turn to fat. Your muscle cells will shrink, as with any other "use-it-or-lose-it" situation, but they cannot transform into different cells.

Muscular Endurance

Muscular endurance is the ability of any particular muscle or muscle group to do continuous activity at low intensity. Examples are found any time you exert against light weights many times, as with leg lifts, pedaling a bicycle, swimming, or walking. Training is simple. When you have progressed to where you can easily continue for a set number of kicks, strokes, reps, or minutes, increase them gradually. Alternate easy and hard workouts, rest adequately, and don't overdo. The long-duration, low-intensity, large-muscle aspect of training for muscular endurance also increases cardiovascular endurance to varying degrees.

Power

Power is the product of strength and speed. Lifting a weight takes strength. Throwing a weight takes power.

You increase your muscular power any time you move faster against a given load, get stronger, or both, in varying combinations. To develop power, lift or move a weight (a package, a dumbbell, or yourself) that you customarily need to lift or move, but do it more quickly. There are special weight machines specifically made for power training.

Be careful when training with weights for power. Potential for serious injury while throwing weights around is high. Never lean over and lift quickly unless you really want to ruin your back.

Developing power for swimming or running is safer. Increase your swimming or running power by swimming or running hard every few laps. Rest with easy laps. Be sure to be well warmed-up before beginning power laps. While you're at the pool, you can practice throwing a rescue line to increase your throwing power. Lift yourself out of the pool without using the ladder to improve your lifting power. It can also be a cool-looking way to get out of the pool.

Flexibility

Stretching increases the range of joint motion you need for daily mobility, not just for sports. Tightness contributes to poor posture, and can make you stand and walk funny. There is good evidence that good flexibility prevents muscle injuries and reduces back pain.

Although stretching for flexibility can reduce injuries, stretching wrong can produce them. Many people don't have the flexibility they need to stand up straight, but make things worse by forward-stretching their already rounded backs and shoulders, making the rounding worse. Forced stretching past a certain range can destabilize your joints until they don't seat well, increasing wear and tear, and predisposing you to sprains and dislocations. Unstable shoulder capsules may allow the bones of your shoulder joint to slip out of place from forces that healthier joint capsules tolerate. Good forward and backward ankle flexibility is important for general pain-free walking, and for many sports, particularly swimming, but excess looseness on the outsides of your ankles increases your chance of ankle sprains because your ankle can bend at a high angle sideways if you stumble. Chapter 6 details what you need for healthy flexibility and gives you bad stretches to avoid and good stretches to do.

> Proper flexibility reduces your chance of muscle and joint injuries and reduces back pain.
>
> Bad stretching can increase your chance of pain and injury by destabilizing joints and reinforcing already poor posture habits.

Several well-known stretches hold your joints at an angle that puts too much weight and pressure on ligaments. The hurdler's stretch is a major example. It twists your knee sideways. Instead, keep the nonstretched leg in front of you with your foot on the floor. Clasping hands behind you, then lifting your arms, strains the front, and weakest part, of your shoulder capsule. Squatting on your heels is tough on knee ligaments because it pulls the knee slightly apart, particularly if you have heavy legs. Full squatting can damage the small cartilaginous cushions in your knees, called meniscus. The bad knees of professional baseball catchers come from chronic squatting. Avoid neck ligament stretchers like the "plow," which involves lying with your legs in the air over your head and much weight on your neck, lengthening it forward. A stretch that puts too much weight on your spine occurs when you bend over from a stand for toe touching, or worse—bounce while bending over for toe touching. The groin stretch, sitting with knees bent and soles of the feet touching, can overstretch the side of the ankles if the sides of the feet are left on the floor, rather than kept in line with the lower leg.

- Avoid stretching in one direction without countering the stretch in the other. A common example is stretching forward through toe touching and abdominal crunches, without stretching the other way by arching backward. Chronic forward bending, particularly with no countering backward stretching, is tough on the discs in your spine. A typical result of unbalanced stretching is often seen in dancers who stretch their legs outward without equal stretching inward. The outside of their legs gradually tightens and shortens while the inside loosens until they walk like ducks. Later, their hips and knees succumb to early wear. Another example you've probably seen is round-shouldered muscle men. They build up the chest without stretching it, and neglect the back, except to allow it to stretch through slouching. A problem results called stretch-weakness. Their weak, overstretched backs allow their tight fronts to pull them into round-shouldered, poor posture.

- Warm up enough to sweat before you stretch. Then stretch by slowly easing into, then holding, the stretch. Don't bounce. Micro-injuries can result.

- Keep the limb you're stretching in line with the joint to stretch the muscle, not the ligaments.

- To stretch your hamstrings without hurting your back, lie on your back and straighten one leg overhead, keeping the other leg, your shoulder, and your head loosely on the floor without straining.

- To avoid posture problems and back pain from unequal stretching, stretch your upper back, lower back, and hip in each direction. Don't overweight your neck by putting your body weight on it. Do lying-down stretches instead of standing, bent-over stretches.

- During the rest of the day, avoid sitting and standing with a rounded back. That's stretching, but it's not good stretching. Keep the normal inward curve of your lower back, and don't hold your upper back rounded.

Details on flexibility and how to stretch for posture and mobility are in Chapter 6, "Stretching and the Eight Great Stretching Mistakes."

> Don't stretch hamstrings by bending over to touch your toes from a stand. It is tough on your discs and promotes poor posture. Stretch lying down instead. Keep neck and shoulders on the floor. Lift one leg, keeping it relaxed instead of yanking it. Keep the other leg flat on the floor to stretch the front of the hip.

Size

Increasing muscle size to the extent that bodybuilders do is not a specific aspect of fitness. Since the topic of gaining size is of high interest, both to those who want it and to those who worry that exercise will make them big, it is covered here.

An unfortunate number of women, and even men, shun weightlifting and its associated health benefits on the assumption they will grow huge. But gaining an appreciable amount of size takes a lot of work—more than many people are willing to do. You can lift weights to get strong, build endurance, gain power, and become healthy. You will get firm and look good, but you won't bulk up big without specific and intense work.

One look at power lifters and you know they're strong. Yet they look different from bodybuilders. Power lifters train for strength; bodybuilders maximize size and visual effect. Two things bodybuilders do differently are to increase volume of work and muscle definition.

> Power lifters and bodybuilders look different even though they both train by lifting heavy weights. They train differently and get different results for that reason.

Volume is the product of how much weight you lift and how many times you lift it. To maximize volume, do more reps and more sets. Lift more slowly than you would for strength or power. You still need heavy weight, but to be able to do more reps, use less weight than for strength training. Use a weight you can lift 12 or so times before muscle failure stops you. Do more sets and take only short rests between those sets. When you can easily lift four sets of 12, increase the weight and, later on, add another set. Definition comes from losing fat under the skin that covers your nooks and crannies.

> Bigger muscles don't always mean a stronger person.
> Small muscles can be strong too.

Someone with large muscles may not always be able to lift as much weight in a single effort as a smaller person who trained specifically for strength. It's difficult to make true assessments about the strength of women or older men, or anyone for that matter, purely on muscle circumference.

Firmness

Like size, body firmness is not a component of fitness, or necessary for health. But since most weightlifting will firm you, and so many people's primary goal in exercising is "toning" or "firming" their bodies, the information is presented here.

Firming your body is easier than working for strength, endurance, or size. You don't have to push it; however, more work makes more firmness. Just going running or doing aerobics classes by themselves may burn fat, so that you have better muscular definition, and they can work your leg muscles, but they won't firm your entire body. You need to work each area that you want to firm, through resistance exercise. The resistance can be your body weight, weight machines, or free weights.

Balance

Balance is directly and immediately helpful to improve your fitness, to prevent injury from slips and falls, and to maintain independence and mobility. Most people never practice balance. Without practice, balance skills diminish. Balance will also be off in an injured limb. A vicious cycle develops when people fear moving in fun ways or for independent living because of poor balance, and deliberately decrease their activities and outings.

You don't need to go to a gym to practice balance. Most gyms don't have balance programs or incorporate balance exercises into classes or workouts. Stand on one foot for increasing lengths of time. Practice shifting your weight slowly from foot to foot, keeping good leg and back posture. Then try more quickly. Try these any time you are standing around—washing dishes, folding laundry, waiting for buses or elevators. Throw and catch things standing on one foot. Practice balancing on one foot, one knee, or one knee and hand, for example, while on the floor. Put your clothes on standing up. Shoes and socks too. Practice in a safe area without risk of falling onto objects, down stairs, or onto hard surfaces. Details on how to improve balance with fun exercises are described in Chapter 8, "What Exercises Do You Need to Be Fit?" and Chapter 9, "Good and Bad Exercises," in the section on good foot exercises.

How to Improve Your Different Aspects of Fitness

Cardiovascular Endurance (aerobic capacity). Long-duration, low-intensity, large-muscle activity like walking, running, skating, dancing, cross-country skiing, or swimming. Comfortable intensity.

Anaerobic Capacity. Short-duration, high-intensity activity like sprints, whether on land, in the water swimming or finning, or on a bicycle. Alternate short, hard exertions with easy ones. Work hard enough to get out of breath, rest briefly, then sprint again.

Strength. Weightlifting. For general strengthening programs, carefully find the heaviest weight you can lift 8 to 12 times. That may even be your own body weight. For serious strength building, do 4 to 8 lifts (reps). Work up to three sets of repetitions. Take long rests between sets. Don't skip major muscle groups; train them all so you can avoid orthopedic problems from unequal strength ratios.

Muscular Endurance. Do continuous repetitions of lifts or motions, with light weight and no rest between repetitions. Vary to avoid overuse, and maintain good posture to prevent injury. More on posture in the two back pain chapters.

Power. Weightlifting or other activity involving moving a heavy or light object (including yourself) quickly. Fast execution of each lift or motion. Long rests. Great care to avoid injury.

Vary Your Workout

If you do the same exercises all the time, your body becomes efficient, working less and less to do the same task. Repetitive strain injuries grow more possible, and the routine itself can become stale. You burn fewer calories to do the same workout, and your fitness gains plateau.

Vary your workout. Regularly shake up your routine and stimulate your muscles and brain (your brain is important to your health) by working in new and different ways. It's healthy, increases your breadth of fitness, and keeps results coming.

When you're a child, you're told, "Sit Still! Be Quiet! Eat Everything on Your Plate!"

As an adult, it's suddenly, "Get Moving! Don't Eat So Much! Say Something Profound!"

Now is the time to learn that activity is health, and eating when not hungry is not. Don't wait to teach good habits or learn them yourself.

Flexibility. Remember that slouching is a stretch—but a bad one. Your back becomes overstretched and rounded. Don't add to that with continued forward stretching. Don't bend over from a stand to stretch your legs. You know that picking things up that way is bad for your back. It doesn't magically become good for you by calling it an exercise. Stretch legs lying on the floor. Don't force your joints into such looseness that they no longer seat properly. After each stretch in one direction, stretch in the opposite direction. More on flexibility in Chapter 6.

Size. Weightlifting. Four sets of 12. Heavy to moderate weight. Short rests between sets. Exercise and eat low fat so muscles can't hide beneath fat stored under your skin.

Firmness. Regularly lift a comfortable weight a comfortable number of times, for example 10 repetitions, building up to one to three sets. Work each area that you want to firm.

Balance. Balance is easily and highly trainable, but often neglected. It is crucial for ease of movement, independence, variety of activity, and preventing dangerous slips and falls. Stand on one foot while on the phone or washing dishes, for example. Increase the challenges with fun and varied balance games. Put on and take off pants, socks, and shoes standing up for a combination balance and flexibility workout. More on balance in Chapters 8 and 9.

Can You Have It All?

To improve a specific sport or activity, you need to develop the systems used in that particular activity. For your health, work on all your different aspects of fitness, rather than working on any particular one and neglecting the others.

Do safe and sane weightlifting to develop strength, endurance, and power. Regularly walk, jog, cycle, swim, row, roller-skate, play, and dance to develop cardiovascular endurance. Do regular stretching and stand up straight to develop healthful range of motion and reduce injury potential. Challenge your balance to keep you agile and mobile.

Check with your physician before starting any program. Get instruction and start easy, even too easy in the initial weeks of a new program. Get the feel of it first. Then, and this is important, get to like it. Progressively work up. Exercise does not have to hurt to be effective. If anything hurts, stop, and find out why. You can have gain without pain. You can have it all.

4

What Does "Aerobic" Really Mean?

A friend of mine runs marathons. He always talks about this runner's high. But he has to go 26 miles for it. That's why I smoke and drink. I get the same feeling from a flight of stairs.

— Larry Miller

When are you most aerobic?

    a.   Sitting in a chair

    b.   Doing 50 sit-ups

    c.   Swimming 200 yards

The answer is (a). You have more aerobic than non-aerobic processes going on when you are sitting in a chair than when you are either doing 50 sit-ups or swimming 200 yards. To understand why, you need to know what "aerobic" *really* means and how it relates to aerobic exercise.

A Quick Overview

"Aerobic" is not just a type of exercise. It is a way your body makes energy, not only to do exercise, but to be alive at all. *Aero* is a Greek word meaning air, and *bios* is another Greek word meaning life. You need the oxygen in air all the time to manufacture the energy to stay alive, for all your body functions at rest, and for moving around. Using oxygen to burn food to make energy is called aerobic metabolism.

Although not an exact example, aerobic metabolism uses oxygen and the breakdown products of food the way a carburetor or fuel injection system mixes oxygen with gasoline to combust into energy and combustion by-products. In your body, the combustion is much slower than in automobile engines. Also, unlike a car with only one energy manufacturing mode, you have three different energy-generating systems. Only one of these systems is aerobic, the one using oxygen. The other two are *an*aerobic. *An* is a prefix meaning "without." Anaerobic processes make energy without oxygen. They use stored fuels and don't need oxygen.

You use your aerobic system just about all the time—sleeping, sitting in a chair, right now while reading. That's why you breathe just about all the time. It's when you begin physical activity that you need the boost from your two *an*aerobic systems as well. Your three systems contribute in different proportions during different length and intensity activities. That means that some activities use more aerobic than anaerobic processes, and so are called aerobic exercises; other activities use more anaerobic processes, and so are not aerobic exercises. But all three of your systems work to do the same thing—to make an energy-giving molecule called ATP.

Aerobic Metabolism Is Not the Same as Aerobic Exercise

Your body makes energy to stay alive using three systems; one is aerobic, the other two are anaerobic (not aerobic). You use all three in different amounts, depending on what you are doing. You need your aerobic system all the time. You are using aerobic processes right now reading this, and even when you sleep.

You need a boost from your two non-aerobic systems when you exercise. When an exercise uses the aerobic system the most and gives you cardiovascular benefits, the exercise is called aerobic exercise, but the term is often misused.

Your Universal Energy Molecule

A special body molecule called ATP is the universal energy molecule. ATP fuels the activity and life processes of all living things, from bacteria, to plants, to bats, to you.

You can't eat ATP. Your body makes it using oxygen and the breakdown products of the food you eat. You don't store much ATP in your body, you mostly make it as you go. The fitter you are, the more you can make, and the more energy you get to do your activities.

You need oxygen to "burn" your food fuel to make ATP. Your body can use only so much oxygen—determined by how fit you are, not by how much you breathe.

If unfit, you can't do as much exercise to use stored carbohydrate and fat fuels. You also can't move as much oxygen to your muscle cells during exercise to burn the food fuel. Getting fit makes you better able to move the oxygen with more blood cells, blood volume, blood vessels, and cellular enzymes.

ATP is short for adenosine triphosphate. It's called *tri*phosphate because it has three phosphates. The third phosphate is held on with a lot of energy (a high-energy bond). Breaking off the third phosphate releases that energy. Think of ATP like one of those toy spring-snakes in a can. When you undo the latch, the snake springs out all over. The latch is the high-energy bond—just a little thing, but holding back much energy. When your body needs energy, it uses a bit of water and an enzyme to undo the latch of ATP, and zing! Out springs energy. You have billions and billions of ATP molecules doing this all the time. Zing! Zing!

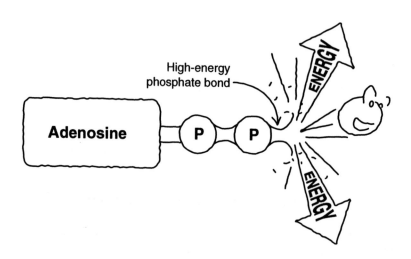

Figure 4.1. You get energy from millions of molecules of ATP by breaking their high-energy bond. You store a little ATP in your body and make the rest all the time using oxygen and the foods you eat.

All three of your energy systems (two anaerobic and one aerobic) work toward the same final common event—to make ATP. Your aerobic, oxygen-using system makes large quantities of ATP from fat, carbohydrate, and sometimes protein. It can make ATP for long periods of time. That's a good thing—you need to fuel your body processes even when you are asleep. But your aerobic system just can't make all that ATP very fast.

Sometimes you begin an activity so quickly and intensely that you can't supply your body with enough oxygen fast enough. So the first few seconds are fueled by your first anaerobic system of stored ATP. You don't have much stored ATP, so you run out quickly. If you continue your activity, your body has to change over to your second system, also *an*aerobic, where you make ATP by breaking down glucose and another carbohydrate called glycogen that you store in your muscles and liver. This second system is also limited in how much ATP it can make. After several more minutes of continued activity, your third system, the aerobic energy system, begins to contribute more and more to the energy needs of your cells.

When you exercise above the fitness of your aerobic system, your body can't make the switch back to aerobic metabolism to make the energy to do your exercise. Without aerobic metabolism, you have to continue using the quick-and-ready glucose and glycogen. One problem is you can't make much ATP that way, so you get tired. Another problem is that without aerobic metabolism, your body can't remove lactic acid and other products that build up during *an*aerobic metabolism (more on this in a bit). So you feel a burning sensation. All of this forces you to slow to a pace that can be supplied with ATP energy aerobically. If you don't slow down, you are soon halted in your tracks, gasping and burning—anaerobic. In short, the harder and faster you work (or the more it hurts), the more anaerobic. The steadier, or more relatively comfortable the pace, the more oxygen, and the more aerobic. But remember too, the more you push your limit, the further you push back the dividing line, and the more you can work hard and remain aerobic.

> Although people often equate hard exercise with aerobic exercise, the harder and faster you work, the more anaerobic processes you use. With a more relatively comfortable pace, you can use more oxygen and be more aerobic.
>
> The more in-shape you are, the harder you can work and still be comfortable and aerobic.

	System 1	*System 2*	*System 3*
System Name	ATP-CP	Glycolysis	Oxidative
Type	Anaerobic	Anaerobic	Aerobic
Method	Stored ATP	Makes ATP from stored glucose and glycogen	Makes ATP from carbohydrates, fats, and sometimes protein
Uses Oxygen?	No	No	Yes
Duration	Very short—seconds	Short to medium—minutes	Long—hours
Intensity of Activity	Very high	High to medium	Medium to low

A Closer Look at Your Three Energy Systems

You use your three energy systems for different intensity and duration activities ranging on a continuum from quick power, to speed and strength, to long endurance. Here's a closer, but still simplified, look.

System 1. ATP-CP. The original earth atmosphere was oxygen-free. The first living things made energy using only anaerobic processes. Several kinds of your cells, including muscle fibers, retain that anaerobic ability. Nerve cells can't work anaerobically, so they are sensitive to oxygen shortages. But muscle cells work both aerobically and anaerobically, so they have a great capacity to vary metabolic rate—more than any other body system.

Extremely brief, high-intensity bursts of activity lasting less than about 10 seconds are anaerobic and use stored ATP in your muscles to give you immediate energy. This is the realm of power movements, like opening a window, hitting a home run, doing football sprints, lifting a suitcase or grocery bag, putting the shot, leaping for a tennis ball or basketball, or kicking and punching in martial arts.

ATP stores energy until you need it. Biological energy is measured in calories. One mole of ATP can break apart to give you about 7 to 12 calories of energy to spend as you like (a mole is a chemical measurement of an awful lot of molecules—see the glossary). ATP gives you energy by breaking off its third phosphate. But then what happens to it? You still need to make energy, and without the third phosphate, adenosine triphosphate becomes only adenosine *di*phosphate, ADP, with just two phosphates. The low-energy bond of the second phosphate is as much use to you as a nearly run-out battery. You need to recharge it.

As rapidly as you break up ATP for energy using this system, another stored molecule called creatinine phosphate (CP) puts it back together. CP sits around in your muscles until you need it to give up one of its phosphates. CP sticks one of its phosphates on ADP to make ATP again. Because ATP and CP work together, the ATP system is also called the ATP-CP system, or phosphagen system. But now, how can you make more CP?

Your supply of CP is limited. When you are doing intense exercise and run low on CP, you must slow down enough to be aerobic again, using oxygen. Then oxygen helps make and replenish your ATP and CP stores, a process taking only a few minutes. The energy repayment comes mostly from the calories in your next meal. Being in shape with good aerobic ability increases the rebuilding of anaerobic energy stores, aiding the anaerobic recovery process.

How to Improve Your Anaerobic Capacity. You need anaerobic training like sprint swimming to increase the enzymes that are part of the ATP-CP cycle. Eating these enzymes to increase performance won't work, no matter what the health food claims tell you. All enzymes are proteins and are mostly destroyed by digestion if eaten. That's the job of digestion. They won't automatically reassemble back into enzymes on the other side of the intestinal wall (Chapter 14, "Nutrition Myths"). Only power and speed-specific exercise, and plenty of it, builds this system.

System 2. Anaerobic Glycolysis. When you continue activity past the point where your CP stores run low, your cells switch to energy system 2. This system breaks down glucose to make ATP. Breaking down glucose is called glycolysis (*lysis* means "breaking down"), pronounced gly-COL'-ih-sis. This system needs no oxygen, so this process is alternately called anaerobic glycolysis.

Anaerobic glycolysis can make ATP quickly, just not very much of it. For comparison, glycolysis can make about two molecules of ATP for each molecule of glucose, while your aerobic system can make 36 ATPs. (Actually, glycolysis makes four molecules of ATP, but uses two ATPs to do it. Everything takes energy.)

When Do You Use Glycolysis? Glycolysis lets you do longer activities than those using your ATP-CP system, but not as long as with aerobic energy-making processes. Since glycolysis can make ATP quickly, it allows more intense activity than aerobic processes. This is the strength and speed domain. Efforts of one to three minutes, like a 400-meter run, a 100-meter swim, climbing a hill carrying a load, carrying someone out of a burning building, or bringing a couple of boxes up from the basement, rely heavily on anaerobic glycolysis. Since this system is anaerobic, you can do many of these activities holding your breath, like swimming underwater. The extent of glucose and glycogen use depends on whether your exercise is continuous and long, or intermittent and exhaustive, and varies greatly with intensity.

Glycolysis and the Food You Eat. Only carbohydrate, not protein or fat, can be turned into energy without oxygen. Your body can store a fair amount of glucose by chaining glucose molecules together into molecules called glycogen, which you store mainly in your muscles and liver. When you need more glucose for glycolysis, your body just breaks apart the glycogen. Glycogen is broken down to glucose in all cells, but this process is most active in muscle and red blood cells.

Restoring your muscle and liver glycogen stores after hard exercise depends on how much carbohydrate you eat and how soon after activity you start eating. The optimum time for restocking is in the first 30 minutes after exercise, and the second restocking "window" is in the next two hours or so. If you don't eat much carbohydrate in this time period, you won't have as much glycogen, even as long as five days later, than you would have if you ate right away.

You can increase your muscle glycogen stores by eating carbohydrates regularly, particularly right after exercising. Don't overdo or the extra will have to store as fat. You also need to exercise regularly enough to convince your muscles they have a reason to store more. It's not food, but exercise, that principally trains this system.

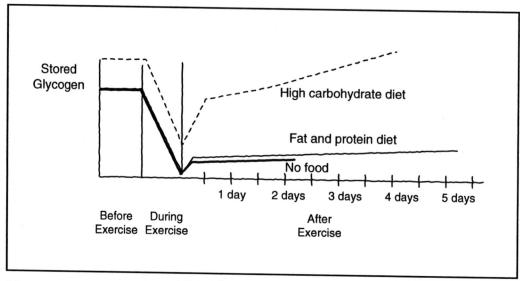

Figure 4.2. How much glycogen energy you can store for your next activity depends on how fit you are, how hard you work, how soon after exercising you start eating, and how much carbohydrate you eat.

What (Really) Is "Go for the Burn"? Breaking down glucose to make ATP so that you can live and move takes 12 steps. The end product of glycolysis is pyruvate (or pyruvic acid). After pyruvate forms, it can go two ways. Without enough oxygen to carry off the hydrogen ions that form when you are working anaerobically, they stick onto the pyruvate, making it into lactate (or lactic acid).

Your body produces lactic acid all the time. That isn't bad by itself. Lactic acid has a few important functions; then your body processes it, using oxygen, so that it doesn't build up. When you work above your aerobic capacity, more lactic acid is produced than you can process, so it builds up too high. All the acid products cause a burning feeling. "Go for the burn" indicates you are *an*aerobic. It's not beneficial, it's just waste products like lactic acid and extra hydrogen ions making your body acidic and stimulating your pain receptors to say "ow."

The better shape you're in, the more lactic acid you can process because you make a large number of body changes that supply more oxygen to your cells to remove it. Breathing in more oxygen (on a tank, for example) won't work. Your body can't use it. But with exercise, you grow more lung capillaries to take up oxygen, more red blood cells to carry the oxygen, more and bigger blood vessels to convey it, and more enzymes in the cells to uptake and change oxygen into energy. Remember too that feeling a burn with intense activity doesn't necessarily mean you are out of shape. Olympic athletes gasp and pant after their events too. It means they are giving their top effort.

Many secret potions have been tried to reduce lactic acid on the premise that you can work harder without the pain stopping you. Most involve stopping and taking the pill or potion. The pain goes, not from the potion, but because you stopped working. Some experiments have been tried with making the blood more alkaline to offset the acid produced. Results are marginal to nil for most exercisers. Nothing works better than just getting in better shape.

In summary, there are two main ways you reduce lactic acid. Lower your intensity to where available oxygen can supply your needs, so oxygen can turn the lactic acid back to pyruvate by carrying off the hydrogen ions and combining with them to form water. Also, you can get into better shape and be able to work at a higher level and still process the lactic acid into pyruvate. In both cases the pyruvate becomes available for your third, and last, system—your aerobic system.

> "Go for the burn" is lactic acid building up and stimulating your pain receptors—a signal that you are working above your aerobic capacity. It means that you are not aerobic.
>
> Working at a lower level reduces lactic acid to a level where you can process it. But getting into better shape lets you work at a higher level and still process it.

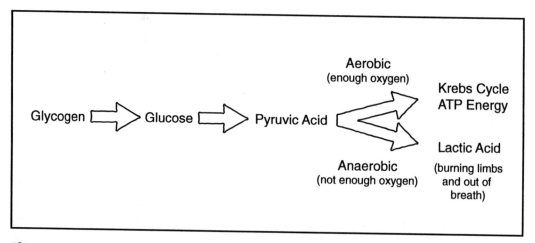

Figure 4.3. When you break down stored sugar to make energy while working very hard (anaerobically), the process stops with lactic acid because there is not enough oxygen for how hard you are working. When you work aerobically, the lactic acid doesn't build up but can turn into pyruvate, which you use for more energy.

System 3. Aerobic (Oxidative) Metabolism. When the duration of your activity is long, and intensity is low enough to be met without your anaerobic systems, your body signals your cells to begin the gradual change back to your aerobic system. Endurance events are primarily aerobic and use oxygen (oxidative metabolism) to produce energy. Aerobic metabolism can make a great deal of ATP to carry through long events. Be happy you're not a lizard. Reptile and amphibian hearts and lungs are not developed enough to use aerobic (oxidative) metabolism. They rely on glycolysis. Lizards don't win many long races.

Aerobic metabolism uses stored carbohydrate, fat, and protein if necessary, in two interesting pathways to make ATP. The first pathway is the Krebs cycle, and the second is the electron transport chain. For more detail on these pathways, see the glossary. You make most of your ATP in the electron transport chain. The electron transport chain takes the hydrogen ions formed in the energy-making process and, by combining them with oxygen, makes lots of ATP instead of allowing the ions to stick onto pyruvate. The extra ions turn pyruvate into the burning lactate. With lactate, you can't get into the Krebs cycle, so you lose a large portion of your ATP production opportunities. Having oxygen makes the difference between stopping your energy-making processes with lactate (while you gasp and rub burning limbs) or restoring lactate to pyruvate, so the pyruvate can enter into aerobic energy-making processes.

The Difference Between Aerobic Metabolism and Aerobic Exercise

Your aerobic metabolism goes on all day and night, even when you're sitting around or sleeping, making a distinction between aerobic metabolism and aerobic exercise. Not everything that predominantly uses your aerobic system is aerobic exercise. What does "aerobic exercise" mean in light of the fact that you are aerobic even when you are sleeping?

The word "aerobic" describing a type of exercise was coined by Dr. Kenneth Cooper, "Father of Aerobics." The intensity must be high enough to give a cardiovascular training effect, or it is not aerobic exercise. The intensity must not be so high that you are primarily using your non-aerobic systems, making you out of breath or with burning muscles. The key here is that with low fitness levels you have to work at a low level to stay aerobic. That doesn't make it better because it is aerobic. If you push it, you could raise the level where you can work and still stay aerobic.

What About Walking? It's true that slow walking mostly uses your aerobic system. It does not invoke much of your *an*aerobic systems because it is such low intensity. In this case, energy is supplied aerobically, but it is not aerobic exercise. Faster walking may qualify as aerobic exercise depending on how high you raise your heart rate and how long you walk. Walk so that you feel you are moderately exerting yourself for at least 10 to 20 minutes a few times each week to start gaining health benefits. Walk longer and harder, and add other forms of exercise for fitness benefits.

What About Running, Swimming, and Biking? Nothing is very aerobic if you do it so fast that you are out of breath and have to stop. Then you are exercising primarily *an*aerobically. That does not mean that it is bad, just that you're working too hard to last long enough to give you cardiovascular (aerobic) training effects. One way to use this is to do intervals. Go hard and fast, rest a short bit, then go again before your heart and breathing slow to below your training level. To run or jog aerobically, try a pace that you can maintain for at least 10 to 20 minutes and that feels comfortably hard. To swim or bike aerobically, do the same.

What About Football? Short, high exercise intensities decrease the ability of your aerobic system to meet the demand of your activity. Football games may be long, but the actual exercise is extremely short. A few tens of yards and tackles at most. This does not mean that football is not a hard sport, just that it is not an aerobic one. It is non-aerobic precisely because it can be so intense.

That introduces an interesting tidbit—a common sight is players clapping oxygen masks over their faces, believing it will help performance and recovery. The practice will not hurt them, but neither will it physically help. Football moves do not use oxygen for energy—the exercise bouts are just too short. Players use anaerobic fuel stored in their muscles. Oxygen supplementation increases blood levels only minimally since blood already carries almost all the oxygen it can hold. To put it technically, your oxygen saturation is usually around 97 to 98%. Plus, any small increase in blood oxygen saturation with bottled oxygen will be gone by the time players get back to the field and aligned in formation.

What About Sit-ups? During short, anaerobic exercises, you use stored ATP, CP, and glycogen. That's why doing the 50 sit-ups mentioned at the beginning of this story is not aerobic, and is metabolically less aerobic than sitting in a chair, where all your processes are just about 100% aerobic. Swimming 200 yards is not long enough to switch back to primarily aerobic metabolism.

If you are out of breath and your heart is pounding, you are more anaerobic than aerobic. Although you are breathing in plenty of oxygen, your body can't deliver and process it fast enough. Lactic acid builds. When you exercise aerobically, oxygen changes lactic acid back to pyruvate, which can be used to make ATP.

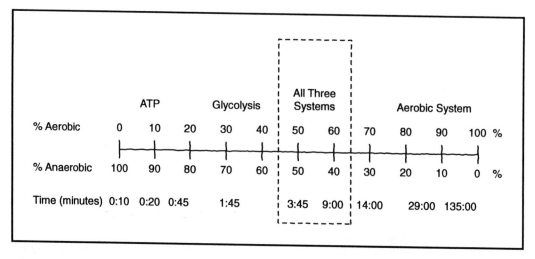

Figure 4.4. You have three energy systems—ATP-CP, glycolysis, and aerobic. Each contributes in different amounts during different intensities and durations of exercise.

What About "Fat-Burner" Classes? A popular fad exercise class is the "fat-burner." Fat-burner classes are lower intensity than regular exercise classes, yet advertising for these classes states that participants burn more fat. The reasoning given is that during high-intensity exercise, glycogen is the primary fuel, but with lower-intensity activity, more fat is used as a primary fuel. A little knowledge of "aerobic metabolism" seems to be a dangerous thing.

Fewer total calories are burned in these classes than in more vigorous classes because the intensity is lower. Even though fat would supply a greater percentage of the energy in a low-intensity class, not as much in total would be mobilized over the same period of time. High-intensity activities, done for the same period of time, burn more total fat and calories.

That does not mean that overweight, beginning exercisers should start with high-intensity exercises. Prolonged low-intensity exercise is a safer start for a weight loss program. An easy class now and then isn't so bad. Even regular exercise at only 50% of your maximum ability helps reduce risk of high blood pressure, diabetes, and cardiovascular disease.

Eating for Aerobic Exercise

Your body's preferred fuel for aerobic metabolism is fat. That does not mean you have to eat it, but that your body uses it from its stores. A trained endurance athlete's body will begin the change to fat-burning from glycolysis sooner than an out-of-shape person's body can. The in-shape body wants to preserve muscle carbohydrate stores as long as possible, because more carbohydrate allows exercise to continue longer. Preferentially using fat instead of glycogen is called glycogen sparing, and it is a training adaptation that delays fatigue.

It is popular to market foods that "give you energy." Since the main energy fuel for aerobic exercise is fat, will just eating lots of fat give you energy for aerobic exercise? Eating an oxidative fuel like fat isn't the way to increase your aerobic ability. You need aerobic practice, like regularly swimming long laps. See the previous chapter, "Improving Your Fitness," for more on how to get in shape, and Chapters 14, "Nutrition Myths," and 17, "Ergogenic Aids," in Part II for more on foods that do and don't help your physical abilities.

An Aerobic and Anaerobic Bike Ride

Now you know enough to follow the three simplified metabolic pathways through a sample physical activity—a bike ride.

You're sitting quietly, oxidatively aerobic. You decide to go out for a bike ride, so you stand up and walk over to get your bike, with the help of some ATP-CP stored in your legs.

You lift your bike in another burst of ATP-CP and carry it out the door and down the steps, rapidly shifting to anaerobic glycolysis.

You catch your breath and begin your ride, first an easy warm-up, then up a nearby hill. As you pick up the pace, your bodily processes speed up to manufacture more ATP for energy. You breathe faster to take in more oxygen to help make ATP. But there's a limit to how fast your body can deliver oxygen to your cells and how fast your cells can process oxygen in oxidative energy production. In your uphill ride, your energy demand exceeds the oxidative supply. Your cells rapidly switch to a mostly anaerobic glycolytic system. You begin to pant. Had you regularly worked out and gotten in better shape, the energy demand would be within range of your aerobic system. You would now be comfortably supplying your leg muscles with oxidatively stoked energy, not likely to run low soon.

But your cells are switching to your energy production processes that don't need oxygen. These processes can make energy for only short periods of time. Without enough oxygen to carry off extra hydrogen ions that attach to the pyruvate that forms from anaerobic metabolism, the pyruvate becomes lactic acid. Hydrogen ions accumulate, dropping your pH to the acid. Your legs burn.

The terrain changes and the hill levels off. You drop intensity and slow your pedaling. After several more deep breaths you "pay back" your debt to your anaerobic system and allow oxygen to turn lactic acid back into pyruvate. You settle into a comfortable aerobic pace. After 10 or so minutes of continuous pedaling, you are about 50% aerobic and 50% glycolytic anaerobic. After another 10 to 20 minutes of exploring, the aerobic percentage might have risen to about 60 to 70% or so. If your fitness level is high, it can climb higher, a response of a well-trained body to help spare muscle glycogen and delay fatigue.

You reach the halfway point, turn around, and pedal back, now mostly aerobic. You reach the hill, and enjoy the effortless coast downhill. Your energy needs are still supplied aerobically, even more than during your uphill and level-terrain ride, although you are now doing almost no exercise. This does not mean that you are burning as many calories. Remember, you have to exercise more to burn more. During the aerobic portion of your ride, your body has been busy replenishing much of your stored muscle CP for your ATP-CP system, but not glycogen. For restocking glycogen, you need to eat and drink. Oops! You went too far downhill and missed the turnoff. You turn around and pedal back uphill, with a rush of ATP-CP. Seconds later, your body shifts to primarily anaerobic glycolysis, but there's not as much glycogen stored as before. These few minutes seem much harder than the first strong pedals at the start of your ride. There's your street, and then the steps. Up the steps in another ATP-intensive effort.

You put your bike down and take off your jacket, using all three systems. Sitting quietly after your ride, you are primarily running on aerobic metabolism again. You get a snack of raw walnuts and fruit to begin restocking muscle and liver glycogen. The phone rings. You would jump up, but your anaerobic fuel stores are low, and you are tired. It's been a fun day of exercise.

5

What Does "Warm-Up" Really Mean?

Now King David was old and stricken in years; and they covered him with clothes, but he got no heat. Wherefore his servants said unto him, Let there be sought for my lord the King a young virgin: and let her stand before the King, and let her cherish him, and let her lie in thy bosom, that the lord the King may get heat.

— I Kings 1:1-2

Getting warmed up for exercise doesn't mean stretching or deep breathing. Even some common activities done for warm-ups in exercise classes are not warm-ups.

What Is a Warm-Up?

"Warm-up" means doing enough muscular work to raise your body temperature several degrees. People usually call just about any preparatory activity a warm-up, but the term literally means to get warmer.

You are like an automobile engine that heats up with use. Not all the fuel you put into your car goes to move the car. Most of the fuel energy to move the engine parts is lost as heat. In you, about 75% of all the energy you use for making your heart beat, for digestion, and for every other body process, turns into heat, too. Human energy inefficiency works in your favor to heat you to 98.6° F (37° C) at rest. That's good. If it didn't, your chemical processes wouldn't go as quickly, and you wouldn't be able to move around as easily. Muscular work using your large muscles converts even more mechanical energy into heat, raising your temperature even further.

> "Warm-up" is not synonymous with any old preparation for exercise. It specifically means to raise your body temperature, making exercise safer.

What Is Not a Warm-Up?

You won't raise your body temperature with deep breathing, arm-waving, or small muscle activity. Many exercise classes start by having you rise up and down on your toes, supposedly to warm up your calves. Or alternately bending and straightening your elbows. Or worse yet, with stretching. These are not warm-up activities. Your biceps and calf muscles are too small to contribute enough heat to warm your body. Starting out with small muscle activities will only poop you out before you can start some real exercise. Stretching doesn't warm you—there is not enough large muscle movement going on. Moreover, stretching while you are still cold can microtear and weaken your muscle fibers. People injure themselves with many stretching mistakes. One is not waiting until you are warmed up before stretching. Read more about stretching in Chapter 6, "Stretching and the Eight Great Stretching Mistakes."

> Stretching is not a warm-up. You need to warm up first using continuous, large muscle exercises, before stretching. Stretching before you are warmed up can injure you in several ways.

Why Warm Up?

Warming up changes your body in several ways that make exercise orthopedically safer, and lessen your chance of overdoing things with your heart. By raising your resting body temperature, your muscles become more pliable, more injury-resistant, and can work faster. Warmed-up muscles can stretch more, and endure more force without tearing. Increased body temperature improves diffusion of oxygen, carbon dioxide, and metabolites to and from tissues. Blood viscosity lessens and blood vessels widen, slightly reducing resistance to blood flow in muscles, including the heart. Abruptly beginning intense activity without adequate warm-up can leave you without enough blood and oxygen to your heart. In a study of men with chest pain accompanying exercise because of narrowed heart blood vessels, warming up increased the length of time they could walk before onset of chest pain.

Benefits of Warm-Up

- Muscles can stretch farther without tearing.

- Muscles become more injury-resistant.

- Muscles can work faster.

- Blood viscosity lessens.

- Needed chemical reactions in your body speed up.

- Blood vessels widen, reducing resistance to blood flow.

- Blood and oxygen can get into your heart and muscles more easily.

- Carbon dioxide and waste products can get out of your tissues more easily.

How Does a Warm-Up Work?

Your body's chemical processes are sensitive to small temperature increases. The enzyme reactions in your cells that produce energy and control body functions speed up proportionally as your body temperature rises. A 10° C rise would double the rate of enzyme reactions. This is called the Q10 Effect. Of course, your internal temperature could never change 10° without severe health consequences. But the few degrees that a warm-up raises your temperature use the Q10 Effect to boost your athletic performance.

Who Doesn't Need a Warm-Up?

You won't benefit by warm-up exercises if you're a lizard. Lizards are cold-blooded, meaning they can't change body temperature on their own. They have to lie in the sun to warm up. Their internal temperature changes as their environment changes, so they are called poikilotherms (POY'-kill-oh-thurms), which means "variable temperature." Warm-blooded beasties like us maintain a remarkably constant internal temperature at rest, so we are called homeotherms (HOME'-ee-oh-thurms), a word meaning "same temperature." Like lizards, scuba divers are another group that may not benefit by warm-up activities, but for different reasons. Warmer body temperature allows more nitrogen to get in and out of you. Lower temperature inhibits nitrogen uptake and elimination. Studies found that divers who spent their entire dives cold were less likely to get decompression sickness. But a diver starting a dive warm would absorb more nitrogen. If that diver then chilled, which is common during a dive, eliminating that additional nitrogen slows, increasing decompression sickness risk.

Other activities benefit from warm-up. The more strenuous the activity, or the more range of motion you need, the more you need a warm-up. Even a not-very-strenuous activity like golf needs a good range of motion of your back, shoulders, and hips, making warm-up important.

How Do You Know When You're Warmed Up?

You're warm when you break a sweat. It takes 5 to 10 minutes of exercise to increase muscle temperature, so give your warm-up at least that long.

What to Do

You can warm up for activity in three ways:

- Active direct warm-up

- Active indirect warm-up

- Passive warm-up

An active direct warm-up is the same activity as the actual exercise, but at a lower intensity. For example, fast walking warms you for jogging. Slow jogging warms you for running. Slow cycling warms you for faster cycling. Slower swimming (not just sloshing) is a good warm-up for pool training.

An active indirect warm-up uses any large muscle activity, such as pedaling a bicycle. In an exercise class, look for rhythmic leg motions that use the large muscles of the leg, not small muscle activity, such as arm movements and heel raises.

For active warm-ups, start with large muscle exercises that move upper legs and hips. Large muscle activity converts more mechanical energy into heat. Start off easy, then gradually increase the work. If anything hurts or doesn't want to move where you're moving, slow down.

For a passive warm-up, get in a sauna, steam, or conventional hot bath. Your body temperature rises with passive warm-up, although passive warm-up lacks the circulatory benefits of active exercise. That's not to say passive warm-up isn't useful. Hot, steamy showers give people with arthritis or other injuries the head start on muscle heat they need to reduce pain and increase range of movement enough to start exercising actively. Just drink extra water to avoid dehydration.

Spend 5 to 10 minutes warming up, and continue until you break a sweat. Don't stretch until after you're sweating. Most important, have fun so that you'll look forward to the next time.

Important Points for Warm-Ups

- Start with large muscle exercises that move your upper legs and hips.

- Gradually increase the tempo.

- If anything hurts or doesn't want to move where you're moving, slow down.

- Spend 5 to 10 minutes to warm up.

- Break a sweat.

- Put off stretching until you're sweating.

- Don't overdo.

- Have fun so that you'll look forward to the next time.

6

Stretching and the Eight Great Stretching Mistakes

One learns to itch where one can scratch.

—Ernest Bramah

Have you ever started to fall asleep while sitting up in a chair? You struggled to stay awake. When you lost the battle, your head slumped forward, only to jerk suddenly back up again. Pulling your head back up was not a voluntary move. It was a reflex that resulted from stretches and bounces. This chapter will tell you more about it, and how that relates to stretching right.

This chapter also covers the "Eight Great Stretching Mistakes." Although flexibility can reduce injuries, some stretches produce them, and even create and promote poor posture. How can this be? Bouncing on stretches increases flexibility but can cause injuries. Stretching isn't a warm-up. You need flexibility, but you also have a few bodily structures you should not stretch at all.

Benefits of Stretching

Where does poor posture come from? From not holding your body weight up with your muscles. Your body weight slumps onto your joints. Tight chest and shoulders pull you forward. Weak and overly stretched upper back muscles don't counter it. Standing bent forward or "knock-kneed" are also poor postures from weak, loose muscles on one side, and tight muscles on the other.

Many people are too tight to simply stand up straight. With proper stretching, your joints can line up properly, avoiding wear and tear. You can stand up with good posture and without turning your legs and feet in or out.

> Tight chest and shoulders contribute to round-shouldered posture. Tight hips are hard on your back and inhibit normal standing, walking, and running. Tight hip and calf muscles and Achilles tendons contribute to walking "duck-footed" or toe-out. This can wear on your ankles, knees, hips, and big toe.

Although not all studies show stretching prevents sports injuries, the reasoning has good basis. Your muscles can lengthen more before reaching the point where they tear. If you move in a way that surpasses that range, you may strain or tear the muscle and the tough fibrous structures called tendons that attach the muscle to the bone. The range of motion to strain tight low back muscles is small, accounting for many painful backs after a day of fun. Your Achilles tendon at the back of your lower leg attaches your calf muscle to your heel. Tight calf muscles and Achilles tendons can lead to tendonitis, knee pain, and foot pain, if you don't wind up with an outright tear. Tight soles of the feet contribute to foot and heel pain, foot cramps, plantar fasciitis, and heel spurs. More on feet in Chapter 9, "Good and Bad Exercises."

Tight hamstrings are prone to pulls and contribute to low back pain because they change the normal angle of the hip and low back. Sadly, an indirect way that tight hamstrings contribute to back pain is when people kill their backs to stretch their hamstrings. More on this follows.

Tight hip muscles, common in people who sit a lot, change the normal angle of your hip and low back, adding a large share of low back pain. Tightness limits the range of hip and leg motion, preventing efficient bending and reaching, or even standing, sitting, and walking normally. Tight hips are sometimes a hidden cause of shoulder pain. Many people with tight hips habitually stand bent-forward at the crease where the leg meets the body. This area should be able to straighten completely to let you stand upright, but can't when tight. During overhead activities, the shoulder overcompensates reaching by straining and rotating too far back. The repetitive strain on the shoulder during weightlifting, tennis, football, and overhead activities, like combing and washing hair and reaching shelves, can produce shoulder pain that is hard to rehab if you do not also stretch the tight hips that are causing the malalignment in the first place.

Many people think flexibility training means wrapping your foot around your ear or bending over forward to touch your toes.

But many people don't have the upper back, shoulder, and neck flexibility simply to lie down flat without a pillow. They are too rounded forward. How can they possibly stand up straight all day? Flexibility training needs to address normal posture.

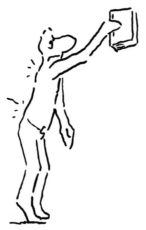

Figure 6.1. A little lack of flexibility can contribute to a lot of problems. Tight hip muscles change the normal angle of your hip and low back, and limit the range of motion you need for normal walking, running, and even reaching overhead. Tight shoulder muscles mean arching your back to reach and craning your neck.

The Eight Great Stretching Mistakes

Stretching Mistake #1: Promoting the Original Problem

You wake up and sit hunched at the edge of the bed, bend over the sink to wash, sit round-shouldered at breakfast, while commuting to work, and at a desk. You lean and bend wrong all day by bending at the waist. At the gym, you do crunches and toe-touching. You bend over the dishes, the lawn mower, and the vacuum cleaner, and slump to watch television. You go to sleep for the night with your head pushed forward by pillows. You are mystified when your back, neck, and shoulders ache. You call it stress. You go to someone and say, "My back hurts, can you give me a stretch to fix it?" They suggest bending over to touch your toes, or bringing your chin to your chest, your knee to your chest, sitting on the floor and leaning over to touch your toes, sitting in a chair and leaning forward with your chest on your thighs, touching your elbows in front by rounding your back, curling up in a ball, or other stretches that promote more rounding and more pressure on your back and discs.

Doing more of what caused the original problem is not what you need. To feel better, your poor, weakened, overstretched back and neck muscles need to stop getting overly stretched. Then you need specific stretches in the other direction, specific strengtheners to be able to hold yourself up straight, and posture exercises to know where and how to hold things consciously.

> People hunch forward all day, then do more forward bending for exercise. Their weakened, over-stretched back and neck ache. They call that "tension" and do more forward bending to "fix it."

Just doing a stretch doesn't fix a problem. You need five things:

- Know where the right posture should be.

- Have the body awareness to know how to move the body part to the proper position.

- Have the flexibility to be able to move the body part to the proper position.

- Have the muscular strength and endurance to hold the body part in the proper position all the time, even when you are doing other things.

- Consciously hold the right posture. Like manners, it doesn't automatically happen by itself.

> When your muscles are so weak and tight that good posture feels unnatural, that means you need to strengthen and stretch to be comfortable, not slouch to be comfortable.

Stretching Mistake #2: Not Stretching What You Think You're Stretching

Overhead stretches that don't stretch the shoulder. Quadriceps stretches that don't stretch your quads. Back extension that doesn't extend the back. Toe touches that don't stretch the hamstrings. How is all this possible?

Shoulder. It's common to see someone stretching their arm overhead by arching their back. Their shoulder angle is often no more than reaching to eye level. Many "shoulder stretches" in this way add to mysterious low back aches and never target the shoulder.

Try this:

- Stand up and reach your arm overhead, letting your back arch. Bend your elbow so your hand can reach your back, as if to scratch between your shoulder blades.

- With your arm in the same position, flex your trunk forward, as if to start doing a "crunch" to straighten your torso. Lift your elbow to the ceiling.

- Feel the stretch move to your shoulder and triceps.

Quads. Same mistake as with the shoulder stretch. People arch their backs.

Try this:

- Stand on one leg and arch your back while you grab your other foot behind you. You won't feel much stretch in your thigh.

- Still holding your foot, straighten your torso and push your behind forward.

- Drop your bent knee down next to the standing knee. Feel the stretch move to your thigh.

Read the next chapter on abs to learn more on how to use your abs to stabilize your body while reaching overhead or moving your legs.

Back. Often only one easily movable vertebra in the low back moves during a backward arching stretch, with the rest of the back held straight as a board. A hypermobile vertebra can wind up hurting from all the strain. Like constantly bending a spoon, the bending point eventually wears out.

Try this:

- Lie facedown and push your upper body up by pressing your hands against the floor near your shoulders. Notice where your back is bending. Is it mostly from one "crease" in your low back?

- Rest on your forearms. Push your forearms against the floor and distribute the stretch evenly up your back, making a graceful C-shape curve.

With the retraining above, and the ability to hold your body weight during an arch with your abs, as described in the next chapter, you can properly learn backward arching stretches while standing.

Hamstrings. Your hamstrings are the muscles in back of your thigh. Hamstring stretches are commonly misunderstood and abused. People bend their neck forward, round their back, hunch their shoulders, tighten their quadriceps, and do just about anything except stretch their hamstrings. Hamstrings attach to your sit bones—the bumps you can feel when you sit. Most people sit with their back rounded and hip tilted under, so that their sit bones tilt to the front, shortening their hamstrings.

Many people can touch their toes and still not put much, or any, stretch on their hamstrings because they bend from everywhere else. They never tilt their hips back so that the hamstrings lengthen. They can pass a flexibility test but still have mysterious aches and pulls from tight hamstrings, plus a hunched posture. Or maybe they can't touch their toes and don't understand why, since they stretch all the time.

Try this:

- Sit on the floor, knees bent out to the side cross-legged, and let your hips tilt back with your back rounded. Pull your ankles with your hands to straighten your torso. Rock your hips so that you arch your back. Many people are so tight that their hips are practically fused. Rocking may take a bit of effort to do. When your hip can move, even a little, let it rock back and forth until it moves easily.

- Straighten your legs in front of you. If your hamstrings are tight, your hip will tilt back under and your back will round again. Lift your ribs and arch your back to lengthen your hamstrings. Put your hands behind you and press them against the floor. This alone should give you a respectable stretch on the hamstrings. Don't lean your upper body forward. For many, leaning forward automatically means rolling the hip under and rounding the back.

- Let your hip rock under again and feel tension on your hamstrings release. Rock the other way again and feel the hamstrings lengthen again, without leaning over forward or rounding your back.

> Most people don't have the hamstring flexibility to sit properly without their hip tucked under and back rounded.
>
> Instead of stretching their hamstrings to sit properly, they sit rounded because tightness makes it more comfortable that way.

- Now, try this stretch standing up. Prop one heel on a low chair. Keep your standing foot facing straight forward, or it takes the stretch off your hamstring. Hop in close. Keep the raised leg straight in front of you, not out to the side. Keep your hips straight across the front, not tilted toward one side. Arch your back to lengthen the hamstring. Push down on the hip of the raised leg. Practice rocking your hip forward and back to feel the length of the hamstring change. Keep your body upright and chin in.

- The best way to stretch your hamstrings is lying down. Lie on your back and raise one leg up without lifting your head or shoulders from the floor. This keeps your back straight and the pressure off your discs. Experiment with arching your back. Don't let your behind lift off the floor. To stretch the hip of the other leg, keep the other leg flat on the floor. For more on leg and hip stretches, see Chapter 21 on back and neck pain.

Stretching Mistake #3: Stretching Before Warm-up

Stretching cold muscles is one way to injure yourself. At cooler muscle temperatures it takes less force and stretch to tear the fibers. "Warming up" literally means increasing your body temperature. Activities that warm you enough to safely begin exercise are large muscle exercises like pedaling a bicycle or slow jogging. Stretching doesn't raise your body temperature, so it's not a warm-up. Wait to stretch until after you warm up. When you've exercised enough to get sweaty you're warmed up enough to stretch. See Chapter 5 for more on warm-ups.

What about yoga and stretch classes that begin right away by bending right over to touch the floor? That is also stretching without a warm-up. It does not magically become all right because it has a mystical name. A venerated yogi in India was asked why yoga would begin right away with stretching instead of warming up first. He replied, "Because in India, it is veddy, veddy HOT."

- Stretching is not a warm-up.

- Stretching before warm-up can lead to muscle tears, cramps, and other injuries.

- Warm up at least 5 to 10 minutes before stretching.

- You're warmed up when you begin to break a sweat.

Stretching Mistake #4: Stretching Ligaments, Not Muscles

Ligaments are fibrous bands that hold your bones together so you don't rattle around. Ligaments normally are not supposed to stretch much. They retain their length, within a range, to hold your bones in position, so the bones glide past each other along anatomically healthy paths.

Your joints need to be flexible, but not too loose either. When injury or chronic improper stretching forces ligaments to lengthen, they do not readily go back to their former length. Technically speaking they are *plastic*, but not *elastic*. Stretched ligaments hang shapelessly loose like worn-out underwear waistbands. What's so bad about that?

Stretched ligaments don't hold your bones in line, allowing them to rub and grind at unhealthy angles. The friction contributes to degenerative changes over time and all the pain and disability that accompanies it. Ligament instability predisposes to sprains and dislocations. For example, too much looseness on the sides of your ankle increases your chance of ankle sprains. Lax shoulder capsules may slip out of place from forces that healthier joint capsules tolerate. People with overly lax joints need strengthening exercises for the supporting musculature, to offset the potential for injury.

Everyone has different amounts of natural ligament looseness. Men generally have less natural flexibility than women, but can attain healthy flexibility with regular stretching. Some people have too much flexibility. Extreme ligament laxity is a common problem among dancers, and sometimes swimmers who overdo shoulder stretching. Although dancers need extreme flexibility for their art, and swimmers get better reach and range, it is not always healthy for them. With the increasing popularity of exercise classes, ligament damage from improper stretching instruction is becoming common in the general population. These people need strengthening programs to compensate for their acquired structural problems and the damage that can result.

There are several things you can do to avoid stretching ligaments when you really want to stretch muscles. Two are most important:

Keep the limb you're stretching in line with the joint. Several well-known stretches hold the joint at an angle that puts too much weight and pressure on ligaments. The "hurdler's stretch" is a major example. It twists your knee sideways. Instead, keep the non-stretched leg in front of you with your foot on the floor. Forcing your arms high up behind you strains the front, and weakest part, of your shoulder capsule. There's no need to stretch your arms like that.

Avoid constant pressure on joints over extended periods of time. An example is continuously sitting with a rounded back. Slouching overstretches the long ligament running up and down the back of your spine called the posterior longitudinal ligament. A chronically overstretched posterior longitudinal ligament weakens your back, and can lead to disc trouble. See Chapters 20 and 21 on back and neck pain. Habitually standing with your head forward stretches the back of your neck, with similar results. Squatting on your "haunches" pries knee ligaments apart, particularly if you have heavy legs. Continuous, long-term squatting damages the small discs of cartilaginous cushion in your knees, called meniscus. The bad knees of professional baseball catchers come from chronic squatting.

- Ligaments normally are not supposed to stretch much.

- Stretched ligaments don't hold your bones in line, allowing them to rub and grind at unhealthy angles.

- Avoid putting weight and pressure on ligaments, such as in the "hurdler's stretch" and pulling your arms high up behind you.

- Avoid positions that place constant pressure on joints over extended periods of time, such as slouching, which weakens muscles and joints and pressures the discs.

Stretching Mistake #5: Putting More Weight on Joint Capsules Than They Can Stand

Your joints are places where your body crams many structures into little space. Because of that, it's easy to do things that squash, tear, and abrade your joints. Joint cartilage and ligaments have a poorer blood supply than other body parts. Low blood supply means slow repair that may not keep up with each small, destructive incident. Some damaged joints never heal, forcing their owners into surgery. Damage usually occurs slowly without your knowing it is happening and can, over time, injure your joint to the same degree as can a single accident. Chronic mistreatment slowly thickens a joint with fibrous scar tissue. Scarring makes the capsule less mobile and more uncomfortable as small abuses gradually accelerate the normal wear and tear of aging.

Examples of well-known stretch-intensive activities that can damage your joints are squatting on your heels and duck walks, both of which force the knee joint open. Avoid neck manglers like the "plow"—lying with your legs in the air over your head and all your weight on your shoulders and neck.

A stretch that puts too much weight on your spine is bending over from a stand for toe touching, or worse, bouncing while bending over for toe touching. Stretches like that do more harm than good. You don't need them. To stretch your hamstrings without hurting your back, lie on your back, bend both knees, then leave one foot on the floor and straighten the other leg overhead. Most foolhardy of all is bent-over weightlifting like straight-legged dead lifting. See Chapters 20 and 21 on back pain.

- It's easy to squash, tear, abrade, and scar your joints when you put more weight on them than they were designed for.

- Examples of stretches that overweight your joints are the "plow," duck walk, standing toe touch, and straight-legged dead lift.

- Damage can occur slowly without your knowing it and can injure your joints over time as much as a single accident can.

Stretching Mistake #6: Unequal Stretching

It is common to overdo stretching in one direction without countering the stretch in the opposite direction of movement. An obvious example is dancers who stretch their legs outward without stretching inward. The outside of their legs gradually tightens and shortens, the inside loosens, until they walk like ducks. Later, their hips, knees, and big toe joint succumb to early wear.

Another easily recognized example is round-shouldered muscle guys. They build up their chest without stretching it, which tightens and shortens it. Their back cannot counter the pull of their strong and shortened big chests. Their chests pull them into a round-shouldered posture. This posture can slowly cause back and neck pain. Often, the shortening is so extensive that it pulls on the shoulder where the upper arm attaches. The upper arm rotates so that their thumbs face inward, sometimes even backward, rather than forward. Check for thumbs facing each other on all your friends. Check yourself.

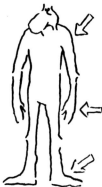

Figure 6.2. It is common to stretch too much in one direction and not enough in the other. You may overstretch your back but not stretch your front, so you become round-shouldered. Some people do this so much that their arms rotate inward. You may work the inside and outside of your legs unequally, which allows them to turn in one direction more than the other. These postures can cause early wear and tear on your joints.

The most common example of unequal stretching is when ordinary people chronically round their back and hip all day long by sitting, standing, and walking with poor posture. The only stretching they do, if any, is more forward motion during toe touches, sit-ups, leg lifts, and chest exercises. Damage builds up gradually. The consequences of an overstretched back and a tight chest range from poor posture, pot belly, and shallow breathing, to back pain and disc injury. This is also the least recognized example. It is so common that it looks "normal."

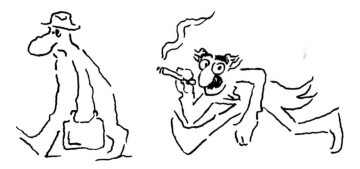

Figure 6.3. An overstretched back and tight chest are so common they look normal. The bent forward postures that result can lead to back pain and disc injury.

After stretching in one direction, stretch the other way. (Check with your physician before beginning any new exercises.) After each half hour or so of sitting, get up and stretch backward or lie facedown, propped up on your elbows. When standing or sitting, keep your ear centered over your shoulder, not in front of or behind it, to keep your neck from overstretching. See Chapters 20 and 21 on back pain for more on this important issue.

- Stretching in one direction without countering the stretch in the opposite direction can make you stand and walk funny, and lead to injury.

- Stretching shouldn't mean doing strange contortions; it should address the posture you need for daily life so you can stand up straight.

- Examples of unequal stretching are stretching forward for toe touches, chest exercises, ab exercises like crunches, and standing round-shouldered all day, but never stretching and strengthening backward. Poor posture and back pain commonly result.

Stretching Mistake #7: Bouncing

Bouncing forces your muscles to an unsafe length before your pain receptors have time to signal you not to do such a thing. Bouncing can increase your flexibility, but at the cost of microinjuries; it is one of several reasons you sometimes get sore after exercise. Bouncing is called ballistic stretching. By contrast, slow stretches called static stretches are not usually associated with delayed-onset soreness and may help relieve soreness after you've already overdone it. There is some debate whether static stretching ahead of time reduces the delayed soreness of too much exercise. See Chapter 10, "Just Overdo It."

Sense organs all over your body pick up and send information about what's happening to your body. These sense organs are called proprioceptors. *Proprio* means "self," and the word root *ceptors* refers to "receiving information." Proprioceptors tell you about yourself. The most abundant proprioceptors in your body are structures called muscle spindles. Spindles lie embedded in your muscles. Bouncing has an interesting effect on your muscles because of these muscle spindles. When you stretch a muscle quickly, the spindle stretches too, activating its sensory nerve. The sensory nerve carries a message to your spinal cord about how much and how fast your muscle stretched. Your nervous system sends a signal back to tell your muscle not to stretch so much.

An example is maintaining balance. You make thousands of minor adjustments all day without thinking about it, while sitting, standing, and walking. If you lean forward, the spindles in your back and the back of your legs stretch. They signal your spine to send a return message to your muscles; not only to contract, but how much to contract. They pull you back to an upright position, but no further. The muscle stretch-contraction loop is called the myotatic reflex, or stretch reflex.

The sudden stretch of bouncing activates muscle spindles. Your spindles send a sensory message up your neural chain of command, triggering a motor message back down to contract the muscle. Bouncing again during the contract reflex forces the muscle to lengthen against the energy of its own contraction. Damage can occur in the structures that both stretch and resist the stretch.

Remember falling asleep in your chair at the beginning of this story? When the sudden stretch of your head bouncing forward activated neck muscle spindles, the message came back to contract your neck muscles just as suddenly, pulling your head back up again. Now you know it was your muscle spindles at work in a stretch reflex.

- Bouncing while stretching can increase your flexibility but can cause tiny (or large) muscle and joint pulls and tears.

- Bouncing sends your nervous system a signal to make the muscle contract to protect it from tearing, so bouncing can sometimes make your muscle tighter.

- Hold your stretch without bouncing.

Neuromuscular Facilitation

If you'd like to make your receptors work for you to increase flexibility, not against you, try this easy, effective technique. Lie on your back, one leg up in the air. Hold the back of your leg with your hands and press your leg against your hands hard, while counting to three. When you relax the press, you'll usually find you can pull your leg into a further stretch.

This works with all stretches. First push away from the stretch to fatigue the muscle, then relax and pull the stretch a bit further.

Another way to do this is to lie on your back, as above, put your hands on the front of your thigh, and try to push your leg down with your hands. Resist with your leg. When you relax, you may find you can pull the hamstring into more of a stretch. This can be done on all muscles. First, push the opposite muscle while resisting, then relax and pull the muscle you want to stretch without resisting.

Stretching Mistake #8: Stretching Without Strengthening

Being highly flexible, by itself, does not make you a better person, or more fit. It can even create problems. A joint must be able to move, but not so much that it moves out of place, rubs adjacent structures, or jangles loosely during daily movement. Joints that are too loose and not strong can become unstable and not seat well. Like any two surfaces in your car or other machinery that don't seat well, your joints will suffer early wear and tear. There is a difference between flexibility and instability. It is important to keep the musculature surrounding your joints strong, to support your joints, and keep joint angles and movement in healthy directions and ranges.

- By itself, being flexible is not synonymous with being in good shape.

- Stretching a joint without exercising it to be strong may allow it to stretch too far, injuring it, or to become so weak and overstretched that your joints rub and don't seat well.

- Combine strengthening exercises with your stretching exercises.

Protect Your Back and Neck During Stretching

- Avoid the "plow," the "frog," and other shoulder-stand positions where you put your weight on a bent-forward neck.

- Do back and hamstring stretches lying down.

- Keep the normal inward curve of your lower back. Notice if your hip is tipping under, allowing your back to round.

- Don't round your back and crane your neck and call that a hamstring stretch.

- Avoid sitting with a rounded back and a forward head.

- Don't push or force back stretches, and don't let anyone help you stretch by pushing or forcing.

- Stretch in both directions—if you stretch by leaning forward then stretch by leaning backward.

- Make an even arc with your back, rather than just "folding" at one easily moved joint.

What to Do

Don't Add to the Problem. More forward stretching when you are already round-shouldered adds to the problem. Make sure to stretch your neck, shoulder, chest, back, and hip toward the back too, so you can stand up straight.

Stretch What You Think You're Stretching. When stretching one part, don't crane other parts so that you lose the stretch. When stretching your shoulder or hamstring, for example, don't let the stretch come from your back. Keep good posture in the rest of your body.

Stretch Often. Reduce your injury potential by stretching often. Flexibility gains are easily and quickly lost.

Stretch Safely. Warm up enough to sweat before you stretch. Then slowly ease into your stretch, and hold. Don't bounce or you'll activate your myotatic stretch contraction loop, and you don't want to do that. Stretch in a comfortable range, not forced to the point of pain. Forcing stimulates your spindle reflex to give your muscle a shrink, not a stretch. Breathe normally while stretching. Don't hold your breath.

Stretch Evenly. To avoid posture problems and back pain from unequal stretching, stretch in each natural direction. Don't overload your back. Substitute lying-down back stretches for standing, bent-over ones. Avoid sitting with a rounded back. Keep the normal inward curve of your lower back without exaggerating it.

7

Abdominal Muscles— Why You Need Good Ones, and How to Get Them

He was a man of an unbounded stomach.

– Katharine, in Shakespeare's King Henry VIII, Act 4, Scene 2

Your abdominal muscles help your back, but how? Your "abs" have something to do with posture, but exactly what? You know something vague about "support," but what does that really mean? Most people want "ab" exercises but have no idea what the exercises really do or how they translate to "real life." Two exercises popularly thought to benefit abs—sit-ups and leg lifts—often aren't done in ways that work your abs. They are also tough on your back. Why is that? "Crunches" are practically synonymous with ab exercises but are terrible for your posture and don't work your abs the way you need for real life. What can you do instead? What exercises flatten your abdomen, and what if you don't like to go to a gym? Using abs doesn't mean sucking them in or making them tight. Then how do you use them? Did you know that you should exercise your abs standing up? How can you do that?

How Your Muscles Work

To understand how to improve your abdominal muscles, you need to know important things about muscles in general. All muscles originate on a bone, cross a joint, then attach to another bone on the other side of the joint. When a muscle contracts, it pulls on the bones to bend the joint it crosses. That's how you move. It's like a marionette—when you pull the string, the attached part comes with it. In your body, the string is the tendon that attaches muscle to bone. To move your arm, for example, your biceps muscle in front of your upper arm contracts to pull your lower arm bone and bend your elbow. Muscles can only contract and pull. Your biceps cannot actively lengthen to push your arm straight again. To straighten your elbow, another muscle, the triceps in back of your arm, contracts and pulls your lower arm bone straight. Your biceps still keep a certain amount of tension to decelerate the straightening so that your arm straightens with control and stops softly, instead of flinging straight and banging your elbow.

Muscles on one side of a joint pull one way, and muscles on the other side pull the other way. When neither pulls, you don't move voluntarily. There are no muscles at work. But you can still sag under gravity since no muscle is working to prevent that. That is one big reason people slouch—they aren't using muscles to prevent it. When muscles on both sides of a joint pull at the same time, with the same amount of force, you also don't move. Both are working, but neither can shorten to move anything. This kind of contraction is called "isometric," which means "same measure." It is a hugely important way for muscles to work so that you can stand and sit up without flopping over. All your posture muscles need to work isometrically to hold you in healthy posture without sagging.

How Your Abs Work

Abs connect from rib bones to hip bones. The joints they cross are your backbones (vertebrae). They may seem far away from your vertebrae, but they still span them, and control their joint angles from the front. Your back muscles cross your vertebrae from the back and control the curve from the back. When abs contract, they pull ribs closer to hips, bending your vertebral column forward. Abs are the muscles that, like a guy wire keeping a tree from tipping backward, keep you from arching your vertebrae backward and dropping your weight on your low back.

Abdominal muscles are among your main posture muscles. You need to use your abs to keep you upright when standing up, walking, exercising, and just sitting around. Abs help keep your spine and hip bones at healthy angles for the postural control that avoids wear and tear, and back pain.

Using your abs doesn't mean sucking them in or making them "tight." It is not the often quoted, "Press your navel to your spine and contract your backside muscles." You couldn't function normally that way, and that wouldn't specifically help your posture. Using abs means changing the curve of your torso so your upper body weight doesn't arch the weight of your upper back onto your lower back. Few people actually do this.

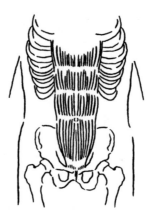

Figure 7.1. Your rectus abdominis muscle runs from your ribs to the front of your pelvic bones. When this muscle is in good shape and is used, it holds your torso from swaying backward by being a guy wire between your ribs and pelvis.

> Using abs does not mean sucking them in, or tightening them, or "pressing them to your spine." It means moving your torso, the way you move any other joints, to control your back from arching backward and flopping your weight on your low back.

In life, your abs need to work isometrically—at one length—to hold your torso upright, instead of leaning your body weight backward onto your low back. Unless you are a Japanese greeter at a department store, you don't repeatedly bow forward. Yet people do crunches, which not only are not functional for daily life but make a person, who likely spends much of their day already hunched over a work area, practice that hunched posture, which may be mechanically promoting the back and neck pain they think they are working their abs to prevent.

> Most people hunch forward for a few "ab exercises," then stand and work in postures with slack abs, which allow ribs to lift up, hips to drop down, and their back to arch, chronically slamming their body weight down on their low back.

How Do Good Abs Help Your Back?

People usually have some vague idea that abs have something to do with helping your back. But abs don't do that automatically. You can have very strong abs and never use them to do anything for your back. So then what exactly do the abs do?

Try this:

- Hold your right hand up in front of your face sideways so that you see your thumb toward you. Your palm (facing left) is your tummy. The back of your hand (facing right) is your back. With your left hand, press against the fingers of your right hand so that they bend backward as far as they will go. Keep your palm upright and perpendicular to the floor—only the fingers arch back. Observe a pinched fold on the back of your right hand at the knuckle. That is your low back. The palm of your hand is your tummy with your abs slack. This represents how your body weight falls on the joints of your low back without using your muscles in front.

- Now bounce against your fingers so that they rock back, and fold, fold, fold. That is walking with your tummy out. Now do it hard. That is running with your tummy out and not using your abs. Ouch. This is what you are doing to your low back every day when you do not consciously use your abs to prevent that kind of arching.

- Now, to represent how to use your abs to prevent arching, with your left hand still pressing the right fingers back, use the muscles in the palm of your right hand to straighten your right hand. Keep the palm straight up as before. The fingers come back up into straight line. That is how you need to use your abs. All day, every day. All the time.

- Use a mirror and experiment with your whole body in the same manner of letting your back arch so that you fold back and stick out your tummy. Do you feel a familiar discomfort in your low back? That isn't an inescapable back condition; that is just poor mechanics. Now use your ab muscles to take out the over-arch; tuck your behind in under you until you stand with a normal small curve and good posture.

- Using abs so that weight doesn't smash your low back is supposed to be done all the time for all normal standing activities. But it is forgotten both during exercise and in "real life."

> Strengthening alone will not fix posture.
> Plenty of people with strong muscles stand terribly.
> It's like having brains and not using them.

> Doing crunches will not heal your back.
> You must learn how to use the strong abs to hold your weight
> up with good body mechanics.

Just doing strengthening exercises has no effect on posture if you don't apply the strength the rest of the day to control joint angles and body mechanics for all your activities. Using abs during a specific exercise doesn't automatically make you know to use them during life. You need to consciously use your abs to control your torso posture during all your activities. Stand and sit well all the time and you'll exercise your abs without working out. See Chapters 20 and 21 on back pain and prevention.

What's Wrong With Crunches?

- Crunches do not work your abs the way you need for real life.

- They do not train you how to use your abs the rest of the day.

- Crunches promote poor posture, even when done properly.

When you exercise a muscle, it gets good at what you make it practice. That means that when you do crunches, you develop your ability to curl your torso forward and back and forward and back. Is that what you really want? When do you need to do that in a day? Chances are that you rarely do that, unless you're a professional Japanese greeter. Even for getting up from lying on your back, it's safer for your back not to sit up directly. Back specialists advise that you roll to one side first.

The most common ab exercise is trunk flexion, also called trunk curls, or crunches, pictured in Figure 7.2. But crunches aren't functional exercises. That is, they don't use your body the way you need for real life. Also, doing crunches does not

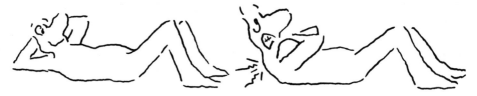

Figure 7.2. "Crunches" are common but don't work your abs the way you need them for real life. Do you do anything in life that looks like this? If you still like to do crunches, or find yourself in classes that still do them, keep your head back, not craned forward. That hurts your neck and promotes poor posture. Instead of lifting your body up by your head, learn to contract your abs first, until they lift the rest of your upper body up with them. That is better training for how to use your abs in life.

automatically make your back supported for the rest of the day. Unless you consciously control your torso angles using your ab and back muscles, nothing to support your back happens, no matter how many crunches you have done.

What Do Crunches Do? To understand what crunches do and what contracting your abs so that you curl forward does, try this:

- Stand up and feel where your abs begin at the bottom of your ribs. Put your other hand on the center-front of your hip bone where your abs end. Check Figure 7.1 for placement. Hold these two points with your fingers.

- To simulate contracting your abs, draw your two hands toward each other, still holding on to where the abs attach at the top and bottom. Your torso will curl forward.

- Hold that position. That is what crunches do for you. They curl you forward. Do you do this much in real life?

- Now, still holding onto your ribs and hip bone, let the distance between your two hands increase to simulate slack abs. Arch back and let your ribs pull up and your tummy curve out. Feel your body weight fall onto your low back? That is what not using your abs allows—an arched back and your weight smashing your low back.

- Now pull your two hands and your torso upright to a straight position, simulating using your abs isometrically the way you need them to stand properly. No more low back pressure and better posture.

You Need Your Abs Working All the Time While Standing

Many people can't imagine using their abs while standing. Yet this is what will keep your back supported and prevent pain and injury during daily activities. To understand what to do to use your abs in real life, remember the example earlier in the "How Do Good Abs Help Your Back?" section, and try this:

- Stand sideways and look in a mirror big enough to see your body. If you don't have a mirror, pay close attention to what it feels like.

- Allow your body weight to sag so that you arch your back and exaggerate your low back curve. Your stomach will curve out in front. Allow your weight to press on your low back. You may feel the familiar ache you often get and don't know why. Many people stand with far too much lumbar curve because they are not using their abs.

- Tuck your behind under enough to reduce the large back arch. You'll keep a small inward curve, but the key here is your weight is held up on your ab muscles and not pressing back and down on your low back.

- Now reach overhead. Did your back arch again? Many people arch their back with no ab support every time they reach. That throws weight on their low back again. Now, still reaching overhead, tuck your behind under using abs to move your torso straight. Feel a new strong middle. Keep that all the time. Use this whenever you reach overhead—from pulling shirts off to reaching in cabinets, to washing your hair, to lifting weights.

> Many people don't use their abs when standing and reaching overhead. Their back arches and their ribs lift up each time they raise their arms. This happens hundreds of times a day— combing hair, pulling off shirts, reaching shelves, waving, putting away groceries, then again in the gym lifting weights and exercising.
>
> People often do plenty of crunches but walk out of the gym without using their abs to stand and walk with supported posture. Their backs are still getting pummeled by all their body weight smashing on it all day.

What Exercises Work Your Abs the Way You Need Them for Real Life?

Other than standing and reaching properly all day every day, what can you do to train good ab use for posture, activities, and good looks too?

The ab exercises you see everywhere in gyms get you good at bowing forward and back and forward and back. But your abs need to work isometrically in real life, not by bowing you forward. So exercise your abs isometrically for postural control when you sit, stand, walk, run, and carry packages, so you don't arch backwards. You can benefit by exercising your abs in the manner in which they normally should work. That means radically different exercises than you commonly see in gyms and on exercise videos.

- Hold the push-up position without sagging and arching in the middle or hiking up your bottom. Many people will droop like an old horse in the middle. Imagine standing up this way. Then use your abs to fix your posture. Tuck your behind under and straighten out your torso. The push-up position is a fabulous postural control exercise—using your "anti-gravity" torso muscles the way you need them for standing posture.

- Now turn to one side, lifting one arm to the sky so that you balance on one arm and still hold your body straight without drooping in the middle. That uses your oblique abs the way you need them for posture—to hold your posture without sagging under packages, shoulder bags, and children carried on one hip. Do this exercise on both sides.

Most people can't do this exercise for more than a few seconds. No wonder their posture sags so terribly after a day. They don't have the strength and use of their abs to stand up straight. Gradually increase the time you hold good posture with this exercise.

> Having stronger abs, by itself, doesn't do anything. You can have a "six-pack" and still stand and exercise with a big arch in your low back, and allow all your weight to smash your low back.

Controlling Ab and Torso Posture When Using Weights

- Lie on your back with your knees bent and feet on the floor. Arch your back up, lifting your ribs high so you know what it feels like. Put your hand on the floor under the arch of your back. Now press your back against your hand so that you feel how to use your abs to control your torso. Don't lift your hips, just use your abs. You'll feel your abs working right under your skin, since ab muscles are shallow. Now put your other arm overhead just off the floor, biceps by your ear. Did your back arch again off your hand? Press it back down. Put both hands overhead, just an inch off the floor, biceps near your ears. Feel your abs contract to hold your torso straight without allowing your back to arch.

- When you can comfortably do this, hold hand weights, making sure your low back does not arch. Your abdominal muscles work hard on this one to control your posture against challenge. Holding the hand weight also works your arms and latissimus dorsi muscles along the side of your back. You get several exercises for the price of one. Remember that your life is multi-segment, not isolated movements, so it's helpful to exercise as you need for real life.

- Now try pulsing the weight fairly quickly—an inch higher and lower up and down without touching the floor. Each time the weight lowers, your back will want to arch. Don't let it. This simulates all the daily life activities where you will either support things you carry or lift by your muscles, or allow youself to drop your weight into an arched back.

- Increase the weight slowly and safely as you improve your abs so that they can maintain your low back in good neutral posture.

- To increase the difficulty of this exercise as you progress, extend your legs so that your knees are less bent. Keep your abs contracted so that your back does not pull into an arch.

- As long as you can safely increase the difficulty, work until you can properly do this isometric ab exercise, with hand weights, with your legs completely straight out on the floor as if you were standing up, and your low back not pulled out of good neutral posture.

- You may need to stretch your hip flexor muscles so that you can straighten your legs without your low back being pulled into an arch.

- Now think of all the exercises involving lifting weights overhead, where people should stand straight, as you have practiced, but don't, and pump the weight up and down with the force crashing down on their low back. When you do standing weightlifting, control your posture with what you learned with this lying-down training exercise.

Note: Anyone with cardiovascular disease and/or hypertension should not do sustained isometric contraction of their upper extremities such as this until their condition is controlled. Since exercise is helpful to controlling blood pressure, consult with your physician. It's better to deal with the blood pressure so you can exercise, than miss the benefits of exercising.

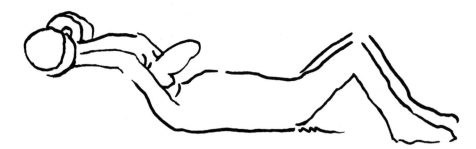

Figure 7.3. Your abs normally work isometrically—at one length—so you can stand, sit, walk, and exercise without arching. In this isometric ab exercise, you don't allow your back to arch, which contracts your abs in a way similar to that needed in life for posture control and normal function.

Controlling Ab and Torso Posture When Standing and Using Resistance

- Stand up and reach overhead. Did your ribs come up and your back arch? First learn to stop doing that with the exercise shown in Figure 7.3. Keep your hip tucked under you. Not exaggerated, but just until your body is straight and supported. Reach overhead again. Wave your arms around. Keep your torso from increasing the arch, no matter what.

- Tie the middle of a commercial stretchy band, pair of panty hose, or stretchy cord securely to a doorknob, pole, or pipe at about waist height. Leave both ends free. Turn around with your back to the tie. Pick up one end of the stretchy band in each hand. Lift both arms overhead, controlling your torso posture with your abs. Step away until there is tension on the band. Don't let your arms get pulled behind you. Try various arm exercises while controlling your torso with your abs. This simulates gravity and the loads you routinely carry in your daily life while moving around. Keep your back from arching.

Using Abs for Throwing, Punching, and Other Arm Activities

When throwing and punching properly, you use your arm for only a small part of the power. Your torso and legs should power most of it. But most people just fling their arm. Shoulder and back injury can eventually develop. When swinging a tennis racquet, for example, by not contracting the abs and using the torso to power the move, you overload your shoulder. When punching, you would shift weight onto your low back.

- Using the stretchy cord tied as above, turn your back to the wall, still holding both ends of the stretchy cord. Keep your arms in front of you and overhead. Don't let the cord pull you into an arch or pull your arms behind you. Feel how to stabilize your body, using abs.

- Do crunches standing up.

- Simulate throwing a ball or a punch by first contracting your abs so that your torso begins curling forward. Only then does the arm come forward.

- Turn sideways and hold your torso stable against the sideways pull of the stretchy cord. Do side curls or walk around and keep your torso stable against the changing pull of the band.

- Have a friend hold the other end of the band and pull you in odd directions while you practice torso stabilization. This simulates walking a dog, and carrying a squirming baby and packages while trying to get in the door.

> Backpacks and heavy shoulder bags don't make you arch your back. Not using your torso muscles to counter the pull so that you stand with good posture is the problem.
> Carrying your bags could be a built-in ab exercise.

Why Don't Sit-Ups and Leg Lifts Work Your Abs?

In the classic sit-up, you raise your trunk toward your leg by bending at the hip. Leg raises lift your legs closer to your trunk, also by bending at the hip. Bending the hip is called hip flexion. The muscles working during sit-ups and leg lifts are your hip flexors. They lie deeper than your abdominals, and they are mostly what you feel working when you do sit-ups and leg lifts.

Your main hip flexor muscle crosses your hip. Your abdominal muscles do not cross the hip, so are not used in hip flexion. If they were, you could work out your abdominals by the most frequent form of dynamic hip flexion—walking.

When doing leg lifts (lying on the back and lifting the legs up), most people allow the weight of their legs to arch their back and pinch their low back. If they used their abs to prevent that, they could use their abs during this exercise. Instead of training the abs, many people are taught to put their hands under their behinds to tilt their hips. That keeps the back from arching but doesn't use the abs. This is a missed ab opportunity and an exercise that works the hip flexors, which usually are pretty strong and tight to begin with. Tight hip flexors cause a variety of problems.

Why Can Sit-Ups and Leg Lifts Hurt Your Back?

Sit-ups and leg lifts contribute to back pain in two ways. Two of your hip flexor muscles attach to your lower spine. Contracting your hip flexors the way sit-ups and leg lifts are usually done pulls on the site of attachment. Your spine was not built to withstand the constant yanking.

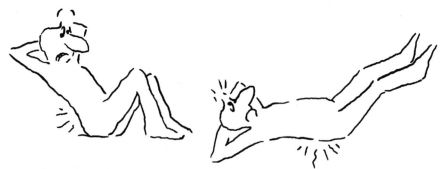

Figure 7.4. Sit-ups and leg lifts done without your abs supporting your torso can contribute to back pain even if you are in good shape.

Another problem with sit-ups and leg lifts occurs when they shorten your hip flexor muscles. This shortening is common in people who sit a lot, and who overdo hip flexor exercise without stretching their hip flexors. Several problems can result:

- Short, tight hip flexors pull your pelvis forward. The shift in the normal tilt is one of several contributors to low back pain.

- Tight hip flexors yank on your back bones with every step you take.

- Tight hip flexor muscles can contribute, surprisingly, to shoulder injuries. Tight hip flexors do not allow full range of motion of your torso, so that when you try to reach overhead, your shoulder has to overrotate.

- Hip flexor muscles can sometimes be so tight that they prevent you from lying flat. When you lie on your back, tight hip flexors can make you arch too much when you straighten your legs against the floor.

> Some specialists recommend that people who sleep on their back keep a pillow under their knees to prevent back pain. With the knees bent up by the pillow, the tight hip flexors cannot pull the back into an arch.
>
> The pillow perpetuates the problem, not solves it. These people need hip flexor stretches so their back isn't pulled up in the first place, not a pillow.

There are better exercises for your abs without the risk sit-ups and leg lifts pose to your back. Unless you need extraordinary hip flexor strength for rugby, ballet, springboard diving, martial arts, or gymnastics; are willing to take extra care to learn ab use during these exercises; and do extra hip flexor stretches, stick with the exercises described earlier in this section. For more on back pain, see Chapters 20 and 21.

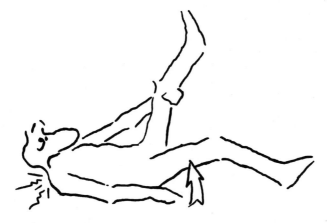

Figure 7.5. When the muscles in front of your hip are tight, the tight leg will come up when you raise the other, instead of lying flat. Tight hip muscles can contribute to several posture and back pain problems.

Arching Isn't the Culprit

Arching by itself is not the problem. The problem is allowing your upper body weight to arch onto your low back. This is often confused, and some people think they must never arch their back. By holding back the weight with your abs you can arch without your weight pressing onto your low back. This supported arch is necessary during gymnastics, yoga, healthy stretching, and sports activities. Many people do not know to use their abs during these kinds of moves, so fold backward with all their weight.

Try this:

- Arch your back with no ab involvement and feel your weight on your low back (don't do this if you have back pain).

- Now lift your weight up and off your low back using your abs as previously described in this chapter.

- Begin to lean back, but use your abs to keep weight off your low back. Don't tilt your head back or pinch your neck. Pull your shoulders back. It should be a good-feeling stretch.

- Now try this while bending your knees to tilt backward further. Don't let your abs "go" or allow your weight to slump. You should feel a nice ab exercise and no back pain.

"Ab-Only" Exercises Are Not Good

Abs create an important support structure for your lower torso and back, but they are not the entire support. Many people mistakenly do only abdominal muscle exercises, thinking it will make their backs injury-free.

Just as your ab muscles, when used, prevent you from arching back so that your body weight hinges on your low back, your back muscles, when used, keep you from slouching and hunching forward—a poor posture that people are usually very good at. This forward-slouching posture slowly puts unhealthy pressure on the vertebrae and nerves that exit the vertebrae. It pressures your discs to bulge out toward the back, and overstretches your back muscles. Keeping your back muscles, or any muscles, lengthened by poor posture weakens them.

Doing ab exercises does not work your back muscles. You need to work your back separately to keep it from being so fatigued at the end of the day that it screams in protest.

Without adding exercises that actively contract your back muscles, you will reach a point where your weaker back muscles can't counter the chronic muscle tension developed in front from your abs. The resulting forward pull encourages your body to slouch forward as your natural state. Because your abs attach to your pelvic bone in front, too much muscle tension from abs, unbalanced by low back muscles, pulls your pelvis into a tilt that adds to back pain.

You won't feel a problem right away. This kind of back injury takes time to develop, so have patience.

> "Ab-only" exercises can contribute to back pain and poor posture.
>
> Add exercises that contract your back muscles, called lumbar extension exercises, to balance the supporting muscles for your torso.

Should You Work Your Abs Every Day or Every Other Day?

It's common for people to debate fiber type and fatigue, and conclude whether to exercise abs daily or intermittently. Flurries of articles are written on this. What is missed is that you need your abs working all day every day. Doing specific moves for an hour and not using your abs for daily life is like couples being nice in a counselor's office for an hour, then screaming at each other the rest of the day, and justifying that by saying harmony was already done for a time each day (or alternate days) and it's too tiring to do it all the time. Plenty of guys have six-pack abs and don't use them for daily life the way they need for posture and back pain control. Like your heart beating, you need your abs working all the time. If you worked your abs all day all the time to control your posture, you wouldn't need to go to a gym to do funny little crunches, either every day, or every few days.

> Using your abs is like the Ten Commandments.
> You're supposed to do it all the time,
> not just during your hour of worship.

How Do You Flatten Your Abdomen?

No exercise selectively removes fat from any target body part. That myth is called "spot reducing." If spot reducing worked, people would have thin mouths from talking, speed skaters would have little legs, and the repetitive act of chewing and swallowing lots of food would make your face thin.

Aerobic exercise burns fat. This fat comes from everywhere it is stored. That means to lose fat, including fat from your abdomen, you need to run, swim, bike, row, dance, skate, jog, ski, or walk. Ab exercises alone will not remove fat from your abdomen. That does not mean that resistance exercise does not have a place in weight control. Weight training builds muscle, which raises your metabolic rate. A higher rate means your body burns more calories every day.

Ab exercise helps compress your abdomen and tone your abdominal muscles. Ab exercise is part of the work you need for the good posture that pulls your back and hips into better alignment, so that you don't stand with your abdomen sticking out. How ironic that many exercises done in gyms mistakenly tighten the hip and ignore the back so that you do just that.

> Why kill yourself working out, but ignore your abs
> the other 23 hours a day?
>
> Stand, sit, and reach well all the time and you'll exercise
> your abs without working out.

How Do You Get a "Washboard"?

You have bands of fibrous tissue called fascia that run across your abdominal muscles at intervals. Doing good abdominal work will enlarge the muscles enough to poke through the facial bands, giving a "washboard" or "ripple" effect. You won't see that if body fat covers everything. The entire package of getting results includes proper abdominal exercise, good posture, adequate complex carbohydrate and water in your diet to fuel good workouts, and reduced fat under your skin to produce a beautiful washboard abdomen.

8

What Exercises Do You Need to Be Fit?

I do not like work even when someone else does it.

– Mark Twain

What is fit? Does it mean just being healthy? Clearly, someone completely out of shape may not have a fun time during a hike or exercise class. Yet fitness is specific to the exercise you use to "get fit." Olympian shot-putters may be fit to put the shot, but not for gymnastics or aerobics class. Some people play tennis as their exercise for the week, but tennis won't get you fit for hiking or swimming, and it won't get all your body parts and systems fit. There are health benefits to the commonly heard exercise "prescription" of three times a week for 20 minutes, but you still may not be cardiovascularly "fit" enough to get you through a day without fatigue, or muscularly fit to get you through a day without back pain.

Chapter 2 explained the different aspects of fitness, and Chapter 3 covered how to improve each different aspect of fitness. Chapter 13 explains that you don't even need to go to the gym if your lifestyle involves varied physical movement as part of your daily real life. So what exercises are good for you to get fit? This chapter covers the different types of exercise to improve the different aspects of fitness, to improve your different body parts, and to avoid injury while you "get fit."

Why Do You Need Different Exercises?

Exercising one body part or system does little to get other parts or systems fit. Stretching every day does a lot for your flexibility, but will not get your cardiovascular system fit. Weightlifting using weight machines improves muscle and bone strength, but doesn't give you good posture. Swimming will help your heart and other muscles, not train your sense of balance to reduce your risk of falls. Getting a good run every day conditions your legs and heart in ways that don't transfer to swimming. That's why good runners often exhaust themselves during long swims, and swimmers, during runs, even though both may be aerobically fit.

Each body part, system, and ability gets fit from different kinds of exercise. The principle is called *specificity*, and explains why you need many different activities to be completely fit.

Fit for a Sport vs. Sport for Fitness

What if you just play one sport and are not interested in other sports? Or any sports? Some people play a sport or do an exercise class just to "get fit," rather than do specific exercises to get better at their sport. For these people, the principle of specificity is still important. What specificity means to you is that if you do only one kind of activity, such as a regular racquetball game or aerobics class, although it is great exercise, you probably will not be getting fit overall. It's like practicing the tuba. It will not make you a good violin player, even though both are musical skills. You need other exercise for overall health and fitness, even if you regularly "work out" doing just one or two activities.

Exercises That "Work" Are
Not Always Good for You

Many common exercises will give you the cosmetic results claimed for them. That is, they will shape your muscles or burn fat. But they may injure your joints and soft tissue. Other exercises work the muscles they claim to work, but not at all in the manner you need in daily life. So they don't do much good, but take up valuable exercise time. You don't need to choose between an exercise that "works" and one that is safe and effective. Plenty of exercises, described later in this chapter, "work," and do it properly and safely.

> Some exercises will make you look better, but are injurious.
> Other exercises will give you the look you want,
> but without risk of injury.

Aerobic Exercises

Do You Need Step Aerobics? Cardiovascular workouts of many types improve health and ability to do physical work. Stepping can be a good cardiovascular exercise with potential to improve strength and muscular endurance of the legs. It also has potential for several injuries.

Stepping down, if not done lightly or close to the bench, forcibly pulls the Achilles tendon, and can produce painful and slow-healing tendon trauma. Banging down hard and repeatedly can also hurt your calf muscle.

Knee injury is common. How can that be, when physical therapists use benches for knee rehabilitation? Specific kinds of stepping can help with rehabilitation of one type of knee injury involving the meniscus (the shock-absorbing cartilage "washers" between your upper and lower leg bones). Yet stepping can be injurious to another knee problem—a poorly tracking kneecap that grinds with each step.

Normally, your four quadriceps muscles all pull equally on your kneecap when you move your knee. That makes your kneecap slide up and down in a narrow track in the front of your knee. Stepping can preferentially develop the outer quadriceps muscles more than those on the inside. When the stronger ones on the outside pull more than the weaker ones on the inside, it makes the kneecap track poorly and rub and grind in its groove, causing pain.

Exercisers often step down with a straight knee, rather than bending their knee for shock absorption. It is easier to throw the jolt onto the joint than to use the thigh muscles. But it is bad for the joint and you get less exercise. Bend your knees and use thigh muscles with any step down, not just in an exercise class.

Two more knee problems come when using a step that is too high. The high degree of knee bending with stepping brings your kneecap in contact with your upper leg bone (femur), even in knees without tracking problems. This can grind your kneecap against your upper leg bone with every step. High benches also magnify impact when stepping down. Many rehabilitation exercises that use a step use a lateral step up, so you step to the side rather than the front, avoiding the compression on the kneecap.

Commonly, people step up allowing their knees to sway inward. This is injurious to the knee over time. Stepping down with all your weight on this angulated knee is even worse. Keep your knee right over the line of your foot. Use the muscles on the side of your thigh to pull outward until your knee stays in place without wobbling all over. When you do this, you'll often find that it keeps the arches in your feet from rolling in and flattening. The feet may roll in on their own, too. In either case, use the muscles on the sides of your ankles and thighs to keep your leg lined up, not slumping.

Standing and moving with your feet facing toe-out like a dancer (duck-foot) or turned inward (pigeon-toe) is a common bad posture habit, often ignored as normal. Standing toe-in strains the foot, knee, and hip, and affects normal gait. Standing with your feet "turned out" contributes to much hip and knee pain and is often mistaken for "flat-foot" because it puts your weight on the inside of your foot and smashes your arches. Both bad foot postures can make you stand and move "knock-kneed," which is another bad posture, not a normal trait you just happen to be born with. Putting weight on the inside of your knees slowly pressures and strains them, wearing out the cartilage and interfering with normal muscle use and kneecap tracking.

> If your tires are crooked, they will wear.
> You don't just stop driving or change the tires, and you don't just keep driving that way. You check why they are crooked and fix that. Same with bad knee and foot posture—learn how to hold your knees and feet straight by using your muscles, not just letting them sway and slump.

Step up onto your whole foot, pushing through your heel, not just the ball of the foot. Leaning forward and stepping up onto the ball of the foot throws weight onto the knee joint. Sure, it's easier than using your thigh and backside muscles, but the point of stepping is to use your muscles. Stand and step with your feet parallel, not turning toe-in or toe-out.

How do you know if you will wind up with knee pain or other injuries? One approach is to take a step class and see if it screws up your knees in a few months or years. Another is to modify how you step. Keep your bench low to reduce knee angle. Step up and down lightly and close to the bench. Decelerate on the step down, using your leg and behind muscles; even when jumping down, don't just stomp down. Incorporate more side step-up moves to reduce the pounding and kneecap compression that forward stepping can produce. An interesting innovation to promote more lateral stepping is to turn the bench so that it faces the front the long way. That way your body can face the instructor while you do lateral stepping. Avoid continuous "repeaters," where you touch down behind the bench repeatedly with the same leg. They are tough on your calf muscles and Achilles tendons and can result in tears and strains.

Problems with Bench Stepping

- Repeated banging down to the rear of the bench can injure your Achilles tendon and calf muscle.

- Some people are susceptible to kneecap pain when the kneecap does not slide evenly in its groove, but rubs and grinds. Stepping magnifies this tendency.

- A high degree of knee bending rubs the kneecap against the upper leg bone with each step, even in knees without tracking problems.

- Many steppers allow their knees to sway inward, instead of keeping the lower leg perpendicular, right over the foot. This strains and pressures the knee joint and wears it out over time.

- Standing and moving with feet facing toe-out (duck-foot) or turned inward (pigeon-toe) is a common and destructive bad habit. Unfortunately, it is often ignored as normal or not changeable.

- Leaning your knee forward so that it is past your toe, and pushing off on the ball of the foot transfers your body weight to your anterior knee joint, instead of keeping your weight on your leg muscles.

- Many steppers step heavily and flop down to decelerate without muscle use from the leg still on the bench. Shock transmits to the joints of your ankle, knee, hip, back, and neck, and can strain your calf muscle and Achilles tendon.

The bottom line on step aerobics: It can help and harm. Modify your stepping to reduce injury potential. Have your knees orthopedically assessed if you get knee pain.

Modifications for Bench Stepping

- Step up with weight on your heel, not only on the ball of your foot.

- Step down lightly and close to the bench for better shock absorption. You'll use your muscles more and burn more calories.

- Generate shock absorption with the leg that steps down. Bend your knee as you touch the ground to absorb impact with your muscles, not your knee joint.

- Keep your thigh muscles (quadriceps) strong to support your knee and improve your body's natural shock absorption.

- When stepping down, use conscious muscle control to decelerate. Use the thigh muscles of the leg that is still on the bench to slow your descent. Don't just crash your weight down.

- Incorporate more lateral step-up, stepping to the side rather than the front, to lessen compression on the kneecap.

- Keep the step low.

- Avoid banging down with "repeater" steps.

- Keep your knee right over the line of your foot; don't let your knee sway inward. Use the muscles on the side of your thigh to pull outward until your knee stays in place without wobbling all over.

- Keep your knee no farther forward than your toe. Leaning forward more than that throws weight on the knee joint.

- Stand and step up and down with your feet parallel, not turning toe-in (pigeon-toe) or toe-out (duck-foot).

- Use good foot, knee, and posture mechanics on stair-stepping machines, and when going up and down all stairs and steps, not just in exercise class.

Do You Need Arm Swinging? Many exercise classes emphasize swinging arms repeatedly overhead and to the side. Although swinging is fun, it burns only a few extra calories and can sometimes cause injury.

The common aerobics class motion of endlessly bending and straightening the elbow with no weights is useless for fitness. If done too much it can produce a repetitive motion injury. To increase arm strength, you need something that weighs more than your arm, using fewer repetitions.

Flinging your arms behind your body is tough on the front of your shoulder capsule, which is not supposed to be accelerated that way. It can cause early wear on your shoulder.

The common move of raising the arms repeatedly to the side with the thumbs down, brings a bony prominence at the top of your upper arm bone (the humeral tubercle) crashing into the bony ledge of your shoulder bone above it. That repeatedly squashes structures between them. Ouch. Keep your thumbs turned upward to rotate the bony bump of your humeral tubercle out of the way so that it does not impinge against your shoulder bone above it.

Problems with Arm Swinging

- Repetitive motion injury can occur from endless, uncontrolled bending and straightening.

- Flailing arms behind the midline of the body can weaken and destabilize the front of the shoulder.

- Impingement in the shoulder joint can occur when raising the arm overhead with thumbs turned down.

The bottom line on arm swinging during aerobics: You will make more fitness gains for your arms in the weight room by lifting heavier weights than with repeated swinging. If you enjoy swinging your arms, keep your thumbs facing up, rather than facing down, particularly when you raise your elbows in the "farmer" move. Limit motion backward to no further than the midline of your body. Don't allow momentum to overstretch your shoulders. Lift with control.

Modifications for Arm Swinging

- Keep your thumbs facing up.

- Limit motion backward to no further than the midline of your body.

- Lift your arms with control, rather than speed.

Do You Need Swimming? Swimming is great for your cardiovascular and muscular systems, and is a low-impact, calorie-burning exercise. Swimming does not use all your muscles (contrary to popular belief), but it is an excellent exercise for both upper and lower body. The worse you swim, the more calories you burn, and the more your muscles have to work to do the poor, inefficient stroke. Still, taking a stroke mechanics clinic to improve your swimming stroke can increase your enjoyment, the number of laps you can swim, and teach you to swim more safely and comfortably. It is another myth that swimming does not burn fat. If you only swish around, you won't get enough exercise to burn fat. Done as a vigorous exercise, swimming is a fat burner.

Poor stroke mechanics can create shoulder and neck pain. Bad stretches can hurt shoulders. Many swimmers do not roll their body as needed for good swimming form. Instead, they keep their body level and yank their arms out of the water and crane their neck to breathe. A good body roll puts the shoulder and neck into easy position without strain and promotes a much faster stroke. Poor stroke mechanics combined with extreme distance work can result in neck and back pain from twisting movements or over-arching vertebral segments.

Problems with Swimming

Swimming is such a good, low-impact, relatively injury-free exercise that it is hard to find problems with it. If you want to nitpick, you could say that not everyone has a pool handy, and that with poor hygiene, you can get athlete's foot and swimmer's ear.

Poor stroke mechanics and bad stretches can lead to shoulder and neck pain.

Allowing your back to arch through poor body posture during strokes on your front can strain your back. Use your abs to keep your body from sinking into an arch, which will also improve your streamline. See Chapter 7 on abs for how to do this.

The bottom line on swimming: Go swimming. Vary your stroke to avoid repetitive-strain injuries. Use a smooth body roll, as if you have a pole from head to feet and log-roll around that pole. The body roll lifts your arms from the water safely and smoothly, the shoulder does not exceed normal motion, and you can breathe comfortably to the side without lifting your head forward. Try arm-only and leg-only work as part of your routine, and swimming with fins for variety and additional leg workouts. Don't let your tummy "hang down" by arching your back. Use your abs to keep the normal curve in your back, but no more. Have your stroke checked by a good stroke-mechanics specialist or coach to be able to do more of a workout if you are just a splasher, or to reduce your chance of mechanical injuries if you pile on the laps.

Modifications for Swimming

- Dry your toes and ears after swimming to avoid athlete's foot and swimmer's ear. Wear clean, dry socks. Powder your feet before dressing. Don't remove the protective ear wax that keeps germs out. Ear plugs do not keep much water out of your ears, and there's no need to keep water out. Just dry things afterwards.

- Avoid shoulder-mangling stretches, such as lifting arms overhead behind your body.

- Vary your stroke and workout.

- Use a body rolling technique to improve your speed and form, and to lift your arms from the water without injury potential to the shoulder.

- Use your abs to keep the normal curve in your back without arching.

"Floor Work" Exercises

Do You Need Sit-ups? Sit-ups and other common ab exercises burn few calories, because you do not do them for long enough for aerobic benefit (even if it feels like a long time), and do not remove fat from your abdomen. Done correctly, they strengthen your abdomen for good posture, back pain control, general activities of daily living, and cosmetic appearance. Done incorrectly, they can hurt your back and contribute to poor posture. Chapter 7 has more on abdominal muscles.

Sit-ups, done the traditional way of raising your torso to meet your leg by bending at the hip, work the leg muscles that bend your hip, called hip flexors. The hip flexors lie deep under your abdominal muscles. You get enough exercise for your hip flexors every day by walking. In most people, the hip flexors are already too strong and tight, causing poor posture, and are a common source of back pain. (See Chapters 20 and 21 on back pain.) Sit-ups to develop the hip flexors are useful for sports demanding extreme hip flexor strength—ballet, gymnastics, martial arts, place kicking, but not activities like scuba diving or tennis.

To work your abdominal muscles, stand up properly all day—don't let your back arch and your behind stick out. You need your abs to pull your torso enough to keep you from sagging. Try the often neglected, but excellent, isometric abdominal exercise explained in the previous chapter on abdominal muscles. It simulates how you need to use your abs all the time for standing, reaching, throwing, and healthy posture.

Problems with Sit-ups

- The traditional sit-up lifts the torso from the floor, bending at the hip. This works muscles that yank on the low back, rather than the abdominal muscles, with each repetition.

- Abdominal muscle exercise, done alone with no back muscle exercise to counter it, can contribute to poor posture and back pain.

- Most "ab" exercise does not automatically change your posture or help your back. You must consciously use your ab muscles to hold your posture to reduce strain on the back.

The bottom line on sit-ups: Isometric ab work, not sit-ups, is preferred to improve the abdominal strength and endurance you need to directly benefit your sport, your posture, and part of the support needed by your back.

Modifications for Sit-ups

- Instead of sit-ups, do exercises described in Chapter 7 that strengthen the abdominal muscles and directly coach your posture.

- After doing abdominal muscle exercises, turn over and work your back muscles.

Do You Need Leg Lifts? Leg lifts to the front, like sit-ups, use more hip flexor muscle action than abdominal muscle work (described in the previous section and in Chapter 7). Often, people's abs are so weak that when they do front leg lifts, they let their back arch, and all weight pinches on the low back. One of the hip flexor muscles attaches to the low back, further encouraging people to let their back arch to the point where the repeated pressure and banging around can damage it.

The abs work to keep your back from arching by attaching from the ribs to the front of the hip. Try that now—arch your back and see that the distance from the middle of your chest to the front of your hip bones (above the groin) increases. Now make that space shorter by curling your torso forward. When doing lying-down leg lifts, curl your torso enough that your low back is against the floor. Keep it there while slowly lifting one leg, not allowing your back to arch. That is how to use your abs during leg lifts. It is not the leg lift that uses the abs—it is the abs controlling your back posture that uses your abs.

The same principle applies to standing-up leg raises, for example, "Captain's Chair" exercises. They are often done with no use of abs. In Captain's Chair, you hang in the air with your forearms on two pads on either side of you, with your legs dangling free. You lift your legs with knees bent or straight. People usually use only hip flexors and allow their backs to arch. While hanging, first curl your behind under you using your abs. Then lift your legs, not allowing your back to arch, by using abs throughout the entire exercise. Maintain this tuck even when you swing your legs down.

Leg lifts while lying on your side, to work the gluteus medius muscle so popular in exercise classes, do little unless you are debilitated from sedentary living or injury. Your leg is just too light to give the resistance you need for strengthening. It's a small muscle, so it easily "burns," but that doesn't mean it's working the way you need it. Since you can't spot-reduce fat, the fat on the side of the hip will not be reduced by any amount of leg lifting.

A side leg lift while lying down is not a "functional" movement exercise. That means it is not one that you use for your daily life when you move around, or do sports or recreational activities. Think a minute. When do you use that motion at all? Because of "specificity of exercise," the effects of doing leg lifts to the side on your side hip muscles will be different lying down than standing up. To best work the muscle on the side of your hip, you need to use it during exercise class in the manner that you use it for real. Standing leg lifts to the side are more functional.

When you raise your right leg to the side while standing, the gluteus medius on the side of your left hip must work to keep your hip stable. If not, it drops down when you walk like the walk of a runway model. That jolts the hip with each step, and grinds structures into each other. It is one interesting and often missed cause of hip pain. You need strong medius muscles for posture stabilization while walking, going up and down stairs, running, and any time you need to shift your weight from one leg to the other. That's a lot of reasons to develop your gluteus medius in the way it functions.

As far as leg lifts to the back, if there ever was, as Shakespeare supposed, "a deity that shapes our ends," that patron saint of buns is back leg lifts. Lie facedown with your chin on your hands. Lift one leg up slowly with straight knee, hold, then lower. For a tougher exercise, lift both legs together. This action of prone (facedown) hip extension benefits your low back and behind (gluteal muscles), structurally and cosmetically. Don't lift so high that it hurts. If your back hurts no matter how you try it, stop immediately and call for an appointment to be evaluated for back trouble. Another exercise to improve your low back and gluteal muscles is to lie facedown on a chair, bed, couch, bench, or special back apparatus, bending at the waist so that your legs hang off the edge, toward the floor. Then lift your legs until they are in line with your body.

Problems with Leg Lifts

- Leg lifts to the front use more hip flexor muscle action than abdominal muscle work, and can contribute to poor posture and back pain.

- Side-lying leg lifts, so popular in exercise classes, do little unless you are debilitated from sedentary living or injury.

- Side-lying leg lifts are not "functional" movements—you don't use them for any activities. This exercise doesn't benefit your muscles the way you need them.

The bottom line on leg lifts: Leg lifts to the front are usually not a good abdominal muscle exercise. They use other muscles that pull on the low back. Substitute abdominal exercises instead, as described in Chapter 7.

Prone (facedown) hip extension is an excellent back and bun exercise. Strong gluteal muscles are important for shock absorption, and tremendously important for back and knee health. Lift, don't yank, legs up.

Side-lying leg lifts are not an effective use of exercise time. They do little to get the hip muscle fit, and are not how you use your legs in your daily life. Substitute standing leg lifts to the side.

Modifications for Leg Lifts

- Substitute abdominal exercises instead of leg lifts to the front. Experiment with leg lifts while keeping low back against the floor, then slowly lifting one leg, not allowing back to arch. The abs work to keep back from arching.

- In Captain's Chair exercise, first curl your behind under you, using your abs. Then lift legs not allowing back to arch. Maintain this hip tuck even when lowering your legs back down.

- Do facedown leg lifts for excellent low back and gluteal exercise, important to good posture and back pain control.

- Do leg lifts to the side while standing.

Do You Need Push-ups? The push-up is a bench press upside down, using your body weight for resistance. You might think that since push-ups use the same motion as the bench press, they would have the same training effect. They don't because push-ups use your muscles differently and use more muscles. They are also a wonderful, and usually missed, ab exercise.

In the bench press, your hands move freely, while your shoulders remain a fixed axis. In the push-up, your hands stay fixed against the floor. Your elbows and shoulders rotate around them. The forces in each joint are different in the two situations. The adaptations are close, but separate. Push-ups won't improve your bench press as much as doing bench presses. Specificity again. Your body weight may not be as great as your bench press weight, or the other way around. To increase resistance during push-ups, put weights on your back, or have a friend actively resist your push-ups, or eventually even sit on you while you keep correct posture.

Push-ups have many surprising benefits. Although your principle movers are three arm and chest muscle groups, you need a lot of back and abdominal stabilization—the same stabilization so critical for good posture and back pain control. Even if you don't do complete push-ups, just holding the push-up position properly gets your torso muscles fit for daily life. Tuck your behind under so your back doesn't arch. Hold your body as straight as you would if you were standing up. Don't let your behind stick out. This trains your posture muscles the way you need them for real life. Keep your head up and your back from curving too much up or down. Don't lock your elbows; keep them slightly bent. Sure, it's easier to throw your weight on your poor elbow joints, but it's better to strengthen your arms instead.

The push-up uses so many muscles that, if you are pressed for time and have to choose just a few exercises to work as much of your body as possible, do push-ups.

> Push-ups work more than your arms and chest. They work your torso-stabilizing muscles that are important for posture and back pain control. Don't let your back arch, and you will have a wonderful ab exercise.

If you can't do regular push-ups yet, there are several easy, modified push-ups you can start with to build up to regular push-ups. Start by standing up, leaning against a wall, and pushing away. Then work up to a lower starting position, such as the arm of a couch. Then to the floor, resting on your knees. Then try regular push-ups. When these become easy, and they will with regular work, prop your feet up on a box, then chair, then on the couch arm, then finally you may even work up to standing on your hands, against the same wall you started with, to do your advanced incline push-ups.

Just holding the push-up position is an excellent exercise for most of your body; done correctly, it uses your postural stabilization muscles the way you really need for good standing posture. Don't let your back arch or hump up, or your head hang down. Hold the way you would want to stand with good posture. If you can't do this for more than a few seconds, then no wonder your posture is awful and your back hurts after a whole long day.

The bottom line on push-ups: Push-ups are an excellent exercise and have several health and posture benefits. They improve the musculature of your chest, shoulder, and arm, plus the posture stabilization muscles of your trunk and hip. Push-ups are a good exercise to maintain ability to get up off the floor, more important with every passing year.

Weightlifting

Weightlifting is good for you. Some people reject lifting for fear of hurting themselves or becoming bulky. Done properly, you reduce your chance of later injury from other activities, and look trimmer. Weightlifting increases your ability to do the physical work of your recreational sports and your daily activities, like carrying groceries. Weightlifting strengthens and firms you, and increases muscle that burns calories and keeps you warm. Weightlifting increases bone density, which is important for bone health. Weightlifting is one important part of everyone's fitness plan. It's funny how many women will be taught to shy away from weightlifting as "not right for women," forgetting that they already carry monstrous loads of groceries, babies, dogs, household items, and who-knows-what daily.

> Aerobic exercise alone will not increase your lean tissue. For well-rounded fitness, you need resistance exercises. That means strength training with either weights, packages, or your body weight.

Do You Need the Bench Press? The bench press is a popular lift. In the bench press you lie on your back on a bench, push a weight up from your chest until your arms are straight, then down again to your chest. The bench press works several muscles, including those that keep you from falling off the bench. The three muscle groups getting most of the work are the triceps, which straighten your arm (located in back of your arm); the round chest muscles, called pectoralis major; and the muscles in front of your shoulder, called the anterior deltoid.

The bench press can improve size, strength, and endurance of these three muscle groups, but remember specificity. You are pressing up a weight while lying on your back. How often do you need that? In wrestling, in hand-to-hand combat, or anytime something heavy is on top of you and you want to get it off.

The main hazard in bench pressing (aside from dropping the weight on your neck) is lowering the weight so far that it touches your chest. Many people believe that unless the weight touches the chest, it is not a real exercise. But for most people, the elbows extend too far behind them, stretching the shoulder past a safe range. Such overstretching can lead to strain, chronic shoulder problems, and occasionally, shoulder dislocation. Only the barrel-chested, short-armed power lifters can keep the elbows in line with the body when the weight touches the (large) chest. For the rest of the population, to test how far you should lower the weight, lie on the floor. When your elbows reach the floor, your arms are in line with your shoulder. You may be surprised that the weight is many inches above your chest. But your shoulder joints will not be slowly pried apart.

Problems with Bench Pressing

- Risk of dropping the weight on your neck.

- Possible shoulder trouble from bringing the weight down too far, allowing your elbows to drop too far back.

- Tight hips can allow your back to arch when lying on your back.

The bottom line on the bench press: It benefits your physical condition through the usual benefits of weightlifting. It helps you look and feel good. For maximum shoulder safety, limit the range by stopping the weight before it reaches your chest. Keep your elbows even with your body; don't let them drop lower. Keep your knees bent for back safety and stability while lifting.

Modifications for Bench Pressing

- Lift with a spotter.

- Avoid shoulder trouble by not bringing the weight all the way to your chest. Bring your elbows even with your body, no farther. Practice this by bench pressing while lying on the floor.

- Keep your knees bent for back safety and stability while lifting.

Do You Need the Military Press? In the military press, or shoulder press, you lift a weight overhead. That is an excellent choice for people who hand up boxes and other things overhead, play volleyball, or open windows. There is potential for shoulder and back injury if done incorrectly, a good reason to learn how to do it well. Lifting items overhead is a practical daily life activity. You don't want to hurt yourself putting things up on shelves or opening windows. People with existing shoulder or back injury need to check with their orthopedists before doing this exercise. Lifting a weight overhead compresses the spine, can worsen a disc problem, and can be tough on rotator cuff injury in the shoulder. If lifting with a barbell, the bar prevents a natural rotation of the arms. Dumbbells work better, allowing natural hand placement. Lift with control, and avoid arching your back when doing this lift. Keep a small inward curve of the lower back, without exaggerating it. This is where you use your abs to maintain good low back posture—not by tightening or "sucking in" your abs, but by not allowing the back to arch.

Sitting is very tough on your back, and sitting while lifting a weight is very, *very* tough on your back. It can be much safer to lift while standing, but even more important to have good posture, because you do not have the aid of the bench to stabilize you.

If you hold your head forward of the center line of your body, as many people do, you can interfere with normal shoulder motion when lifting overhead. With each overhead lift, you can be impinging your shoulder. Keep your chin in, not up or down. Find proper position by standing (or sitting) with your back against a wall. The back of your head should be able to touch the wall comfortably. Chapters 20 and 21 on back pain detail all of this.

Even more interesting is the connection between tight hip joints and injury from overhead lifting and reaching. When the front of the hip joint is tight, as it often is in most people whether they can feel it or not, they wind up leaning forward a bit from the hip. To compensate, the back arches when reaching overhead, and even when just standing and walking. The shoulder must overrotate and overcompensate, resulting in rotator cuff injury that is difficult to treat. When the hip is the reason behind the injury, and that is not known or fixed, the shoulder injury keeps coming back, and the back continues to hurt. When the tight hip is found and corrected with stretches, the damage to shoulder and back can stop. The hip bone really is connected to the shoulder bone.

Problems with the Military Press

- Lifting a weight overhead compresses the spine, can worsen a disc problem, and can be tough on the shoulder, particularly when done sitting.

- Lifting with a barbell prevents natural rotation of the arms.

- Sitting while lifting a weight is very tough on your back.

- If your shoulder and hip are tight, it increases injury potential.

The bottom line on the military or chest press: It is a good exercise, with direct benefit to activities of daily life. If you have back or shoulder trouble, check with your doctor before trying the military press. Check your hip and shoulder flexibility to make sure you can lift overhead without overstressing the shoulder. Learn good form and keep your entire body fit and flexible.

Modifications for the Military Press

- Lift standing up.

- Use dumbbells for more natural hand placement and arm rotation.

- Lift with control.

- Avoid arching your back. Keep a small inward curve of the lower back, without exaggerating it. Use your abs to prevent arching.

- Keep your chin in and ear over shoulder. A forward head while lifting overhead can make your arm bone bang into the forward-held shoulder bone, eventually bringing on shoulder and neck pain.

- Avoid bending at the hip. That bends your body forward, creating shoulder stress. Stand properly without sticking your behind out.

Do You Need Squats? The squat is an exercise done from a standing position, by bending your knees to a position that looks like sitting in a chair, but without the chair. It is often done holding a weight across the chest or shoulders. Safety of the squat stirs passionate debate. Some insist it is excellent for your body and knees.

Others state categorically the squat damages knees. The explanation is simple. The squat has benefits and potential for harm, depending on how it's done. You can easily modify for the advantages without harming your knees.

> Some say the squat is good for you; others say it's bad for you.
> What's right? Simple.
>
> Done properly, it's very good for you.
> Done incorrectly, it can injure you.

The squat has many benefits:

- The squat is a multi-segment, full-body activity, meaning it works many body parts simultaneously. The benefit over isolating each muscle group comes from specificity. From standing, to lifting bags, to getting out of bed, to climbing stairs, to most everything you do, your daily activities are multi-segment.

- Squats are good for posture muscles and overall body stabilization.

- Squats raise your capacity for lifting things and accomplishing chores properly. Your back is not made for lifting. The squat trains your legs to do the work. Overall, the squat can be an excellent exercise.

- Squats are "functional" exercises—that is, they train you to use your body the way you really need it for daily life. You know you shouldn't bend over at the waist to pick things up; you should bend your knees properly, keeping back upright, as in the squat.

- The squat uses so many muscles that it is a big "bang-for-the-buck" exercise.

A main modification to safeguard knees is to keep your knees over your feet. Avoid allowing your knees to droop forward past the line of your toe. Many people do this because it is easier to do the exercise this way. It puts your weight on your knee joint instead of having to use muscular strength. But the purpose of the exercise is to get exercise, so learn to use muscles and you'll burn more calories and tone your legs and body quickly. Practice with a mirror. Stand sideways. Begin to squat and watch your knees. They should not move forward. Your behind should move back. You can practice this by putting the front of your knees against something like a wall to prevent them from moving forward. Begin to squat. You'll feel your thigh and behind muscles working. Also keep knees from drooping inward, knock-kneed style. That stresses the knee terribly. Use muscles on the outside of your thigh to keep knees right over the line of your feet.

Another modification to safeguard knees is not to squat down fully, but stop at a quarter or half of the way so that your thighs go no farther than parallel to the floor. One way to ensure this is to put a chair behind you, so that your behind will contact the chair at the end of the squat, preventing further lowering. Full squats put high pressure on your knee cartilage. Rising from a full squat twists the leg bones against the cartilage while exerting pressure. Knee problems are occupational injuries of baseball catchers. Once injured, the nonvascular cartilage will not heal. The inflammation may subside, but other times the tear acts as chronic irritant, inflaming the area until you have surgery. This can be avoided with proper knee posture during squats.

The squat has several variations. One uses no weight at all, except for your own body weight. For many people this is all they need to get a lot of benefit from a simple exercise. While traveling, some people do squats in their hotel room, either with their body weight alone, holding suitcases, or wearing a backpack, for a quick, easy workout on the run.

Many people hold a barbell across the back of their neck and shoulders while squatting. That pushes your neck into back posture and pressures neck and spine structures. Alternatives that are safer for both neck and shoulder include holding weights in each hand, holding the bar across your chest in front of you (better exercise for your arms that way), or using a machine that places the weight on your shoulders like a horseshoe.

Another way to get most of the benefits of the squat with the least work and risk is to use a "leg sled." You could argue that the leg sled is not a squat at all, but a leg press machine while lying down. There are two main kinds of leg sleds. In one, you lie on your back and push the weight directly upwards with the bottoms of your feet. In the other, you semi-recline, pushing the weight away and/or upwards. Both of these leg sleds use the same lower body musculature as the squat, and lack the upper body stabilization of the squat. The leg sled done lying down, pushing the weight directly up, loses the balance practice of standing while supporting weight but keeps most of the compressive forces of the squat off your back, making it a great choice during back pain rehabilitation, and in general.

When returning to the upright position, don't "lock" your knees straight; keep your knees slightly bent. If your leg muscles are so weak that you can't keep the weight on your muscles with knees bent, strengthen them; don't use that as an excuse to wreck your knees. Maintain the natural small, inward curve of your lower back without allowing the weight to pull your back into an arch. Push off your heels, not the balls of your feet. Find a qualified instructor to learn proper form before trying the squat, and start with a broomstick or light weights until you are well-practiced in good form.

Problems with the Squat

- Full squats put high pressure on your knee cartilage.

- Rising from a full squat twists and pressures the knee cartilage.

- Supporting the weight compresses your spine.

- Lifting the heel throws weight onto the knee joint, rather than keeping weight on the thigh and backside muscles.

The bottom line on the squat: Squats can be excellent for general health and improve your ability in activities of your daily life and recreation, if done correctly. Lift with supervision, keep weights off your neck by holding the bar in front on your chest or across your shoulders. Keep your back upright, not tilted far forward, and stay above a 90° knee bend.

Modifications for the Squat

- Use a spotter.

- Hold the bar in front on your chest or across your shoulders, rather than pressing on the back of your neck.

- Keep your back upright, not tilted forward.

- Keep a small inward curve of your lower back, without exaggerating it. Use your abs to prevent arching.

- Maintain less than a 90° knee bend.

- Keep your stance wide to reduce stress on your knees.

- Keep your knees over your feet, not forward past your toes, nor swaying inward.

- Push off your heels, not the ball of your foot. Don't lift the heel.

- Use a leg sled.

- Breathe out with each lift.

Do You Need Leg Machine Exercises? There are usually two main leg machines. The two seem similar, yet can make a difference to your knee health. This topic is one that has seen a lot of debate, and there is still more to learn about how much difference these two different leg exercises make to your knees. Both work your thigh by straightening the knee against resistance. In one, called the leg press, you push the weight with the bottom of your feet. In the other, usually called leg extension, you sit with the weight at your ankle, moving your lower leg up and down in an arc.

Like the bench press and push-up, these two use the same muscles, but with opposite joint dynamics. The second is thought to be tougher on your knees upon full straightening. The first is generally accepted as excellent for your legs without as much burden to your knee joint. The first one is also more similar to the motions your legs need to do in sports, except for kicking things, and is used in all daily life movement like walking, running, climbing up and down steps, and getting up out of a chair or bed.

When using the leg press machine, don't bend your knee too much, or lock it straight. An excellent variation of the first leg extension exercise is the leg sled, where you lie on your back and push the weight with the bottoms of your feet. This exercise works your lower body well, without such stress to your back.

Problem with Leg Machines

- Done improperly, can be tough on the knees.

The bottom line on leg machines: Look for machines where you push the weight with the bottom of your feet, over those where you sit with the weight at your ankle.

Modifications for Leg Machines

- Use machines where you push the weight with the bottom of your feet (rather than machines where you swing the weight up with your ankle).

- Keep knees slightly bent rather than "locking" your knees straight when you push the weight away. It burns more calories to use your muscles and keeps you from smashing the joint.

- Don't bend your knees all the way to your body when bringing the weight back. Keep the weight on your muscles, not your compressed knee joint.

Do You Need Wrist and Ankle Weights? Swimmers, boxers, and martial artists may use hand, wrist, or ankle weights to add to their workouts. There are two main problems with use of these weights.

Wrist weights for swimmers can contribute to shoulder injury. For punching workouts, the main problem with hand, wrist, and ankle weights is that the resistance is in the wrong direction, which builds the wrong skills.

When swimming, you want to increase your ability to pull backward in an S-shape curve. When punching, you want the power of your punch to go forward. Hand weights for boxing or swimming weigh your arms downward. That preferentially builds muscles and neural pathways that raise your arm upward to resist the downward pull, which is not what you want.

Ankle weights for kicking while swimming have similar problems. They throw off your streamline, meaning they throw off your body positioning so that you are no longer horizontal, which reduces your efficiency. Incorrect swimming posture, in turn, makes poor swimming habits by building the wrong neuromuscular patterns. Using weights doesn't really help you swim without them. Tying weights on is also not the safest thing to do in the water, particularly when not wearing a scuba tank.

To improve your swimming or punching ability, you need to increase resistance against your forward progress, not weigh your arms or legs down so that you build patterns that lift upward.

The bottom line on wrist and ankle weights: Don't use them for swimming or punching. They teach you poor form. To improve your swimming, use resistance like tethers, drag suits, and other devices designed to resist your forward progress. For punching skills, use pulleys, or bands that pull your arm directly opposite from the direction you want to develop your punch. If you are punching forward, use a band that hold your arm to the back. If punching diagonally upward, move the band so that it pulls your arm diagonally downward.

Balance Exercises

Who thinks about balance exercises, or even much about balance at all? Your ability to balance while walking anywhere, particularly over uneven ground or ice, can make a big difference to your health, your joints, and your ability to live an active, independent life.

After a three-year study of more than 300 senior citizens, researchers at the University of New Mexico in Albuquerque concluded that people were at twice the risk of suffering an injurious fall if they could not balance on one leg for at least five seconds.

Inactivity decreases your balance skills. Balance is "use-it-or-lose-it." Leg and foot injury also decreases your balance skills. In both cases, balance retraining is crucial to recovery. Poor balance after injury creates a vicious cycle of "wobbling," poor positioning, weakness, poor ability to stabilize the limb, and disuse. Poor balance from inactivity creates a vicious cycle of reducing activities that require balance, which are most activities of independent living, and losing more balance skill.

Many exercises can improve your balance. Do them carefully, in a controlled manner, away from nearby objects, and preferably with supervision. If you have past or present ankle, foot, leg, or other problems that affect your balance, see your physician for a supervised balance program first.

- Put on your pants, shoes, and socks standing up. Take them off that way too. Sitting is hard on your back anyway. Get a free stretch and balance workout.

- Stand on your toes. Keep weight on your big toe and second toe, rather than teetering on the outside of your foot. Then try standing on the toes of only one foot. When you get good, try balancing with eyes closed.

- Stand on one foot for increasing periods of time. Try it when you are on the phone and washing dishes. Remember to do both legs.

- Walk over uneven ground.

- Walk on a line, then walk the line backward.

- Walk the line sideways. Cross your feet, first one in front then the other behind, in a style often called "grapevine walking." Football players practice running like this quickly.

- Hop on the line, then hop the line backward.

- Hop on one foot for increasing periods of time.

- Slalom-hop the line, then slalom-hop the line backward.

- Hold one end of a long stretchy band, such as a commercial exercise band or bungee cord (without the hook), or use panty hose or a stretchy piece of clothing. Have a friend hold the other end and pull on it as you walk, then hop, then hop on a line.

- Practice getting up from the floor and back down in a smooth manner. Then repeat without hands. Then repeat holding a package, then with a friend pulling on the stretchy band, as described previously.

- Go ice skating, roller-skating, and dancing. Try tai chi. In tai chi you practice shifting weight slowly and standing on one foot.

- Do some regular home or work activity while balancing on one leg—filing, cleaning, picking things up, reading, opening mail, juggling.

- Instead of bending over to mop floors, put a rag under one or both feet and skate the floors clean.

- Stand on one foot, pick up things with the other foot, and pass them up to your hand without holding on.

- Get out of chairs without using your hands. Get up and down from the floor without using your hands. Use good leg and back posture. Remember to breathe, not hold your breath, when doing exercises.

More exercises that help balance and stabilization control are in the next chapter, "Good and Bad Exercises," in the section on good foot exercises.

The Bottom Line on 10 Popular Exercises
(and One That You May Not Have Thought About)

Step Aerobics. Can help and harm. Modify stepping to reduce injury potential. The general fitness from this activity benefits your general health directly, and ability in your chosen sports indirectly.

Arm Swinging During Aerobics. Has potential for repetitive strain injury and gives little extra exercise. If you enjoy swinging your arms, keep your thumbs facing up when lifting upward. Limit motion backward to no further than the midline of your body. Lift with control. Don't confuse momentum with strength. To tone or strengthen your arms, you will make more gains through weight training.

Swimming. Good, low-impact aerobic exercise that works both upper and lower body muscles. Use good body rolling for speed and so you don't yank your neck and shoulder joints. Vary your workout and have more fun with fins, kickboards, paddles, and other toys.

Sit-ups. Substitute isometric ab exercises for sit-ups to improve the abdominal strength and endurance that directly benefits your posture, your ability to go long days without back pain, and for sports and recreation. Don't do ab exercises without back exercises. Abs are only part of the support you need. Alone, they can just make you slouch more.

Leg Lifts. Leg lifts lying facedown are a great back and bun exercise. For side lifts, it is better to do them standing than lying down. For front leg lifts, keep your behind tucked under you with your abs, not your hands. Using a band or weight on your legs will improve your leg strength, endurance, and firmness more than using body weight alone.

Push-ups. Use many upper body and torso stabilization muscles. Great for strength and posture if done with good posture—don't let your back arch. More "bang for the buck" than many other exercises.

Bench Press. For shoulder safety, limit the range by stopping the weight before your elbows go too far behind you.

Military Press. Learn proper form for safety. Prevent back from arching. Check with your doctor if you have back or shoulder trouble.

Squats. Squats can be excellent for general health, shaping the lower body, and many sports. Lift with supervision, keep weights off your neck, keep your back upright, not tilted forward, and stay above a 90° knee bend. Keep knees from swaying inward or drooping forward.

Leg Machines. Look for machines where you push the weight with the bottom of your feet, not those that have you sit with the weight at your ankle.

Balance Exercises. Balance exercises are crucial to preventing falls and improving your overall fitness for an active, independent life. Practice with supervision and with no danger of falling onto nearby objects.

Getting Fit Has Many Components

Fitness has many different components. To improve your fitness and health, you need many different activities that work all your different systems, abilities, and body parts. Weightlifters may not be lowering their risk of heart trouble if they never work their cardiovascular system. People who just play tennis need to add weightlifting, stretching, and something with a longer-duration aerobic component. You may be in good shape, yet at risk of falls from poor stability and balance.

Getting in shape for any specific sport or activity requires doing that particular activity and exercising the muscles used in the specific skills. Runners may be in great shape for running, but may easily poop out when trying to swim if they don't train for swimming.

Doing many different exercises doesn't mean drudgery; it can be fun. Doing different things helps liven up old routines and prevent burnout. Make an appointment with yourself, determine a variety of exercises you enjoy for each different system and body part, get out there, and enjoy getting fit.

9

Good and Bad Exercises

He shall not alter it, nor change it, a good for a bad, or a bad for a good.

— Leviticus 27:10

Some exercises are good for you. Many popular moves will make you look good but will eventually injure your joints. Others do nothing at all. How can you know what is good and what is hype? This chapter looks at a few of each, from top to toe.

Your Neck

Your neck has a lot to do all day. It moves constantly and supports the weight of your head. Strength, flexibility, and posture of your neck can make a big difference to your comfort and energy levels.

Poor neck posture from tight, weak neck muscles often brings on pain between your shoulders, under the shoulder blades, around your neck, and down the tops of your shoulders. The most common poor neck posture is standing and sitting with your chin and head forward.

Problematic Neck Exercises. The vertebrae of your neck are not shaped for motion through a circular path. Neck rolls (head rolls) are tough on your neck over time.

Two classic exercises press your neck into extreme forward positions—the overhead bicycle, where you churn your legs in the air with all your weight on your shoulders and neck, and the plow, where you lie with your legs in the air over your head and all your weight on your shoulders and neck. Both of these force the neck too far forward, putting pressure on the discs and overstretching the long ligament down the back of your neck. When ligaments stretch out, they don't return to their healthy length, weakening the neck. A permanent forward head may result, giving you funny posture and upper back pain.

> You're better off without doing the "plow" stretch.
> There are better ways to simultaneously have a stroke
> and herniate discs in your neck.

Other exercises that make a forward head posture worse include pulling your neck forward for abdominal work, craning and tensing your neck while lifting weights, and tipping your neck forward while lifting or pulling a bar in back of your neck. The traditional "lat pull-down" where you pull a bar down in back of your neck forces your neck into bad posture and does not even work your "lats," the large latissimus dorsi muscles of your back and sides, in the line of the muscle fibers. Modifying this exercise by pulling the weight in front of your neck, rather than behind it, changes it into a good exercise.

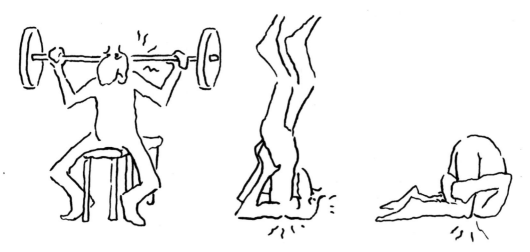

Figure 9.1. Some exercises force your neck into a forward posture, straining your neck. A forward head posture can eventually become a habit. A slouching forward head is not good for you, so why practice it in a gym?

Good Neck Exercises

Strengtheners. To strengthen the muscles of your upper back that contribute to good head posture, lie facedown, arms out at your sides, and gently, slowly, lift your arms and upper body from the floor, and hold. Then slowly lower and repeat. Don't tilt your neck back; just hold it in line. Work up to 10 repetitions at a time. Don't do anything that hurts.

When lifting or pulling weights, keep the weight in front of your neck, not behind it.

Stretches. For healthy neck range of motion, don't roll your head around. Just look down, look up, look left, look right, and tip each ear to each shoulder. The shape of the vertebrae isn't made for rolling around and will grind. Keep your shoulders down, not up in your ears.

Don't put your body weight onto your neck with shoulder stands like the plow. They pressure the discs and overstretch the neck forward contributing to poor posture. Similarly, don't let anyone roll, push, and pull your neck. There have been several recorded cases of death from stroke and from the neck artery tearing.

Posture Exercises. To correct poor head posture, practice pulling your chin in and head back until your ears center over your shoulders. Keep your gaze looking forward, not up or down, just pull back. Try it for 10 counts to start, then learn to hold the good posture all day.

For more good neck strengtheners, stretches, and posture exercises, see Chapter 21.

Your Arms, Shoulders, and Chest

Strong upper bodies look sexy and can carry more things, more easily, with less chance of injury.

Problematic Arm, Shoulder, and Chest Exercises. Swinging the arms in aerobics class was mentioned in the previous chapter. Two shoulder injuries appear most often, the first from swinging your arms too hard and far from front to back. The front of the shoulder capsule, constitutionally too weak to withstand such trauma, forcibly stretches past a safe range. In the second, called "The Farmer," you turn your thumbs down and lift both elbows. This action brings a structure on your upper arm bone, technically called the humeral tubercle, directly under the bony ledge of your shoulder bone, technically called the acromion, squashing the cushiony sac between them, called a bursa. Over time, this can produce what is technically called an "injury," known as bursitis.

When doing the bench press, many people are taught to touch the bar to their chest, but with so many different arm lengths and chest widths, that is not for everyone. For most people, it allows the elbows to lower too far down, harmful to the front of the shoulder.

Swimming is great for your upper body in general but doesn't work all your muscles. Swimming preferentially ignores your biceps and the muscles called external rotators, which turn your arm in a thumb-upward position like a hitchhiker, while building internal rotators, which rotate the arm thumb-downward. The underpowered external rotators may destabilize the shoulder, at times contributing more to swimmer's shoulder than the repetitive action of swimming itself.

Certain stretches can be injurious to your shoulders. Many exercisers seem to reproduce wartime torture techniques. They clasp their hands together behind them and yank their arms up overhead in back. Swimmers routinely do this for a greater range of motion, which can improve swimming speed. The price can be shoulder instability and susceptibility to long-term injury. Ironically, when pain develops, they are often told, "Gee, a shoulder injury and you're a swimmer. It must be the repetitive strain of swimming, so you had better stop the swimming for a while." Meanwhile, it was not necessarily the swimming, but the stretching. The poorly advised person continues to stretch, and no longer has the muscle-building activity of swimming. Strong shoulder muscles help to counteract the laxity and instability that poor stretching technique can produce. The unstable shoulder joint continues to rub, clank, and hurt.

> Sometimes, it's not the shoulder exercise (like swimming) that wrecks the shoulder, but the damaging shoulder stretches done.

Another popular, but problematic, shoulder stretch is forcibly holding your arm in back of your body by pressing the side of your arm against a wall. This overstresses the front of the shoulder capsule, and overstretches parts that are not healthy to stretch. It also does not stretch the front of your chest, a stretch that a majority of people need.

Many people sit round-shouldered, which shortens the muscles, creating a vicious cycle of shortening and round-shouldered posture. This posture can create back and neck pain. The shortening can continue until the person's arms turn inward, so that their thumbs face the body, instead of hanging forward, naturally.

Good Arm, Shoulder, and Chest Exercises

Strengtheners. The rotator cuff muscles of the shoulder are usually neglected. People work their deltoids and chest and back, but it is your four rotator cuff muscles that stabilize your arm and shoulder. Working the surrounding muscles but not the rotator cuff can allow the top of your upper arm bone to push and grind against your shoulder capsule. One good exercise for the rotator cuff is to lie on your left side, with your right elbow bent. Hold a small hand weight in your right hand near your navel. Keep your elbow close to your body, but not touching it. You can use a towel as a spacer and elbow rest. Lift the weight up toward the ceiling, then lower. Then, while still lying on your left side, switch the weight to the left hand and lift. Switch sides after each set.

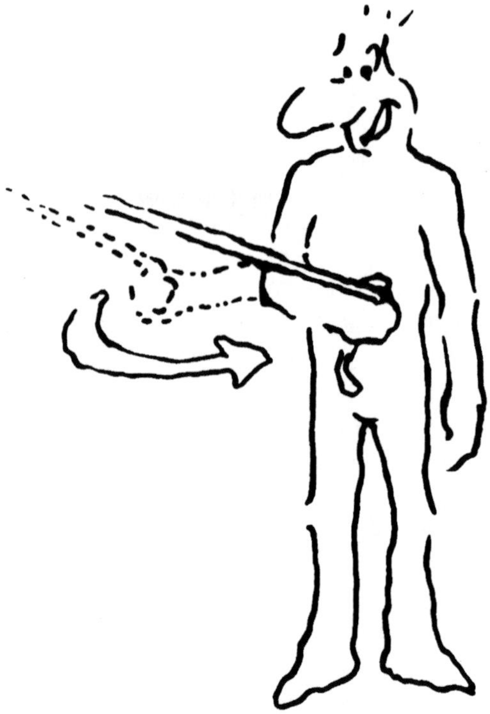

For a good rotator cuff exercise while standing, get a length of rubber tubing and secure it at elbow height from anything that will hold it while you pull. Turn sideways, elbow bent. Use a towel between your elbow and waist as a spacer and elbow rest. Pull the tubing, making sure that you do not pull so hard or so far that it hurts. Turn facing the other way and pull in the other direction. Work up to about 10 repetitions on each side.

The best strengtheners for the upper body use weights—either dumbbells, weight machines, or your own body weight. Waving your arms in an aerobics class won't do it. Your arm does not weigh

Figure 9.2. When exercising your arms and shoulders, remember your rotator cuff muscles. Good rotator cuff muscles are important to the health of your shoulder joint and for normal arm functioning.

enough by itself to provide the resistance your muscles need to get stronger. Try the various machines, or lift dumbbells, packages, yourself, or willing friends, to exercise your biceps, triceps, and shoulder. The upper back exercises, described in Chapters 20 and 21 on back and neck pain, are also good for shoulder stabilization.

When doing the bench press, keep your elbows in line with your shoulders, not lower. A good way to check this is to lie on the floor and lower your elbows until they touch the floor. That is where to stop your bench press, even if the bar does not touch your chest. Read more on the bench press, push-up, and military press in the previous chapter.

Stretches. To stretch your arms, shoulders, and chest, move through a gentle range of motion in all directions. Don't yank your arms up behind you overhead.

Combination Stretch/Posture Exercise. To stretch the front of the chest and shoulder, stand in a doorway and hold your arm out to your side, bending your elbow 90° so that your fingers face the ceiling, hand forward, as if calling someone to a stop. Press the inside of your elbow against the doorway, then gently turn your body away from your arm. You should feel a pleasant stretch in the front of your chest, just below the shoulder. This stretch also brings the shoulder back in line with the body, demonstrating proper shoulder posture. Most people stand round-shouldered, with their shoulders forward of the midline of their body.

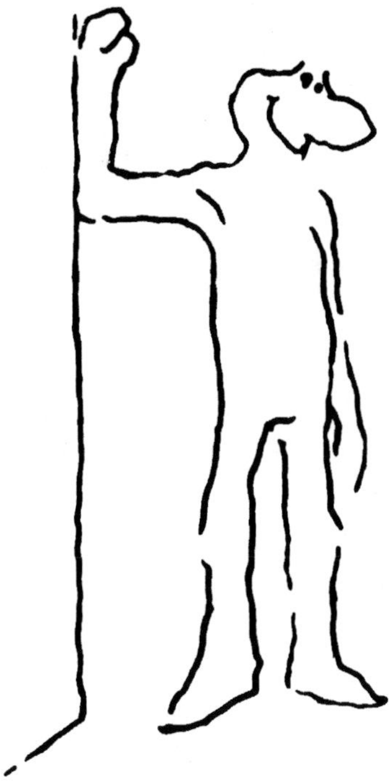

Your Abdomen

Abdominal muscles run down the front of you from your ribs to your pelvic bones. One of their duties is to hold some tension all the time to keep you from arching too far backward during normal standing and sitting. Muscles running along your back work similarly to keep you from slouching over forward. Weakness in your back and/or ab muscles allows you to sit and stand in ways that slowly injure you without you knowing it. Benefits from improved abdominal muscles and specific abdominal exercises were covered in Chapter 7.

Problematic Abdominal Exercises. Leg lifts and full sit-ups don't use your ab muscles as much as they use another set of muscles that bend your hip. Overworking these hip flexors is tough on the back.

Another problem with ab exercises occurs when you strengthen your abs too much until your weaker back muscles can't counter the pull from the front. Abs create an important support structure for your torso, but they are not the entire support. When you exercise your abs, also work your back muscles with the exercises described in the earlier paragraphs on backs, and Chapters 20 and 21 on back pain. Without adding back exercises to your ab routine, your tight abs can pull you too far forward, resulting in poor posture and back pain. That's why "ab-only" classes, although popular, are not as helpful as you would think. These classes need to incorporate back exercises as well.

Leaning sideways from side to side while holding hand weights is not an ab exercise. It does not benefit your back and does not tone or reduce your midsection. The muscles in play here are called "hip hikers," used in walking to keep the swinging leg from dragging on the ground.

Figure 9.3. For a good chest and shoulder stretch, brace the inside of your bent elbow against a doorway or wall, then gently turn away from that arm so you feel the stretch in your chest, not shoulder joint. This is good for improving posture. Do this instead of yanking your arms up behind you, which is tough on your shoulder joint.

The standing torso twist from side to side is not an ab exercise. Holding a weight on the shoulders and twisting can generate momentum greater than the supporting structures of your back and knee can safely absorb.

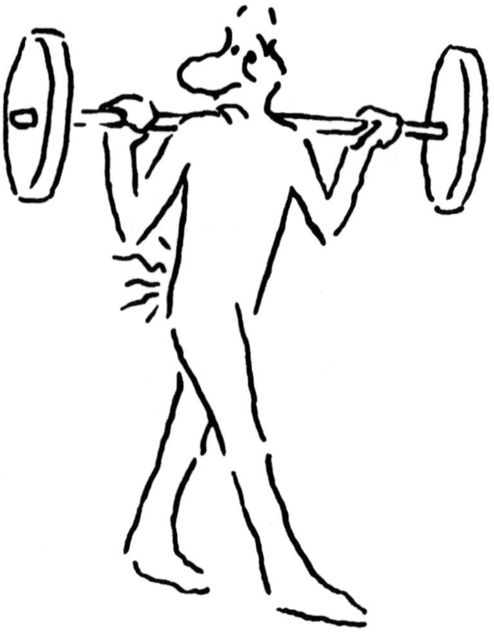

Good Abdominal Exercises. Crunches, almost synonymous with ab exercise, are not the best ab exercise. They encourage bad back and neck posture and don't use your torso muscles the way you need them for real life. Even better is a much neglected, but needed, isometric ab exercise. This exercise and others are fully described in Chapter 7 on abdominal muscles.

Your Back

A common medical prescription for back pain—"Gee, you should get more exercise"—is true, but vague. Many exercises popular at gyms and exercise studios cause more harm than good, and can directly injure your back over time without you being aware of the harm in progress. See Chapter 20 for more on why your back can hurt and Chapter 21 for what exercises to do to prevent back pain.

Figure 9.4. The torso twist is not an ab exercise and can be hard on your back by using your back bones instead of trunk muscles to decelerate the load.

Problematic Back Exercises. A few bad exercises now and then usually do little damage, but give it time. Like smoking, the repeated, forced nature of the exposure can harm at a rate faster than your body can repair.

Some tough-on-your-back exercises are weightlifting while leaning over unsupported from the waist, straight-leg dead lifting, forced repetitive back arching like "donkey kicks" that swing the leg overhead from a hands and knees position, and forced repetitive back bending like toe touches from a stand or swinging elbows down to opposite knees.

Leaning over at the waist for toe touches stretches your back and hamstrings, but it is not a good stretch for regular use. Although it feels great when back muscles are tight, it is tough on your back in the long run.

A bad exercise, like straight-leg dead lifting, may not hurt when you're doing it, but can still injure you over years.
Just give it a chance.

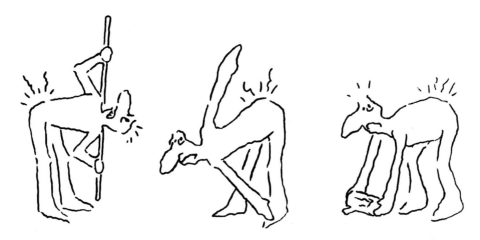

Figure 9.5. Some common exercises can be hard on your back even if you are in good shape. You know that bending over to lift is bad for your back, even more so with straight legs. It does not magically become good for you in a gym, even as a stretch. It can cumulatively stress and damage your back. Straight-legged deadlifting, although popular, has more risks than benefits. Don't lift packages like this either.

Good Back Exercises. You can do many things in your daily routine to make your back more injury-resistant. Strength, posture, and stretching for the back are so important that two chapters in this book are devoted to explaining everything in detail. See Chapters 20 and 21.

Important points to remember when exercising your back are to keep the natural inward curve of your lower back. Don't let it reverse into the shape of the letter C when sitting or lifting. For example, when rowing with pulleys or a rowing machine, don't sit and pull with a rounded back.

When using free weights, don't lean over unsupported. When lifting dumbbells, support your body weight by resting one hand on your knee, and lifting with the other hand, or by leaning against an incline bench.

Good range of motion in all of the directions that your back bends helps to prevent back pain. Stretch through your back's range of motion slowly as part of your regular routine. A safer way to stretch your back than standing or sitting toe touches is to lie on your back and bring one bent leg to your chest at a time.

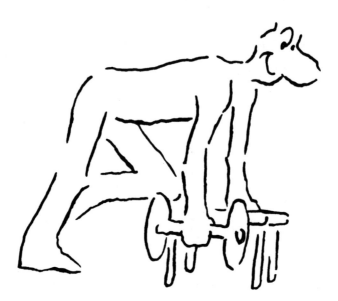

Figure 9.6. When doing back or shoulder exercises, don't bend over unsupported. Always support your upper body weight on a bench or your other thigh. It's not wimpy, and it's not just for people with back problems. It's for anyone who does not want to have a back problem.

Your Legs

You need strong legs for your daily life activities. It's important to exercise your legs until they are strong enough to lift things, instead of using your back. Doing regular leg exercise dramatically reduces the effects of aging. You may have seen aged people too weak to rise from a chair unaided. This is not an inescapable feature of aging; it is usually an avoidable problem of deconditioning. These people benefit greatly from weight training, and are able to dramatically improve their mobility and independent living.

Your legs have posture. This posture is not just something you are born with. You can change your leg posture so that it is good or bad. Bad leg posture can increase wear and tear on your knees, ankles, and hips.

You need to use your leg muscles for proper standing, and for walking posture called "gait." Many people don't hold their weight up on muscles, but let their hips, knees, ankles, and feet sway and bend to the end of the joint range, letting hips tilt, knees sway inward, arches flatten, and knees "lock."

Develop better musculature in your lower body to hold you properly and, very importantly, to decelerate on each step for good shock absorption. Walking lightly is part of that. Without this natural built-in shock absorption, you wham down with each footfall, jolting your spine and joints, and wearing out structures like your Achilles tendon. Poor balance is one often-missed factor in walking heavily. Combine balance exercises, described later in this section, with strength training.

> Legs have posture.
> Use your muscles consciously to hold your legs, ankles, and feet without rolling in or out, locking or bending backward, and for stepping lightly, not slamming down with each step. It tones your muscles, saves your joints, and burns calories.

Problematic Leg Exercises. The hurdler's stretch twists your knee sideways with the possibility of knee ligament damage. The double hurdler's stretch is worse. In that still-common stretch, you sit on the floor on your heels, both knees bent, sometimes with both feet facing outward, and lean far backward. This is hard on the back, and worse on the knees. Full squats (sitting on your heels) and duck walks are tough on the knees. They pry the knee joints open, particularly if you have heavy thighs, and can damage knee cartilage.

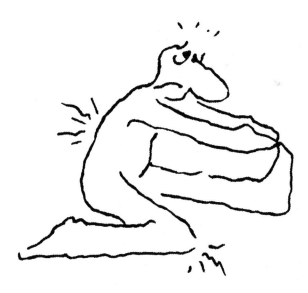

Figure 9.7. The hurdler's stretch is not good for your knees, even if you are flexible. Curling your back forward is also not good for your back. You know that you do not want a round-shouldered, slouching forward posture, so why practice it in a gym?

> The hurdler's stretch is not recommended. It twists your knee.
> Modify by keeping both legs in front of you, one bent at the knee.

Good Leg Exercises. In general, it's easy to exercise your legs.

Strengtheners. People go to gyms to use machines to work their legs, pay trainers, and take classes to do lunges and squats for their legs, then bend wrong to pick up their things to go home, and continue bending wrong the rest of every day, using their back, not legs. You could get an all-day workout and burn many calories just by bending right for all the dozens and dozens of times you bend and pick things up all day.

> Bend and pick up things properly all day—torso upright using a squat or lunge. This is a terrific leg exercise, burns calories, saves your back, and is a free workout. You would get the equivalent of an exercise class with the many dozens of times every day you need to do this in real life.

Walk, run, ride a bike, ski, carry things, take the stairs, swim with fins, get up and walk away from the TV. These exercises use your body weight as resistance. Adding more weight through safe weightlifting further increases leg strength. Weightlifting for your legs can be done with weight machines or other equipment, but don't forget that proper bending and lifting packages in real life can equal taking an exercise class that you say you don't have time for. Your own body weight is a built-in workout if you would just use it.

> If you use your arms to get out of a chair, your legs are probably too weak. This is not the result of aging as much as deconditioning. A great exercise is to just get up from a chair without arms (and without leaning far forward). Work up to 20 or more times in a row.

A fun isometric exercise for your legs that uses your body weight for resistance is called the "ski-sit." Stand with your back against a wall, feet away from the wall. Slide down until you are in a position as if you were sitting in a chair, suspended in space. Make sure your knees are right over your ankles, not past them. Hold. Time how long you can endure. Note that your back is upright and you are using your legs. Train your brain to remember this upright, leg-using posture for your bending.

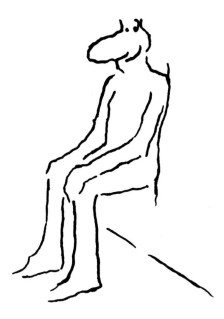

Figure 9.8. The ski-sit is a fun, isometric exercise for your legs. It also reminds you that good squatting posture—which you should use every time you bend—keeps back upright and knees in line with your feet.

> Think you can't exercise your legs without equipment? You have plenty of body weight. Practice getting up and down and up and down off the floor using proper lunge mechanics. Vary how you do it for more exercise. This can become a life-saving exercise in later years.

Stretches. To stretch the back of your legs, lie on your back and straighten one leg up overhead and hold. Or stand with one heel propped up on a chair, keeping the inward curve of your lower back, and sticking your behind out. Keep the foot of the standing leg pointing straight forward, not tilted out to the side, or you won't get much of a stretch. Do these instead of the bent-over toe touch, which is tough on your back.

> For hamstring stretches, substitute lying down with one leg overhead, or one leg on a chair and standing upright in good posture, rather than the bent-over toe touch.
>
> Why practice terrible posture with a bending-over stretch?

Another important, but often forgotten, stretch is for your iliotibial or I.T. band. Your I.T. band extends down the side of your hip to your knee. Tight I.T. bands can lead to knee pain and even change the way you walk, which leads to other problems. To stretch your I.T., stand sideways at arm's length from a wall, right hand touching the wall. Cross your left leg in front of your right. Push your hips forward, then toward the wall. Make sure you are not leaning backwards, or you will not feel a stretch. Hold for about 30 seconds, then switch sides.

Posture Exercises. The muscles of your egs can be weak, tight, and overstretched, allowing your legs to turn and slump out of a natural healthy alignment.

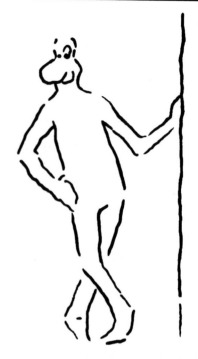

Figure 9.9. Remember to stretch your iliotibial, or "I.T.," band, a fibrous band of supporting tissue that extends down the side of your hip to the outside of your knee. Tight I.T. bands can tug on your knees, leading to pain, and even change the way you walk.

- Stand in front of a full-length mirror. See if your knees slump inside the line between your hips and ankles, or look "knock-kneed." Practice pulling slightly out with your outer leg muscles so that you can hold your knees straight ahead and aligned over your ankle bones when you stand and walk.

- Look in the mirror, standing with both feet straight ahead. See if your kneecaps "look" at each other or face away from each other. Practice holding your knees straight ahead and aligned over your ankle bones when you stand and walk.

- Check to see if you walk toe-out (duck-footed). This is not healthy. It may result from tight calf muscles, tight Achilles tendons, and/or tight hips. In turn, keeping your legs turned out all the time keeps them tight—a vicious cycle.

- Turn sideways and see if you "lock" your knees, or if they appear to bend backward (hyperextend). Locking the knee is when you straighten all the way and put all your weight on your knee joint instead of your leg muscles. Your muscles will lose strength and your joints will wear. Keep your knees slightly bent all the time when you stand, and balance using your muscles. When you walk and run, never straighten your knees so much that they bang the joint. Always use muscles to keep your weight off your knee joint. It's healthy and a free workout.

Letting your body weight slump on your leg joints will wear out your joints and make you stand and walk funny, which further wears your joints.

Warning signs are letting your knees turn in, bend in, or lock, and your feet flatten.

Your Feet

Your feet? Who thinks about exercising their feet? Yet your feet help determine if you will get through your day with easy energy, or limp home hurting and tired. Without strong, flexible, well-balanced musculature of your feet and ankles, problems can occur.

- Standing and walking with poor foot and ankle posture changes how you distribute your weight across your ankles, knees, and hips. That creates extra pressures, shock, and wear.

- Weak ankles are prone to recurring sprains.

- Tight, inflexible feet and ankles may be more likely to cramp.

- If your big toe joint does not bend pliably when walking, it throws off your gait, and pushes the posture of your head and trunk forward. Your low back muscles and discs bear the brunt. Often, if the big toe doesn't bend, the foot will turn out (duck-footed). This poor gait habit causes and perpetuates several problems at once. The pressure against the side of the big toe with each step exacerbates tendency to bunion and means the Achilles tendon and calf don't stretch as they should during normal walking. So they shorten, and continue the cycle, described next.

- Tight Achilles tendons and calf muscles hobble your gait, making you take short steps. They are more likely to strain when you try to walk or run faster. A tight Achilles also can be a reason you walk "duck-footed." Your feet should be parallel and face straight forward when walking and running. Many people "toe-out," putting uneven stresses all over the foot and leg. This produces a variety of effects, from corns, to flattened arches, to knee and hip pain. When you walk toe-out, the push-off place becomes the side of your big toe, instead of the ball of your foot. Over years, it can push the big toe right over your other toes, exacerbating tendency to bunion.

- Injured or weak feet and ankles do not have good motor control or proprioception. (Proprioception means knowing where you are in space.) They cannot react to changes in balance and footing quickly enough to avoid injury. You may turn your ankle before your body recognizes and corrects for it. Good foot and ankle exercises can retrain kinesthetics, motor control, and balance awareness.

- The most common cause of ongoing ankle pain or recurring ankle sprains is incomplete rehabilitation from a previous injury.

- When the bottoms of your feet get too tight, that contributes to a condition where tissues attached to the heel irritate the heel because they pull on it too tightly with every step. This is called plantar fasciitis. *Plantar* means the bottom of your foot (that you "plant" on the ground), and *fasciitis* is an inflammation of the fascia, the fibrous connective tissue spanning the bottom of your foot. Untreated plantar fasciitis can lead to heel spurs. Your heel gets so irritated with all the pulling that, like an oyster, it grows a "pearl" of a bony spur.

- Your feet have posture. Many cases of "flat feet" and "pigeon toes" are not unchangeable hereditary conditions, just poor foot and ankle posture.

- Standing toe-in (pigeon-toe) strains the foot, knee, and hip, and affects normal gait. Walking with your feet turned out like a dancer contributes to hip and knee pain and is often mistaken for "flat-foot" because it can put your weight on the inside of your foot and smash your arches. Both bad foot postures can make you stand and move "knock-kneed," which is another bad posture, not a normal trait you just happen to be born with. Putting weight on the inside of your knees slowly pressures and strains them, wearing out the cartilage and interfering with normal muscle use and kneecap tracking.

- Allowing your arches to roll in and flatten, particularly when one rolls more than the other, which is common, creates a functional leg length difference with every step you take.

> Your feet contribute to your posture and shock absorption, important to preventing back, neck, knee, and hip pain.

Problematic Foot Exercises. There seem to be few problematic foot exercises, mostly because few people bother to exercise their feet and ankles at all. Bad foot exercises haven't had a chance to become popular. Mostly, bad shoes (more common than you would think) and lack of good exercises lead to foot problems. See Chapters 20 and 21 on back and neck pain for more on proper shoes.

One common exercise that weakens the ankle is sitting in a "butterfly position" with the soles of your feet touching, but with your knees high. Another is sitting cross-legged with one foot bent over the opposite knee. The ankle should be straight, but many people sit with the ankle bent. These two bad habits stretch the sides of your ankles too far, loosening them. The loose, destabilized ankle becomes prone to recurring sprains.

> Ankle sprains, particularly recurring ankle sprains, usually come from ankles overstretched on the sides, allowing too much movement. Weak or injured ankles do not have normal "knowledge" and control of balance. They cannot correct for a sudden slip quickly enough. Instead of righting you, these weak, slow, overstretched, and "unaware" ankles let you fall.
>
> You need balance exercises, good motor control exercises, and real strengtheners more than high-top shoes, ACE® bandages, and ankle stretches.

Good Foot Exercises

Strengtheners. More successful than high-top shoes, taping, orthotics, and bracing in preventing ankle sprains, are strong ankle muscles. Most sprains come from rolling over the outside edge of your foot, so that the outside edge turns down. That motion is called *inversion*. While sitting with no weight on your foot, identify that motion. That's what you want to avoid in stretching and exercising. The opposite motion, where you lift the outside edge of your foot up, is a motion called *eversion*. (Don't confuse eversion with pronation, where you let your arch flatten). Your everter muscles are the main muscles you need to strengthen.

- Loop a short rubber tube or bungee cord (without the hook) around both feet. Roll the outside edges of your feet outward and upward, and hold. Repeat. Gradually increase the number you can do, and how thick the band.

- With the same tube, keep your heels together and point your toes away from each other, resisted by the tube. Hold and repeat.

- Repeatedly press the outside of your ankle upward against a wall, as if you are resisting an ankle sprain (which is what you are doing) and hold for 10 counts. Repeat at different angles.

- Get a towel and any 5- to10-pound weight, even a big book. Set the weight on the towel, and your bare foot next to it. Pivot on your heel to slide the towel with your toes. Do both directions, pivoting inward and outward.

- Pull a weighted towel (or whatever you can grab) toward you by scrunching it with your toes.

- Pick up things with your toes while balancing on the other foot. Bend at the hip to lift the object to your hand.

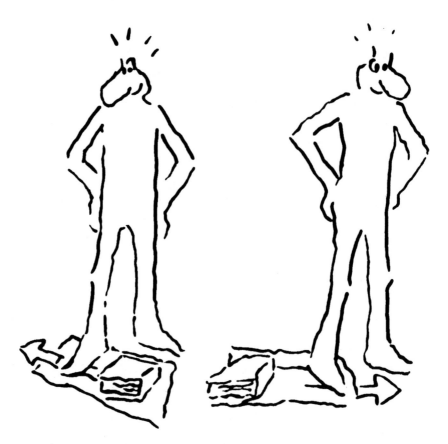

Figure 9.10. Good foot exercises can do a lot for your overall health. The strength and posture of your feet and ankles has a big influence on your chance of some kinds of foot, ankle, knee, and hip pain, and your risk of ankle sprains. Using good foot mechanics when walking reduces pressure on the arches and the big toe, helping to prevent bunions.

Posture Exercises. Some people allow their arches to sag too flat or, occasionally, roll to the side until they are too arched. Others might have weak leg muscles, allowing their stance to toe in or out.

> Think of your feet as the front end alignment of your car.
>
> The tires are your feet and can have posture problems in three directions—caster, camber, and of course, toe.

- Look in a mirror and see if your feet tilt, making your arches too high or low. Practice pressing and lifting the arch while keeping the rest of the sole on the floor. See how the muscles work on the inside and outside of your leg to do that.

- Look in the mirror and see if your toes point in or out. Practice walking with your toes straight ahead.

- Walk properly—an important and effective exercise. Walk and run by rolling heel first, through to the toe. Keeping your heel up "tiptoe fashion" shortens your calf muscle and Achilles tendon, creating poor gait and injury potential. Toe-walking throws weight on your joints rather than the muscles. Keep your feet pointing straight ahead, parallel to each other, not toe-in or toe-out. Step lightly, and use muscles to decelerate to come down lightly; don't just slap down your weight. Good shock absorption uses your muscles and burns more calories than sloppy walking habits.

Don't be fooled by just looking at the bottoms of your shoes for wear patterns. It is true that the bottoms of your shoes can tell a lot if they are completely worn on one side. But it is natural to heel-strike slightly to the side first, then roll to an even position. Shoes with slight wear on the outside heel do not necessarily mean that you are not walking "squarely." To determine that, you need to watch yourself in a mirror or, better yet, have a trained gait mechanics specialist give you a full walking evaluation.

Balance/Kinesthetics Exercises. Among many balance and kinesthetic exercises you can do, here are a few:

- Stand on your toes. Walk on your toes. Walk backward on your toes. Keep your weight on your first two toes, not wobbling on the outside of your little toe.

- Balance on one foot. Repeatedly rise to the toe and lower, then bend the knee and rise again. Try this when you are waiting for things, and while on the phone. When you get good at this, try it when using your arms, as for vacuuming.

- Bounce and catch a ball while standing on one leg. Or throw an object in the air and catch it.

- Catch a ball thrown against the wall and ceiling.

- Walk on a line. Walk backward. Walk sideways.

- When your strength and balance have progressed, hop on one foot along a line on the floor.

- Hop backward on one foot. Hop over things. Hop on things. Hop from one mark, crack, or designated object to the next. Hop, hop, hop. Use your muscle shock absorption; don't just come crashing down on your foot. Bend your knee when you land.

- If hopping is too much, work up to it by leaping softly. Push off one foot and land lightly on the other foot at a designated spot. Then leap backward to the first spot. Change sides. Try this in all directions—forward and back, sideways, and diagonally. Land lightly.

- Try to slalom the line hopping. Make it fun. Play hopscotch on sidewalk cracks.

More balance exercises are explained in the previous chapter, "What Exercises Do You Need to Be Fit?"

Floppy Foot Exercises. It is important to learn how to avoid "holding" tension in your feet and ankles, because it leads to cramps and rigidity, and reduces shock absorption. The floppy foot exercises are explained at length in Chapter 30 on leg cramps. To summarize here, they consist of being able to separate your foot from muscular control until you can take your ankle in both hands, and shake the foot so that it flops with each shake.

- Try it with your hand first, which is easier. Take one wrist in the other hand, and shake it.

- Now duplicate the floppy, tensionless movement in your feet. It will pay.

Stretches. Flexible feet allow healthy range of motion when walking, and reduce chance of strains and tears.

- An important stretch keeps your toes, particularly your big toe, flexible. Stand with one foot in back of you, and lift that heel as you do in walking, bending the toes. Hold and repeat. Then stretch your toes in the other direction by pressing the tops of your toes against the floor behind you, or on your hands.

- You can stretch your Achilles tendon and calf several ways. Carefully stand backwards on a step, let one heel hang off, and press downward. Do this with your leg bent, with it straight, and with the leg straight and your body leaning forward, sticking your behind out. You can also stand facing a wall, one foot in back, toes straight ahead, and lean your hips toward the wall. Don't let your behind stick out in back. An easier stretch is just to stand facing a wall closely, and put the ball of your foot against the wall with your heel on the floor. You can stretch the whole foot, then put your foot lower, and only stretch the toes against the wall. Do both sides.

- Remember to stretch in the other direction—stretch your shins too.

- Point and bend your ankle up and down to increase range of motion.

- Stretch the bottoms of your feet by pulling your toes back firmly and holding. This is a good one to do in the morning to help treat and prevent plantar fasciitis, and to get your feet ready for the day.

Work All Sides for Stabilization

When you work one muscle group, it is important to work the opposite muscles and nearby muscles. That way, you don't overpower your body in one direction, leaving you vulnerable to poor posture and strains in the long run.

Many workouts remember to do "both sides" but forget you have more than just a front and a back—you have sides too. A workout that balances work in each direction is sometimes called a "push-pull" workout. When you push one way in lifting, you also do exercises that pull the other way. It's not necessary to immediately follow each "push" exercise with its corresponding "pull." Do them in the same day's workout. Balance going forward with going backward. Then side to side.

- When you work your arms, work both your biceps and your triceps for front and back. Then remember your rotator cuff. Working only arms and shoulders creates a situation where the arm bone can get too pulled up in the socket. Rotator cuff was covered in the section "Good Arm, Shoulder, and Chest Exercises."

- Match bench presses with rows (pulling the weight toward your chest to work your back) and side exercises.

- Balance lateral arm raises with lateral pull-downs. Then side to side.

- When you work your legs, do exercises for the quadriceps muscles in front, and your hamstring muscles in back. Lift your legs inward and outward.

- After working your calf muscles, remember exercises for your shins. People often forget shins. Sore shins result when they cannot absorb the decelerating shock of walking and running. Your calf muscles push you off, but you need capable shins to "catch" you. Put your toes under something (or someone) and tap your toes. Add lifting your foot toward the little toe to strengthen the side muscles that help prevent sprains.

- When you do ab exercises (explained in Chapter 7 on abs), also do back extensions and exercise for your sides (explained in Chapter 21 on back pain).

- If you do wrist curls, do one set toward your palm and another set toward the back of your hand. Then remember to go side to side too. Add range of motion for your wrist. Wave at people. Don't forget people.

Choose Good Exercises

This chapter barely touched on a few of the good, the bad, and the peculiar of the many exercises you may encounter. See your physician before starting your exercise program. Lift weights with supervision. Remember that your daily life can be more exercise than a gym if you use your body properly and use your muscles, instead of letting your posture sag, walking heavy, and bending wrong. Improve your health and fitness by choosing good exercises for the hour you are in the gym, and using good postural and daily life habits for the rest of your day. Then stick with them. Have fun.

10

Just Overdo It
and
What to Do When You
Do Too Much

First, don't smoke to excess; second, don't drink to excess;
third, don't marry to excess.

– Mark Twain

Usually, the problem is getting people to exercise at all. Occasionally, the opposite is true. Doing too much physical activity once in awhile is fun, often productive and exciting. But what if you do too much, too soon, too often? Sore muscles, injury, and burnout are possible when you "Just Overdo It."

Just Overdo It

Sedentary people just deciding to get in shape typically begin an exercise program with happy expectations. They expect a year's results in a few frantic weeks. That approach is not without its place. The initial infatuation with exercise gets you started. But rather than softly making exercise a lifetime friend, overenthusiastic new exercisers sometimes pound themselves mercilessly. A few weeks later they are tired, irritable, and maybe even injured. Their plan is not novel or fun anymore. They've had enough pounding and enough proof that exercise wasn't for them anyway.

Some people exercise regularly, and every now and then do far more than usual. Others try to do too much all the time. Still others don't exercise at all. They occasionally lug a heavy cooler in and out of their trunk to go play softball, or go skiing. Monday morning they don't call in sick to work because they're too sore to pick up the phone.

How Much Is Too Much?

How do you know if you're overdoing it? According to basketball coach Dean Smith, "If you make every game a life-and-death proposition, you're going to have problems. For one thing, you'll be dead a lot."

Usually, clues are not so obvious. With any unaccustomed exercise, you can overdo, even with activity that seems mild to a more conditioned exerciser. Being out of shape for the activity, insufficient warm-up, and too little rest between exercise sessions are contributors. Exercisers may not eat enough, hoping to increase weight loss. Or you may be in great shape for one activity but not another that uses different muscles and ranges of motion. Warnings may include the phrase, "I used to be pretty good at this...," said just before participating in activities enjoyed long ago, with no conditioning since then.

The Short-term Overdo

Soreness. Anyone can be sore after activity, even trained athletes. Soreness begins the day after activity, so it is called delayed onset muscle soreness (DOMS). DOMS isn't usually dangerous and isn't permanent. It just sometimes feels that way. There are many complicated theories about the mechanisms and consequences of DOMS. In brief, unaccustomed mechanical stress leads to a cascade of events, including damage to the proteins in your muscle fibers, and a big inflammatory response. You're stiff, sore, and weak for one to three days. You've just overdone it.

Acute Injury. Sometimes, an injury is from an external event, like a Frisbee in the face. Other times, you can injure yourself. An activity more intense than you are used to can strain muscle fibers, or you may twist your joints into positions that harm them.

The Long-Term Overdo

Physical and Mental Decline. Up to a point, regular physical exercise enhances health, athletic ability, and feelings of energy. Findings from mental health research indicate positive mood change, increased intellectual function, and improved self-concept, although causal links are not known for sure.

Overdoing exercise reverses the situation. Athletic ability, energy, physical health, and state of mind suffer. "Fatigue," Napoleon observed, "makes cowards of us all."

Diminished physical performance sometimes drives frustrated exercisers to push harder to offset the decline. The overtraining cycle of fatigue, depression, and overdoing continues.

Chronic Injury. Overtraining overloads your musculoskeletal system. In plain English, you wear something out. The resulting injury can cause other injuries later on. Injuries that throw off how you walk and stand eventually stress previously healthy structures into new injuries. Some injuries you might not be aware of. These unrecognized injuries quietly build, decreasing performance and increasing long-range orthopedic consequences. Other, painful injuries, although outwardly more worrisome, can be helpful because they limit further overdoing (except in the pleasure-impaired).

Immune Decline. Studies of immune function seem to show a trend where moderate exercise possibly helps immune function, but intense overtraining can suppress the immune system. Most of the changes so far identified are small, variable, and temporary. It is still not known if these changes increase your risk of recurrent infection or other diseases during periods of extreme ultra-training.

Obsession. The exercise-obsessed person panics at the thought of missing a workout. They are certain that missing their day's pounding means undoing years of hard work. (This phenomenon is not limited to exercise. It includes just about any activity that you overdo.) Although their bodies and physical progress would be better off with rest and recovery time, they go at it every day. Their lack of progress spurs them to further excess. A frustrating cycle perpetuates of obsession, not enough recovery time, overdoing, and lack of progress.

Burnout. We've all done it. Some have done it plenty of times—start out great guns, then fizzle. The burnout syndrome can be summed up by the following: "Tri-weekly, try weekly, try weakly."

How to Just Not Overdo It

Sunday soldiers and chronic exercise abusers are well-researched in sport science, in part because they're so common. The literature reports several strategies to avoid overdoing.

Identify Problems. The point where "doing" becomes "overdoing" is difficult to define. What aspect of your activity do you overdo? Have you built up slowly to the task or did you just plunge in? Is your activity too intense for your abilities? Is your intensity level all right but without enough rest? Do you rest and train moderately yet still suffer injuries? In that case, it may not be overuse, but improper use. Not making progress? Is it lack of rest or not the right exercises? If you're still tired and miserable given an appropriate and safe program, you may need to change the kind of exercise you do. Try a different activity. This time make it one you like.

Modify. If it hurts when you do it, don't do it. Reduce the mileage, the amount of weight, the frequency, the intensity—whatever makes it too much—and then keep moving, but in a safe and sane level.

Avoid Misuse. Were you too out of shape to carry the cooler or haul up the anchor, or did you just lift wrong and screw up your back? Injury may stem not from overdoing, but from misuse, bad gait, poor lifting technique, or problematic exercises. Read about a few of these problems in Chapter 9, "Good and Bad Exercises," and Chapters 20 and 21 on back and neck pain. If misuse is the problem, modify your technique, equipment, or gait. Figure out which injuries you get from overuse and which from misuse.

Train in Cycles. Do you work out too much? The sport science literature is pretty clear that rest is crucial for physical improvement. With rest between sessions, you avoid the problems of overdoing, while increasing your physical ability more than possible by training every day. Alternating days of exercise and rest is called exercise cycling and periodization.

Top athletes don't work out every day. Athletes successfully training for strength usually lift three or four days each week. They don't practice their major heavy lifts like the press, pulls, or squat more than two days per week. During competitions they then cut back overall training to one to three days per week. Top runners allow days of rest between long runs and taper their mileage before races.

Get in Shape. Maybe you don't work out enough to be in shape for the occasional activity you do. Developing some semblance of fitness increases the variety of activities you can do without later paying the piper. Stick with at least a mild exercise program all year, not just in sports season.

Warm Up. Do you fling into activities without warming up? Well, warm up first. Warm-up, just as it sounds, means raising your body temperature. Warm-up is not stretching, arm waving, or rising up and down on tiptoe. Those activities do not raise body temperature. Use large muscle rhythmic activities like walking, slow jogging, swimming, or cycling to warm up. Be warm enough to sweat before you stretch or begin activity. See Chapter 5 on warm-ups.

Enjoy Yourself. Do you enjoy the exercise you do? A major point to consider is "Are you happy?" Make your program one that satisfies your soul along with your body. If you hate your program, chances are you won't stick with it, however well-intentioned.

At the other end of the continuum are those disciplined beings that slog through misery for the results, never mind the painful journey. Try enjoying yourself. Find aspects of exercise that you like. Incorporate rest periods. You'll find your performance improves with a day off in between exercise bouts.

If, on the other hand, you enjoy obsessing, go ahead and obsess. Identify and modify aspects that injure your body, social life, or happiness. Then, if overdoing is really for you, then just overdo it. Remember to reassess periodically. At least go see a movie sometimes.

Summary—How to Just Not Overdo It

Identify Problems. Have you built up gradually enough? Does your intensity level suit your fitness level? Do you get enough rest? Do you like the exercise you do?

Modify. If it hurts when you do it, don't do it. Reduce the mileage, amount of weight used, frequency, intensity, or whatever parameter makes it too much.

Avoid Misuse. Is it overuse or misuse? Bad gait? Poor lifting technique? Bad exercises?

Train in Cycles. Rather than training every day, rest between sessions. You'll avoid the problems of overdoing, while increasing your fitness.

Get in Shape. Developing some semblance of fitness increases the variety of activities you can do without later paying the piper.

Warm Up. Warm-up, just as it sounds, means raising your body temperature. It is not stretching, arm waving, or rising up and down on tiptoe. Be warm enough to sweat before you stretch or begin exercise.

Enjoy Yourself. Make your program one that satisfies your soul along with your body. If you hate your program, chances are you won't stick with it.

Top 10 List for Injury Prevention

1. Optimize. Do the least workout that will maximize your capabilities.

2. Variety. Cross-train. Change routines that have repetitive forces.

3. Get enough rest.

4. Avoid errors in technique. It's estimated that about two-thirds of all injuries come from training errors.

5. Get good nutrition. Most people don't drink enough water. Drink more water.

6. Remember total body fitness. Train for strength, flexibility, and endurance of all your body.

7. If your resting pulse in the morning suddenly goes up more than four beats per minute over normal, that is a sign of overtraining.

8. Listen to your body. It has a lot of good things to say.

9. Alternate hard days with easy days.

10. Customize your program to suit your body, rather than copying an off-the-shelf program from a book or a trainer.

(Source: Dr. Stanley L. James, University of Oregon, 1997 meeting of the American College of Sports Medicine)

What to Do When You've Already Done Too Much

Diagnose. You've done it. You're hurt. Not sore from a good workout, but injured. Go get a complete and accurate diagnosis of the injury, or injuries. There is usually more than one by this point. The key is not to treat until you know the cause, so that proper treatment may follow. Get an accurate diagnosis from a physician specializing in orthopedics. The Greek word *gnosis* means "knowing or recognizing." *Dia* is a word element that, in this context, means "completely." It's helpful to "know completely." Getting rid of pain and the disability that goes with it means treating the cause.

Treat. Don't let any practitioner treat you without first knowing what's wrong. It is easy and effective, at the time, to treat the symptoms, but without knowing the cause, you can't change behavior and practices that will probably bring back the injury and turn it into a chronic problem.

First Aid. Not discounting the importance of accurate diagnosis, many injuries take similar first aid. The first letters of the words *rest, ice, compression,* and *elevation* spell RICE, the acronym for treatment of almost all acute orthopedic injuries. Rest doesn't mean exercising even if it hurts, but it doesn't mean sitting around, getting out of shape so that you injure yourself trying to get back into shape. Rest includes gentle range of motion and activity for the injured area, according to your physician's instructions. It doesn't mean letting the rest of your body go to seed in the interim. Work other areas. Gradually get back to speed, always working below what it takes to reproduce the pain.

Use ice, not heat, for the first few days to reduce pain and swelling. You can continue to use ice even later if it helps to reduce pain. After about 48 hours, you can decide whether ice or heat is better for you. Until then, use ice. Bags of frozen peas or corn make good, pliant ice packs if no others are available. You can freeze a mixture of one-third rubbing alcohol with two-thirds water in a zip lock bag to make a nice cool slush bag.

Compression with ace bandages reduces swelling in limb injuries. Elevation means raising the injured part above your heart, not just propping it on a low chair. Anti-inflammatory medications like aspirin or Motrin® help with pain and inflammation. Tylenol® has no anti-inflammatory action but is good for pain if you can't stomach aspirin.

Stretch. Stretching helps alleviate delayed-onset soreness. Warm up gently, then, just as gently, stretch the affected muscle slowly. A good place to stretch sore muscles is in a hot bath or shower. Don't stretch in a way that causes more pain.

Recharge. Most muscle soreness is not an injury and is nothing to worry about. It will go away by itself. It's a good sign that you are out having a good time and are living, and were exercising enough to have effects. A helpful prescription is a hot bath, bubbles, candles, chocolates, and massage for seven to ten days. The soreness won't last that long, but who cares?

Summary—
What to Do When You've Already Done Too Much

Diagnose. Get a complete and accurate diagnosis of the injuries.

Treat. Treat the cause of the injuries, not just the symptoms.

First Aid. You can treat most injuries with rest, ice, compression, and elevation. Take anti-inflammatories to help reduce pain and inflammation for the short term.

Stretch. Gentle stretching alleviates delayed onset soreness.

Recharge. Hot bath, bubbles, candles, chocolates, and massage.

How to Do Without Overdoing

An exciting area of sports medicine research is devising screening and training programs that maximize physical potential without killing the exerciser. The amount and kind of exercise is different for everyone. Don't be dissuaded from exercise. It's much more common to rust out from inactivity than wear out from overdoing. Here are a few things to try:

Start Easy. For beginners, a twice-a-week program is often enough for the first months. Improvements in a previously sedentary or overweight person will be substantial. Weight loss occurs, waistlines shrink, fitness level and capacity for strenuous exercise improve, as does ability to tolerate heat and cold. Gains from twice-weekly exercise occur more slowly than from a three- or four-day-per-week program, but exercise is more likely to become part of a lifestyle, less likely to be skipped, with less chance of burnout.

Define Your Goals. Do you want to get stronger? Bigger? Smaller? The right exercises are different for each goal. See Chapters 2 and 3, "The Different Aspects of Fitness" and "Improving Your Fitness," and Chapter 8, "What Exercises Do You Need to Be Fit?" for more about the right workout for each desired effect.

Exercise Without Going to the Gym. Why ignore life by going to a gym all the time?

Make your daily activities your exercise. Take stairs instead of elevators; personally deliver messages instead of using interoffice mail.

Make adventure your exercise. Take reconnaissance walks around your neighborhood. Carry packages for people. Help your local club lug things around. You might learn things, meet people, and work out all at once.

Make romance your exercise. You can walk in the park to feed geese as easily as going out to eat a fat dinner. Carry each other piggy back (observing good back mechanics). Walk all over town to find just the right flowers for a surprise. Walk to the post office often to mail frequent, friendly notes. Dates are more memorable when you do fun things, not just sit and eat.

An important concept to "lifetime fitness" is that you don't have to stop your "real life" to go get exercise. Bend properly! You know you shouldn't pick things up by bending over at the waist; you already know you should bend knees and keep your torso upright. Done properly it's great exercise for your legs, burns calories, and saves your back. You probably do several hundreds of bends a day just doing housework, picking things up, tying shoes, arranging papers, and getting things off shelves. That could easily be equivalent to going to a gym and doing squats and lunges for an hour. But you already may have done that during a normal day.

Remember the Rest of You. Your body is not the only part of you that needs exercise. Exercise your sensibilities. Exercise your smile muscles. Exercise your imagination. Exercise your mental abilities. Exercise your funny bone. Exercise your love of life. Many things improve with exercise. Nice and easy.

Summary—How to Do Without Overdoing

Start Easy. For beginners, a twice-a-week program is often enough for the first several months. The gains occur more slowly than from exercising three or four days per week, but exercise is more likely to become part of a lifestyle, less likely to be skipped, with less chance of burnout.

Define Your Goals. Do you want to get stronger? Bigger? Smaller? The right exercises are different for each goal.

Exercise Without Going to the Gym. Make your daily work your exercise. Make having fun your exercise. Make romance your exercise. Why ignore your life and your mate by going to a gym all the time?

Remember the Rest of You. Exercise your sensibilities, your smile muscles, your brain. Exercise your imagination. Exercise your funny bone. Exercise your love of life.

11

Getting Out of Shape
and How to Avoid It

We can now prove that large numbers of Americans are dying from sitting on their behinds.

– Bruce B. Dan

You may not be an exerciser. Or you may have started a program, and then got tired of it, or went on vacation, or got caught up with work. You may have worked hard to get in shape at one time, but gave it up. After a layoff from exercise, your problems are more far-reaching than just gaining a little weight.

Loss of strength, endurance, and flexibility make packages seem heavier, runs longer, shelves harder to reach. Where did all those improvements you made go? Why should you care? What can you do?

How to Get Out of Shape

After long periods of not exercising, weights seem heavier than they used to. Following weeks of weightless space flight, astronauts come home with less muscle, blood volume, and bone than they left with. Even after only a day or two in bed with flu, you get up weak and dizzy even though you're not sick anymore. The principle of "Use It or Lose It" is technically known as "reversibility." Physical performance gains made through exercise reverse with inactivity. The deterioration of your physical condition is technically known as deconditioning.

There are several ways to decondition. Just sitting around for the winter is one. Holiday gatherings and family obligations leave less time for the gym. Winter weather decreases routine outdoor excursions and recreational opportunities. These are technically known as "excuses."

Periods of inactivity often follow injury or illness. Deconditioning may be local as in a limb in a cast, or a global problem of whole body inactivity. The common mechanism is disuse. An immobilized limb dramatically decreases in size, strength, and endurance. Bed rest severely reduces the mechanical stresses your entire body needs to stay healthy. Bed rest so effectively deconditions you that aviation scientists use it to study physical decrements following zero gravity in space flight.

What Goes Bad?

Getting fat is only the tip of the pathologic iceberg of getting out of shape. Deconditioning seriously affects the functional state of your entire body. Strength, cardiovascular capacity, blood, mental skills, and even your bones and immune system suffer.

Muscle. Without use, muscles decrease strength, endurance, and size, and lose blood vessel and nerve associations. They become less able to extract and use oxygen to do work, not only because your entire body's oxygen-carrying and delivery system declines, but for chemical reasons of their own.

In-shape muscle is able to burn more fat as fuel than out-of-shape muscle, which uses more carbohydrate. Deconditioned muscles lose intracellular fluid, stored carbohydrate, and contractile protein, contributing to loss of muscle tone. Your body gets soft. Eating extra protein will not stop muscle protein loss. Only exercise does that. The bottom line is that when muscles decondition, you may not look as good, feel as good, exercise as much, or even do as much around the house.

Cardiovascular. A deconditioned cardiovascular system can't process, deliver, or burn enough oxygen to do intense exercise because several of its components go to seed with inactivity. The total amount of blood your heart pumps per minute decreases, probably from an overall decrease in blood volume in the initial weeks of detraining. You lose oxygen-carrying molecules called hemoglobin.

The size and contractile force of your heart diminishes. The maximum rate your heart can beat doesn't change, yet it has to beat faster and work harder to do the same work you could easily do when you were in better shape. More lactic acid builds up than if you weren't deconditioned. Cardiovascular deconditioning even lowers your ability to regulate body temperature in the heat and cold.

Bone. After your mid-thirties to forties, you usually begin losing bone if you don't exercise, no matter how much calcium you eat. To maintain mineral density, bones need the mechanical stress of muscles pulling on them. Bone loss is a major problem of space flight. As yet, no countermeasures completely halt bone loss while weightless. On earth, sedentary lifestyle is a major risk factor for osteoporosis. Once osteoporosis develops, it is not reversible.

Body Composition. Although you may or may not avoid overeating during the winter holidays, without exercise you'll lose lean weight and put on some fat. Changes in body composition over time include higher body fat percentage and less lean muscle, even with no change in weight.

Cholesterol. One of several reasons regular exercise decreases risk of coronary artery disease is a favorable change in blood cholesterol. High-density lipoprotein cholesterol (HDL), popularly called good cholesterol, increases. "Bad cholesterol," or low-density lipoprotein (LDL), can decrease.

One study of male runners accustomed to 30 to 40 miles per week found detraining of only two to three weeks resulted in a 12% reduction in their aerobic capacity and a 7.7% reduction in good cholesterol. For more about good and bad cholesterol, see Part III.

Memory and Coordination. Sports skills not used over a winter dull and fade from active memory. Both memory and specific skills, like hand-eye coordination and fine motor coordination, appear to involve physical and chemical connections that require practice to stay sharp.

Flexibility. Inactivity, not exercise, reduces flexibility. As joints tighten and your range of motion diminishes for normal, daily activities, you become more likely to pull or strain a muscle, particularly your back and hamstrings. Weak, tight back and trunk muscles are the most usual cause of most back pain.

Balance. You quickly lose balance when you are inactive. Your risk of slips, falls, and injury soars. You do less because of fear of falling. A vicious cycle develops.

Reaction Time. The time it takes you to mobilize a response to something is another skill that you can improve with training and lose with lack of use. Reaction time, coupled with good judgment, allows you to react well in dangerous situations like oncoming traffic and falling objects.

How Long Does It Take?

Even brief detraining periods remarkably reduce physical ability. After only days to weeks of stopping exercise, your capacity for exercise decreases. After longer periods of weeks to months, you can become a complete lump. Gains made from a summer in the gym and pool can disappear over a sedentary winter.

The more drastic your inactivity, the greater and more rapid your losses. Complete bed rest for a week can decrease your capacity to use oxygen, your strength, hemoglobin count, and blood volume by up to 7%. It would take several weeks to deteriorate to the same extent without bed rest even if you didn't exercise.

Does It Hurt?

In one sense you could say getting out of shape doesn't hurt. Deconditioning isn't physically painful. You won't even notice it's happening at first. The harm comes from the fact that getting out of shape is more serious than just gaining a little weight. The global physical decline not only hinders specific sport activities, but activities of daily living.

Capacity for routine walking, lifting, and carrying dwindles. You slowly weaken and as a result do less and push it less. Your sense of balance dwindles. In turn, you decondition further. A negative cycle self-perpetuates. Risk of cardiovascular disease, falls, back pain, obesity, musculotendinous strains, and certain cancers may increase. For these reasons you could say getting out of shape hurts a great deal.

In older people, deconditioning often continues to the point of severe and even dangerous weakness. Getting out of chairs and ordinary daily activities become too much. A serious handicap results, not from aging, but from preventable and reversible deconditioning.

These people, under physician supervision, benefit by regular weightlifting and conditioning programs. Several studies of exercise for populations debilitated by what we formerly called "aging" found dramatic reversals after simple weightlifting and activity programs. These people no longer needed canes or wheelchairs; they decreased medications they took for high blood pressure, arthritis, or diabetes; and they went back to unaided daily activities.

How to Prevent Getting Out of Shape

At Least Do a Little. If you must take time off from exercise, try cutting back, not out. You can hold on to physical fitness, even with less frequency of exercise, if you maintain the intensity. According to some studies, cutting back from three regular days of exercise to two maintenance days can completely preserve oxygen-carrying capacity. Substituting one day for three will not prevent, but can reduce the consequences of detraining.

Avoid Bed Rest. In many instances, the original illness or injury is worsened through the physical degeneration resulting from bed rest. Sometimes, irreversible problems develop. Current treatments for most illness and injury involve early ambulation.

Get Active, Stay Active. If you exercise, stay as active as you can all year, every year. If you are sedentary, find some kind of regular activity you enjoy and get started. The older you get, the more beneficial exercise, including weightlifting, becomes. Exercise can at least partially counteract the physical deterioration of aging. A few table push-aways won't hurt either.

Stay in Shape

Getting out of shape is more serious than just gaining a little weight. It sabotages your cardiovascular condition, strength, endurance, bone health, blood fat status, body composition, and joint range of motion. In a short time, these decrements can become the functional equivalent of aging many years.

Serious problems can result from a vicious cycle of deconditioning, weakness, and poor health. This cycle is easily preventable. Staying in shape once you are active is easier than getting back in shape. You don't have to take care of your entire body, just the parts you want to keep.

12

Exercise Gimmicks

The actress Billie Burke was dining in a restaurant where a man at the next table was obviously suffering from a bad cold.

"I can see you're very uncomfortable," she volunteered. "So, I'll tell you what to do for it: drink lots of orange juice and take lots of aspirin. When you get to bed, cover yourself with as many blankets as you can find. Sweat the cold out. Believe me, I know what I'm talking about. I am Billie Burke of Hollywood."

The man smiled and introduced himself in return: "Thank you. I am Dr. Mayo of the Mayo Clinic."

It seems to be common for exercises to be taught, and health and fitness products promoted, by Hollywood stars and other self-proclaimed experts. Many humorous and outright wrong ideas and statements become commonly accepted.

"Lose fat while you sleep by drinking miracle liquid, not available in stores."

"Watch TV while motorized stomach vibrator burns more calories than 500 sit-ups a day."

"Shrink your waist with secret device known for years to scuba divers."

You've probably seen these catchy ads via tabloids, magazines, and late-night television. Are they true? Yes. Is there a catch? Yes.

Regarding the first claim, everyone burns fat when they're asleep. When they're awake, too. Metabolizing stored fat is part of your round-the-clock energy production for body functions, whether you drink "miracle liquid" or not. See Chapter 4, "What Does 'Aerobic' Really Mean?" for more on the issue of fat burning, and Chapter 14, "Nutrition Myths," for more on how potions get sold by carefully worded, but false, claims.

The second advertisement compares the relative number of calories burned in a longer time frame to a shorter one. In two hours sitting in front of the television you would burn more calories than during the theoretical 15 to 30 minutes it would take to do the sit-ups, with or without a vibrator strapped to your abdomen. That's just your normal metabolism at work.

Claims of Continued Fat Burning

Some products claim to give a workout so intense that you burn fat for hours after you finish. You burn fat 24 hours a day as part of being alive. It is also the case that during vigorous exercise, you increase your metabolism to meet your energy needs. Of course, it slows when you stop exercising, but takes a while to return to your resting values, sometimes up to a day. So any product can truthfully claim to produce increased calorie burning after a workout. A nice run or swim will do the same, although some evidence points to longer bouts of raised post-exercise energy expenditure after resistance training than after aerobic exercise.

Aerobic Benefits by Just Increasing Heart Rate

Many activities like to promote themselves as beneficial for your cardiovascular system. Not everything that increases your heart rate or blood flow gives you aerobic benefits. For example, it is sometimes stated that the yoga position of standing on the head or inclining head-down improves circulation and oxygenation to the head, and therefore confers aerobic benefit. Or that a specific stretch that is difficult to hold and raises heart rate therefore gives aerobic benefit. Neither improves aerobic capacity.

There is more to aerobic exercise than increasing blood flow and heart rate. Many things increase heart rate—for example, fear—without having anything to do with cardiovascular improvement. Increased heart rate from stage fright, for instance, is termed *neurogenic*, meaning it is produced as a nervous system effect, not *cardiogenic*, a cardiovascular system effect. Just moving the legs of a person lying in bed raises heart rate. It is a neurogenic increase, as that seems to be the body's way of preparing for exercise. Taking a long, hot shower or sitting in a hot tub increases heart rate because your skin blood vessels open up to try to dump the extra heat from your body. The vasodilation lowers your blood pressure, and your heart usually must speed up to keep enough blood pumping around. There is no aerobic benefit to overheating. Even massage has sometimes been falsely promoted as beneficial to the cardiovascular system on the basis of increasing blood flow. That doesn't mean that massage is bogus or not helpful, just that it doesn't benefit your cardiovascular capacity. True aerobic benefit comes from a collection of effects that you can get only through long-duration exercise, repeated regularly over time.

Ab Isolators

Several products on the market claim to better isolate your abdominal muscles, and therefore somehow give you the same, spectacular abdomen as pictured on the package. The true way to get a trim, well-defined abdomen is to lower your body fat through long-term exercise, eat healthful meals on a regular basis, and do exercises to improve the size and shape of the abdominal muscles, whether you use an "isolator" or not. There is nothing in an isolating device that you cannot do without the device. For instance, the advertising for one device claims to hold your feet and legs in the specific position required for crunches. You can easily do that yourself without the device.

Other various devices on the market add resistance to the abdominal exercises. More resistance increases the muscle-unit activation you require to do the exercise, the same as carrying extra packages adds more weight to your arms. There is nothing secret or scientific about doing more work to get more results.

Dr. Steven Fleck, sport physiologist formerly with the U.S. Olympic Training Center, reminds us, "The value of these devices is their novelty. If they get you to exercise areas that you wouldn't normally exercise, they might pay for themselves." But remember that the fine print on the packaging mentions that these products need to be combined with healthy eating and regular exercise.

Secret Scuba Device

What is the secret scuba device mentioned at the beginning of this chapter? Neoprene. You've probably seen neoprene bands to wear around the waist and thighs. Yes, they shrink your waist, and yes, it's another gimmick. It has nothing to do with sweat loss. Ever notice when you take off your socks that there's a darkened dent around your leg? The elastic compressed your flesh, leaving you temporarily smaller. You return to normal circumference soon enough. It's healthier, more economical, and longer lasting to just get in shape.

13

How to Get Started
Getting in Shape

A man ought to have a doctor's prescription to be allowed to use a golf cart.

– Paul Dudley White

You know it's good for you, and you know you should get started. Some people are experts at starting an exercise program. They've done it hundreds of times. The trick is staying started.

Lifetime Activity

You don't have to go to a gym to get exercise. You don't have to do push-ups or jumping jacks, or run. You can develop fitness through an active lifestyle. Being active for fun, and for things you have to do anyway, is the concept of lifetime activity.

Your daily activities become more active in a natural way, instead of a sedentary life that has to be made up for by going to a gym. Shake up your concept of exercise from a hated mandatory session with strange rules about heart rates, intensities, and minimum calories to burn, into a daily life exercise playground—yard work, shopping, cleaning, painting. Lift right all day. Stand up straight all day. That's work? Good. Make opportunities to burn calories as part of your normal daily routine. With a little imagination you could burn several hundred extra calories a day. You'll lose two to three pounds a month without doing any special exercises or diets. That may not sound like much, but it's a clothing size every three to four months, and 20 to 30 pounds by next year.

Goal-Specific Exercise

Your plan of attack depends on your fitness goal. For a sedentary beginner to increase aerobic capacity, a three-times-a-week effort is a good starting place.

For disease reduction, three 10-minute walks a day can reduce your risk of early death by disease by 60%, according to the Cooper Institute for Aerobics Research in Dallas.

For fat reduction, start out with long, low-intensity cardiovascular sessions and weightlifting. Weightlifting doesn't burn many calories during the workout, but increases your own lean weight, a helpful calorie burner. Food items are not worked off in single death bouts. Small caloric expenditures multiply over time. A 150-calorie walk per day translates into just over 15 pounds a year. As with many other new physical activities, see your physician first.

Daily Fun, Not Specific Exercises

A key to getting fitter is finding activities you love to do, and making your daily routines more active in general. Some people want the same routine each day. Others need variety. But rather than think of fitness as intentional exercise at set periods for specific body parts, enjoy an active life. If you're heavy or haven't had a recent physical, see your physician before starting. Enjoy yourself. Don't overdo. Here are some ideas:

- Do you like to go dancing? Find a club and live it up weekly for a fun cardiovascular session. Drink water and whole juices for beverages through the night.

- Walk or bike to the market, carry bags home, and help put away groceries. That's both aerobic and muscular endurance, and depending on weight of the bags, some strength work, too.

- Try bicycling for errands or scenery for aerobic endurance and muscular endurance of the legs. Maybe even commute by bike or walk or jog instead of driving for short to moderate distances. It can be quicker and cheaper than driving and paying for parking.

- Take nature walks.

- Plant a garden.

- Vacuum the house.

- Lift right all day—bend your knees properly and that will strengthen them. Use your legs, not your back, to save your back. You'll burn twice the calories or more with each bend, all day every day.

- Wash your car by hand and have fun getting your helpers all soapy.

- Take a walk and feed a few expired parking meters for strangers.

- Park farther away and walk the extra distance. But not everyone has time for that. Where possible, try biking instead.

- Instead of swimming laps, play in the water with beach balls, foam floats, and kickboards.

- If you hate jogging, play Frisbee, tag, catch, or badminton instead. They may not always be as much exercise, but it is a way to get started and have fun.

- Why endure an impatient minute for an elevator when you can improve your legs on the stairs in half the time?

- If you work on a high floor, take the elevator a few flights and walk the rest of the way.

- Hand-deliver interoffice mail.

- Help your local club or group with chores.

- Forget the golf cart and walk.

- Use a push mower instead of a power mower, a walk-behind mower instead of a ride-around mower.

- Hide the remote control.

- Give a friend a piggyback ride.

- Play with children.

- Be a hero and carry things for people.

- Take housebound neighbors' dogs for walks and romps.

- Carry groceries with your arms and good posture, not a cart.

- Walk through instead of driving through.

- Take reconnaissance walks all over your neighborhood. Drive to beautiful nature trails if none are close by, and take a walk.

Some Lifestyle Exercises

Light Exercise:	Moderate Exercise:	Vigorous Exercise:
Less than 280 calories an hour	280 to 420 calories an hour	More than 420 calories an hour
Walking or strolling around 2 miles per hour	Fast walking: 3 to 4 miles per hour	Fast walking up a hill, or with a load
Golfing with a cart	Golfing carrying clubs	Racquet sports
Home care, like vacuuming	House cleaning	Moving furniture
Mowing the lawn with a riding mower	Mowing the lawn with a power mower	Mowing the lawn with a push mower

Your Fitness Future

Make your daily life active and fun, and you never have to go to a gym if you don't want to. Find activities you like to do anyway, and make them a part of your daily life. There are many things you will find that you like, or used to like, that would make your life better if added back into the day. Sit down and plan them. Then get up and do them. Enjoy.

Part II

NUTRITION

How strange a creature is man, who will at times go to such extremes to preserve his life, only to shorten it at the dinner table.

– William H. Gordon

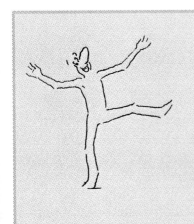

14. Nutrition Myths

15. Calculating Food Fat

16. Sport Drinks

17. Ergogenic Aids—Does Physical Enhancement Await on Your Plate?

18. Healthy Eating

19. How to Lose Weight Without Dieting

14

Nutrition Myths

You believe easily that which you hope for earnestly.

– Terence (Greek-born Roman playwright, second century B.C.)

Nothing is so firmly believed as that which we least know.

– Michel de Montaigne (16th-century French essayist)

If you heard of a nutrient your body requires to transmit nervous system signals, manufacture sex hormones, and is a precursor of the bile that handles ingested fats, would you eat lots of it?

It's cholesterol.

Would you run out and buy a substance your brain can't do without to process decisions and retain memory?

It's sugar.

Do you avoid a common practice using a chemical that constricts brain blood vessels, reducing cerebral blood flow?

It's breathing oxygen.

Descriptions in isolation can mislead. That's how nutrition myths begin. Ordinary food items become income producers to the slick packager. Nutrition myths are no exception. This chapter explores just a few.

The "Isolated Aspect" Myth

Oxygen, in high concentrations, is toxic to every life form on the planet. If you breathe high levels for long periods, you will suffer ill effects. But you don't avoid breathing oxygen in the air around you. You use it for other characteristics in its favor, like staying alive. In similar ways, vitamin and food supplement advertisements divert your focus to and from isolated aspects of their product. They concentrate on problems occurring only from excesses or deficiencies, or on only one effect of the substance, usually exaggerated.

Claims:

- A powdered carbohydrate supplement for weightlifters and athletes advertises that it is insulinogenic. The suffix -gen comes from a Greek word meaning "producing." In other words, it encourages insulin production. The advertising states that insulin is instrumental in getting the building blocks of protein into your muscle cells, and since this product is insulinogenic, it therefore builds muscle. Wouldn't that be great?

- Another product uses exactly the opposite property of insulin for marketing. A popular high-protein diet promotes the idea that you must avoid nonprotein foods because they stimulate insulin. Since another property of insulin is to promote fat storage, these people say to eat only high-protein, non-insulin-stimulating foods, in order to be in a fat-burning "zone."

Critical Reading:

- Insulin has several functions. It transports amino acids into your cells for protein synthesis. It also activates enzymes, which stimulate fat cells to synthesize and store fat. That's just part of how you digest food. So insulin helps you store fat. They don't say that on the labels for insulinogenic muscle-building supplements. They tell you only about storing protein, leading you to believe that their product will increase the normal amount of protein that you use to build your muscles. It doesn't.

- Protein synthesis goes on all the time to replace the continual turnover in your cells. It doesn't construct a bigger muscle and bulge it through your skin. (See The "More The Merrier" Myth to understand why.)

- Almost all food is insulinogenic, particularly sugar. Every time sugar enters the nondiabetic bloodstream, it stimulates insulin release. There's nothing special about the "insulinogenic" product. It's just a sugary food.

- The high-protein diet claims are misleading and potentially unhealthy. High-protein diets "work" to produce weight loss because they are low-calorie, not because of any insulin-stimulating or suppressing quality.

The "More The Merrier" Myth

Most of your brain is water. Almost no one would expect to get more brain by drinking more water. (I say "almost no one" with great optimism.) If you eat an extra amount of something, your body doesn't always use it to do what you hope. Here's where the myths go wild. The most flagrant examples involve protein and calcium supplements.

By themselves, protein and calcium won't grow muscles or strengthen bones. Your body continually "turns over" the protein in muscle fibers, calcium in bone cells, and fat in fat cells. That means it uses some for body function, recycles some, and takes small amounts of incoming material from food for rebuilding. The constant breakdown and resynthesis is called modeling. Modeling doesn't grab extra protein or calcium and add it on to you. It takes what it needs to keep you the same as before and discards the rest, unless you give your body a reason to make you different than before. That reason is resistance exercise, also called weightlifting. Weightlifting will make your body add more protein to your muscles, and calcium to your bones. But just eating a food will not. For more on calcium and your bones, see Chapter 22 in Part III.

Another common place for the "More the Merrier" Myth is vitamins. If a vitamin helps something in your body, then taking more vitamins must do more of that process, right? Wrong. The B vitamins, for example, work as coenzymes. Coenzymes help an enzyme do its enzyme job. The enzyme/coenzyme interdependence is like a lock-and-key relationship. Only one key fits one companion lock. Taking more of a vitamin when your body is not making more of the corresponding enzyme will have no effect. From three wheels you can still make only one bicycle. Taking the companion enzyme in pill form will not help because eating the pills destroys the enzymes, described later in the "No Digestion" Myth.

Here's another example: A precursor of the bile that handles fat digestion is cholesterol. But if you eat more cholesterol, that won't make your body digest more fat. Your body uses what cholesterol it needs and dumps the rest back into your circulation. Too much cholesterol can have tragic effect, bringing us to the "More Can't Hurt" Myth.

The "More Can't Hurt" Myth

Claim:

- Protein builds muscles; therefore, more protein must build more muscle, and after all, more can't hurt.

Critical Reading:

- Extra protein doesn't build extra muscle unless plenty of resistance exercise tells your body that the muscle is needed.

- Even then, your body can use only so much, regardless of how much you exercise.

- Past that amount, extra protein can be harmful.

Problems of Too Much Protein. Extra protein is not stored; it goes several routes. One is through your excretory system, taking water with it to produce urea. With excessive protein intake, you can dehydrate yourself a bit. Another exit route for excess protein is conversion to fat, which can't be turned back to protein later. Another problem with too much protein is that it increases calcium loss through the urine. That means that eating too much protein makes you "pee" out calcium. Epidemiologic studies point to excess protein, particularly animal protein, as contributing to osteoporosis.

What about those high-protein diets that claim you need extra protein to get you into a fat-burning zone? It turns out that if you follow their meal plans, the meals are low-calorie, and for that reason, you lose weight. It does not have anything to do with extra protein, or insulin, or zones. Problems occur because the meals are also low-carbohydrate, which leaves you tired. You need energy to carry out daily activities, and to exercise for weight loss and health. You do need a certain amount of protein every day. Chapter 18 covers the details to figure out how much you will need.

Problems of Too Much Iron. A high blood iron level is also frequently thought to be a good thing. That is not always true. Iron is essential to your health, in several roles. Iron is also involved in certain harmful reactions in your body, involving special molecules called free radicals. (For more on free radicals see the glossary, and the sections on the "No Digestion" Myth and "Reverse Reasoning" Myth.) Free radicals can sometimes be very destructive in your body. That's their job. People with high iron levels have been found to develop high rates of heart disease, possibly from high amounts of free radicals generated from too much iron. Although women are frequently labeled as at a disadvantage for their tendency to have lower iron levels than men, it seems that may have developed to be an advantage. Populations with lower than average iron levels have been found to have lower than average incidence of heart disease. Iron is only one of many factors, not the only factor involved in this phenomenon, but it is not an unimportant consideration. See Chapter 27, "Cardiovascular Disease," for more about the possible connection between too much iron and heart trouble. If that weren't enough, iron supplements are constipating. It is now a common recommendation that people should not supplement iron without physician supervision.

Problems of Too Much Water. Even drinking water can be overdone. It's not common, but extreme prolonged exercise in the heat, with no food or fluid replacement other than large amounts of water, can cause a problem called water intoxication. You just dilute yourself too much.

More is not always better. Philosopher Allen Ross Anderson capsulized maximalist thinking: "We should have our minds open, but not so open that our brains fall out."

The "No Digestion" Myth

More is not always better. Sometimes, more becomes nothing at all. Some health food stores sell pills containing enzymes. The claims are that your body needs these enzymes for various functions, so if you take a supply of these enzymes in their pills, you will get more of the benefits. This does not work at all.

First, there is no way for enzymes to get into your bloodstream by eating them. They cannot pass through your intestinal wall except by breaking down into constituent parts. This destroys them as enzymes.

Broken-down enzymes will not automatically reassemble on the other side of your intestine, so eating enzymes will not raise your body levels of enzymes. Your body makes all the enzymes you need out of the ordinary food you eat. Eating enzymes by themselves, except those that aid digestion (like lactase to digest dairy products), is useless and expensive.

An interesting example is superoxide dismutase (SOD). SOD is an enzyme that is one of several antioxidants your body needs and makes to counter the effects of free radicals, which are generally accepted as being a cause of many physical problems.

Free radicals have an unpaired electron, so they go around trying to get another electron for themselves by taking one from other molecules in your body. Free radicals particularly target fatty acids and proteins, harming them in the process of stealing their electrons. Then the fatty acids and proteins become free radicals themselves, and go around grabbing electrons from other molecules, like a destructive game of tag. Your body has several built-in systems for removing radicals, but can get overwhelmed by too many free radicals, which can then go unchecked in their damage.

Eating SOD in pill form won't do anything against free radical damage or any other oxidative stress in your body. If eaten, SOD, like any other enzyme, is destroyed in your intestine by digestion.

As is often the case with sham cures offered in pill form, there are many research studies that seem to back up the claims. Studies do show that SOD reduces free radical formation. None of these studies involved eating the SOD, but injecting it into laboratory animals under specific conditions. More information on free radicals, oxygen toxicity, and antioxidants is provided in the "Reverse Reasoning" Myth.

The "It Works For Popeye" Myth

People frequently want to know if a food or sports bar advertised as "giving energy" really will perk them up. These products are food, not stimulant drugs such as cocaine or amphetamines. However, many do contain stimulants such as caffeine, ginseng, ma huang, or other substances explained in Chapter 17, "Ergogenic Aids."

Technically, the potential energy in food is measured in units called calories. "High-energy snack" is a euphemism for "high-calorie food" or, in other words, "fattening food." If you eat high quantities of high-energy food, it really will give you potential chemical energy for your activities right now, and plenty more for the future. That stored energy is called fat. Armed with this knowledge, you can now pick out the person who obviously has the most energy at hand (and other places) for activities—an obese person.

What About Vitamins? Vitamins have no calories so, technically, furnish no energy. If you are vitamin deficient in a way that makes you weak, then restoring healthy vitamin levels will restore your normal energy levels. Extra vitamins will not give you "pep." More on vitamins in the "Reverse Reasoning" Myth.

What About Sugar? Sugar makes you feel energetic shortly after eating it. Sugar helps delay fatigue if used during long endurance events where you can't stop to eat. Simple sugars make your insulin levels soar to deal with the sugar, then drop soon after, making you feel tired. That's the problem with eating sugar for energy. Complex sugars (complex carbohydrates) have a steadying effect on insulin, and are a better choice for eating for energy. Regularly relying on simple sugars for "quick fixes" is not the healthiest choice. Although a complex topic, the main idea is to eat smaller, more frequent, low-fat, high-complex-carbohydrate meals every day, and do the work that increases your musculature and fitness. Then you are capable of more energy for exercise. Regular good nutrition and regular exercise, not special energy foods, give you energy.

Claims of enhanced athletic performance and energy from health foods, supplements, vitamins, steroids, caffeine, amphetamines, and others are examined in Chapter 17.

The "Need It Now" Myth

People sometimes ask which vitamins and minerals are removed from your system by sporting activities, and which specific foods have those nutrients, so that they can eat them before exercise. General recreational exercise does not sufficiently deplete any nutrients to affect athletic ability or health. For that reason, after a one-hour hike or game of tennis you don't need to replace specific vitamins or minerals immediately.

Your next good meal will cover you. It is unnecessary to take extra vitamins or minerals ahead of time to offset any loss predicted during your exercise. You don't lose enough to affect performance or fatigue level. Regular healthy eating and hydration assures you don't start your day in an already depleted state. Moreover, your daily requirements of most nutrients typically balance out over days. Minute-to-minute deficits don't matter as much. Drinking water is always a good idea before and after exercise.

Claim:

- It's often said you are in danger of B12 deficiency if you don't eat red meat every day to make up the amounts you use every day.

Critical Reading:

- Only a small number of people can't use the B12 in their diets. These people take supplements. Otherwise, Vitamin B12 is stored in your liver in enormous quantities, sufficient for a three- to five-year period.

The "Reverse Reasoning" Myth

If a deficit causes a weakness, a much-cherished myth is that a surplus will bring strength. But just as the right glasses prescription helps you see better, getting too strong a correction will not make you see even better.

Vitamin E is a good example. A while back, on experiments with rats, researchers removed all Vitamin E from the rats' diets. The rats became bald and sterile. Restoring Vitamin E restored the rats' hair and fertility. Human marketeers got hold of those results, and launched a successful campaign to sell Vitamin E with claims of giving you hair and virility. Of course, Vitamin E does not do that for humans with adequate nutrition. (But bald, sterile rats, take note.)

Claims:

- Vitamin A is often promoted as "Needed for good night vision."

- High-calorie foods are often labeled as "Giving you energy."

- Special powdered mixtures are advertised as "Providing all the nutrients contained in healthy spinal discs," or containing "All the nutrients crucial to healthy hair."

- Free radicals are known to be involved in the various damage to the body caused by their highly oxidative nature. Vitamins C and E are known antioxidant agents against the oxidative free radical activity. People often take extra Vitamins C and E on the presumption that it will reduce their risk of the various damaging effects of free radicals.

Critical Reading:

- Vitamin A deficiency reduces ability to see in dim light. But no amount of carrots or Vitamin A supplements will make adequately nourished eyes see better.

- Calorie deficiency makes you tired. But eating extra calories will not make you energetic; it will make you fat.

- Potions containing the nutrients or component substances of your back and hair don't fix your bad back or grow hair. They're regular food. Countless products line the shelves, truthfully stating they are for skin, nerves, strength, fingernails, or whatever—all just glamorized food. Yes, your body needs specific nutrients to do its job, but eating more of them won't increase the processes.

- Vitamin E is lipid (fat) soluble and protects cell membranes, which have a major lipid component. Vitamin C is a water-soluble antioxidant, having protective effects in blood and the fluid inside and outside of cells. Vitamins E and C work together in their free radical inactivation work. The way Vitamin E inactivates radicals is to accept the extra electron that makes the molecules radical and reactive. When Vitamin E takes that extra electron, it becomes radical itself. Vitamin C then takes the extra electron from E to restore Vitamin E. Vitamin C is special, in that it can accept this extra burden without injury to itself or surrounding molecules.

You need a minimum amount of these vitamins to do their jobs. It's true that many people, particularly those on the typical meat-eating Western diet, may not get enough Vitamins E and C, which are found in vegetables and fruits. But taking more Vitamins E and C than you need has not been shown to increase their usual effects on radicals in the body. If you are vitamin deficient, they may help, but not if you are vitamin sufficient. Taking too much can be injurious.

As an important note, free radicals are not all bad. There are some that perform critically important functions in your body, such as those involved in muscle contraction and in the immune response. You may not want to push your resting levels down, even if it were possible to do so by eating antioxidants. If you got rid of the radicals stored in special cells in your body that fight infection, you would be at serious risk of catastrophic infections.

The bottom line is that eating extra of any particular nutrient will not give you extra abilities. Although protein is a building block of your skin, eating extra protein will not make you grow lots of extra skin. Your body does not use the extra.

The "I Can Eat Anything I Want as Long as It Is Low-Fat" Myth

Eating low-fat and still not losing weight? Forget all the conflicting and confusing articles you've read about needing to eat fat for "zones" or fat burning, or that carbohydrates make you fat. It is the number of calories you eat of those "low-fat" foods that makes the difference. Low-fat cakes, cookies, and candies can easily be high-calorie and full of sugar. Obviously, an entire sack of sugar is nonfat (and a 1,000 calorie block of butter is "sugar-free," too.) Keep your common sense about you. Several hundred extra calories a day of nonfat food will just be stored as fat.

The "I Eat Right" Myth

An average person sits down to an evening meal of steak or burgers; potato mashed with butter, salt, and milk; coffee with cream and sugar; and a small side of buttered vegetables; then has ice cream and/or cake for dessert. A good dinner of protein for muscles, calcium for bones, and energy for exercise? No. The U.S. Department of Agriculture recently surveyed American dietary habits. The findings? Many Americans who think they eat healthy don't at all. The sample dinner is typical of three times too much fat, saturated fat, cholesterol, and salt; double the needed protein; too much simple sugar; hardly any fiber, vitamins, or complex carbohydrates; and not enough water. This kind of eating is increasingly associated with heart and vascular disease, vitamin deficiency, dehydration, calcium loss, high blood pressure, and some cancers.

The "Healthy Eating Is Awful" Myth

Why should low-fat, vegetable-based meals be called drastic, while cardiac bypass surgery, stroke, and colon cancer are considered normal? This is good news, not bad. Good meals need no secret energy foods and no special supplements. They can be delicious and healthy in many ways. Good stuff to eat, and how to prepare it quickly, inexpensively, and make it taste great is covered in Chapter 18, "Healthy Eating."

Escaping Myths

Some nutrition myths don't matter—stomachs don't digest food, that's the job of the small intestine. Some myths stem from mistaken identity—stomachs don't growl, that's the small intestine again. Some myths were just created to sell a product—there never was a real Betty Crocker. Food myths are sometimes like food itself. No matter how thin you slice it, it's still baloney.

15

Calculating Food Fat

I had fried mozzarella cheese. Deep-fried cheese. Oh, there's a cardiovascular dream come true. The cheese doesn't have enough fat—let's give it a cholesterol Jacuzzi!

– Rick Corso

You've been good. You've learned about good eating habits. You're making positive lifestyle changes. You eat less fat because that's how to get slimmer and healthier.

You even order healthy food in restaurants. You ask for salad with dressing on the side; vegetable soup; a potato (no bacon) that you plan to season with lemon-pepper, nonfat dressing, and spices; and spaghetti with spiced red sauce, no Parmesan.

The soup arrives cooked in a beef fat base, thickened with cream, topped with cheese. The potato arrives with a dip of sour cream, cheese, and butter. The entree was cooked with butter or oil. The red sauce is thickened with oil, corn starch, and flour.

The American Heart Association recommends no more than 30% of the calories you eat come from fat. The meal you thought you ordered would have totaled 735 calories, including 185 calories of fat, or about 25% of the calories from fat, and would have been a good tasting, healthy low-fat meal. If you used seasonings instead of dressing, there would have been a mere 50 calories of fat out of 535 total, only 8.5% fat. What you got instead was a 1,558-calorie lunch, with 935 of those calories from fat, or 60% fat. Meanwhile, you thought you were eating low fat, and don't understand why the weight is so hard to keep off.

What You Thought You Ordered:

Item	Total Calories Low-Fat Version	% Fat Low-Fat Version
Salad	50	trace
Thousand Island Dressing	150	86%
Vegetable Soup	90	10%
Plain Potato	145	5%
Spaghetti – No Oil	200	4%
Low-Fat Sauce	100	27%

Total Calories: 735, or 585 without the salad dressing
Fat Calories: 185, or only 50 without the salad dressing
Percent Fat: 25%, or 8.5% without the salad dressing

What You Might Get Instead:

Item	Total Calories Low-Fat Version	% Fat Low-Fat Version
Salad	50	4%
Thousand Island Dressing	150	87%
Creamed Soup with Cheese	322	45%
Potato with Toppings	436	52%
Spaghetti in Butter	300	38%
High-Fat Sauce	300	60%

Total Calories: 1,558
Fat Calories: 935
Percent Fat: 60%

How to Calculate Food Fat

How do you know if a food is high-fat? If it has the words *fried, buttered,* or *rich* in the name, that's one clue. If you put the food on a napkin and it leaves the napkin transparent, that's another.

For most foods, you won't know without looking on the label. The label tells many things, including how many calories and how many grams of fat are in the food. If the label doesn't state the fat percentage, calculating it is not hard. Divide the calories of fat by the total number of calories. If a food has 100 calories and 27 calories come from fat, the food is 27% fat.

To find how many calories of fat there are, multiply the number of grams of fat by 9. Why 9? There are 9 calories in each gram of fat. By comparison, there are 4 calories per gram of protein or carbohydrate.

To Calculate Percentage of Fat in Any Food:

1. Find the number of grams of fat in the food.

2. Multiply the number of grams of fat by 9 to get calories of fat.

3. Find the total number of calories in the food.

4. Divide calories of fat (#2) by the total number of calories (#3).

Two main ways to keep track of the fat you eat are by grams and by percent. The result of each is the same. The method you choose is just a matter of personal preference.

The Percent Method. In the percent method, you try to eat no more than a predefined percent of your daily calories as fat calories. The often-quoted maximum by the American Heart Association is 30%. Several other organizations recommend lower percentages for better health, including 10% fat diets that have a track record of being able to reverse cardiovascular disease. Learn the amount of fat contained in foods you eat and cut back on those with a high percentage.

The Gram Method. In the gram method, you track how many grams of fat you eat per day, and decide not to go over a certain number of grams per day. To know how many grams of fat is right for you, you first need to know how many calories you need every day, then decide what percentage of that you will allow for fat. That tells you how many calories of fat you can have each day. Divide your total calorie need by 9 to find the maximum number of grams of fat. A sample calculation looks like this:

Calorie needs for the average women are roughly 2,000 to 2,300, and for average men, 2500 to 2800 calories per day. These numbers change with activity and body size. If you decide that you will allow 30% of those calories as fat, it's 600 to 690 for women and 750 to 840 for men. Dividing by 9 to find the number of grams of fat would be 66 to 76 for women and 83 to 93 for men.

A rough estimate for the gram method, but without all the math, is to divide your body weight in pounds, or the weight you wish you were, by half. If you weigh 120 pounds (54 kilograms), you can have 60 grams. If you weigh 140 pounds (64 kilograms), you can have 70 grams. If you weigh 160 pounds (73 kilograms), you can have 80 grams. If you weigh 180 pounds (82 kilograms), you can have 90 grams. If you weigh 200 pounds (91 kilograms), then 100 grams of fat per day will pretty much keep you at that weight. If you eat an average number of calories, that will keep your fat percentage just under 30%.

If all of this seems too arcane, remember that the point is to have a general idea of total fat in your diet. Ignore clever advertising. Reduce the grams of fat or the percentage fat to reduce your fat intake.

Why 2% Milk Is Not 98% Fat-Free

Food marketers want you to buy their product. Food labels often state the food is a certain percent "fat-free." Often, that is misleading advertising.

What's important to your health is the percentage of total calories that come from fat. Advertisers often measure the fat by its weight in the product, which is meaningless to you and watching fat. A cup of "2% fat" milk is not 2% fat by calories. A surprising 35% of the total calories are from fat. Here's why:

One cup of 2% fat milk has 121 calories and 4.7 grams of fat. Multiply the 9 calories per gram of fat by the number of grams, in this case 9 x 4.7, or 42.3. So 42.3 calories out of the total of 121 calories are from fat. Divide 42.3 by 121 to get 0.35. One cup of 2% fat milk is 35% fat.

Let's try one cup of whole milk, called 3% milk. It has 150 total calories and 8 grams of fat. Multiply 9 times 8 to get 72. Divide 72 by 150 to learn that whole milk is 48% fat.

What about one cup of 1% fat milk, which is labeled low-fat milk? It has 102 calories and 2.6 grams of fat. Nine times 2.6 is 23.4 calories of fat. Divide 23.4 by 102 to see that 1% fat milk is really 23% fat.

Now try one cup of skim milk, called nonfat milk. It has 86 calories and 0.5 grams of fat. Nine times 0.5 is 4.5 calories of fat out of 86 total. You can see that this is finally low-fat—only 5% fat.

How Low-Fat is Low-Fat Milk?

Milk Product (8 ounces)	Total Calories	Grams of Fat	Calories of Fat (grams x 9)	% Fat (calories of fat divided by total calories)
Whole milk, 3%	150	8.0	72.0	48%
2% fat milk	121	4.7	42.3	35%
1% fat milk	102	2.6	23.4	23%
Skim milk	86	0.5	4.5	5%

(some figures rounded)

The Fat in Your Foods

How Low-Fat Are Common Foods?

Meal	Total Calories	Grams of Fat	Calories of Fat (grams x 9)	% Fat (calories of fat divided by total calories)
Croissant/egg/cheese/ham	475	33.6	302.4	64%
Big Mac	560	33.0	297.0	53%
French fries	220	10.0	90.0	41%
Bowl of oatmeal with cinnamon	145	2.3	20.7	14%
Bowl of pasta and broccoli	223	1.2	10.8	< 5%

(some figures rounded)

Percentage Fat Is Not the Whole Story. A Big Mac and a croissant/egg/cheese/ham sandwich have nearly the same number of grams of fat. The greater number of calories in the Big Mac drops the percent of fat to a deceptively lower figure, while not making the Big Mac the healthier choice. A serving of French fries has nearly the same number of calories as a bowl of pasta and broccoli, but the fries have more than eight times more fat. A meal of whole wheat pasta and broccoli has only 5% or so of fat. A pack of fries, more than 40%. Don't be fooled by percentage of fat only, since sugary junk foods are low-fat but still poor food choices. A raisin bagel is low-fat but is still 400 calories. A bagel loaded with jam is low-fat, but can be 600 calories.

How Low-Fat Are Frozen Desserts?

Dessert	Total Calories (varies greatly, depending on brand)	Grams of Fat (varies greatly, depending on brand)	Calories of Fat (grams x 9)	% Fat (calories of fat divided by total calories)
Ice cream (premium brand)	349	24	216	62%
Ice milk	184	6	54	29%
Frozen yogurt	180	4	36	20%
Sherbet	270	4	36	13%

(some figures rounded)

How Low-Fat Are Movie Foods?

Movie Food	Total Calories	Grams of Fat	Calories of Fat (grams x 9)	% Fat (calories of fat divided by total calories)
Reese's Peanut Butter Cups (2)	250	15	135	54%
Small bag of M&Ms with peanuts	250	13	117	47%
Buttered popcorn (2 cups)	110	6	54	49%
Small bag of M&Ms plain	230	10	90	39%
Box of Cracker Jack	120	3	27	23%
Air popped popcorn (2 cups)	60	trace	trace	< 1%

(some figures rounded)

Snacks

Modern snack foods are loaded with fat. Drinking diet soda with high-fat snacks does not cancel out the calories. The following chart reflects some realistic quantities like handfuls, bars, and small bag-fulls, instead of the commonly listed serving sizes.

How Low-Fat Are Snacks?

Snack	Total Calories	Grams of Fat	Calories of Fat (grams x 9)	% Fat (calories of fat divided by total calories)
Potato chips	316	21.8	196.2	62%
Fritos Corn Wild Mild Chips	150	9	81	54%
Almond Joy	250	14	126	50%
M&M's Peanut	220	11	99	45%
Snickers bar	280	13	117	42%
Hard pretzels	212	3.5	31.5	15%
Plain bagel	350	1.4	12.6	4%
Banana	105	0.5	4.5	4%
Handful of raisins	65	trace	trace	< 1%

(some figures rounded)

What if you added nonfat, but high-calorie, candy to a snack of potato chips? Would that lower the figure for total fat percentage compared to total calories?

Yes, it would. But that will not make that snack a healthier one. You added only more calories and more simple sugars. Total calories count.

Meat

Many people regard meat as only a protein food, forgetting that meat is usually a high-fat item.

How Much Fat Is in Common Meats?

Meat	Total Calories	Grams of Fat	Calories of Fat (grams x 9)	% Fat (calories of fat divided by total calories)
Meat stick, smoked – 1 oz	156.1	14	126	81%
Bacon – 2 slices	72.6	6.2	56	77%
Bologna – pork – 1 slice	56.8	4.6	41	72%
Pork chop – 1	284	22.3	201	71%
Salami – cooked beef – 1 slice	60.3	4.8	43	71%
Hamburger – 1 – baked, not fried	244	17.8	160	66%
Chicken – dark meat with skin – 3 oz	215.4	13.5	122	57%
Ham – 1 slice	40	2.3	21	53%
Meat loaf – frozen dinner	112.3	6.5	59	53%
Hot dog – 1 plain with the bun	242	14.5	131	54%
Chicken – light meat, no skin – 3 oz	147	3.8	34	23%
Turkey – dark meat, no skin	262	10	90	34%
Turkey – light meat, no skin	219	4.5	41	19%

(some figures rounded)

Now compare the calories and fat in real meats to the following imitation meats. These vegetable "meats" can taste surprisingly like the real thing, and are also high in protein.

How Much Fat Is in Common Meat Substitutes?

Meat (made from vegetable sources)	Total Calories	Grams of Fat	Calories of Fat (grams x 9)	% Fat (calories of fat divided by total calories)
Green Giant Harvest Burger	140	4	36	26%
Fantastic Foods Nature's Burger	120	2	18	15%
Morningstar Farms Better'n Burgers	70	0	0	0%
Light Life Smart Dogs	45	0	0	0%

A Few High-Fat Vegetables

Most vegetables are very low-fat. Exceptions are olives at 96% fat and avocados at 86%. Remember when you eat out that coconut is 61% fat, and coconut cream is 93% fat. Nuts have healthy oils and are good to pack for long hikes. But don't overdo. Most nuts are between 60 and 95% fat, and seeds like tahini are 60 to 75% fat. Exceptions are gingko nuts (13%) and chestnuts (8%).

Simple Tips to Cut Back Fats

- Try oatmeal or other grains like millet or amaranth for breakfast instead of croissants or Danish, and trade the Big Mac for a plate of lentils and broccoli for lunch or dinner. In one day you can drop from 60% fat to around 15% for the two meals combined. Don't junk up the oatmeal with sugar and butter. For flavor, try a few almonds, sunflower seeds, blueberries, strawberries, or other berries, and spices like cinnamon, nutmeg, or vanilla.

- High-fat foods, like peanut butter and cake frosting, licked off knives and spoons and tasted from someone else's plate count. Remember them when figuring your totals.

- Cutting out the two tablespoons of thousand island dressing in the sample lunch listed at the beginning of this chapter drops a 27% fat meal to 9%. If you can't do without dressing, use less—one tablespoon instead of the two or four (or more) you use now, or try low- or nonfat substitutes, or seasonings and lemon instead of dressing.

- Many types of meat are usually far above the American Heart Association's recommended fat maximum. Cutting back (and out) on these will greatly reduce your daily fat intake and reduce many other problems with meat-eating.

- List your favorite foods. Find out how much fat is in each. See how many of the foods you like are low-fat. Eat those.

- If you starve yourself, you will not be happy or healthy. Eventually, you will probably rebound into the gooiest, fattiest foods you can find. Have healthy snacks when you are hungry. Then walk away.

- When making omelets, leave out most (or all) of the egg yolks. Or use imitation egg whites.

- Avoid high-sugar, high-calorie items that advertise as low-fat. The sugar calories will creep up on you.

- Grains are usually good bets, as are most vegetable dishes, but that depends on how much oil, cream, and butter you add. Use whole wheat pasta and brown rice. Add spinach, broccoli, lentils, barley, and onions or leeks and chives to the tomato sauce.

- Don't panic if you eat one high-fat food. What counts is your long-term, day in-day out consumption.

- Try more fruit and less pie for your sweet tooth. Make your own desserts and don't add sugar, butter, or oil. You don't need them. Dessert will still be delicious.

- Even if no one sees you eat high-fat food, it still counts.

- Fun, good-tasting ways to substitute good food habits for unhealthy ones are in Chapter 19, "How to Lose Weight Without Dieting."

Resources for Keeping Track of Food Fat

Low-fat Diary by Corinne T. Netzer, Dell Publishing. It costs around $6.95 and has daily pages for recording meals and an index with a good list of fat grams in common foods.

Vegetarian Recipe Archive (www.fatfree.com). This archive has 4,667 fat-free and very low-fat vegetarian recipes, plus information about healthy, very low-fat vegetarian diets. Enjoyable for non-vegetarians too.

16

Sport Drinks

Life is thirst.

– Leonard Michaels

Dehydration is a common, but rarely recognized, factor in fatigue. Dehydration greatly reduces your capacity for exercise and your tolerance to heat. Many sport drinks on the market claim to prevent dehydration better than plain water. Is that so? Sport drinks also state they replace electrolytes. What are electrolytes and why and when do you need to replace them? What do these drinks really do?

What Are Sport Drinks?

You lose water and salts in normal processes all day. You also use up carbohydrates for energy. You need to replace what you lose. The first drink to bring all the needed ingredients together in one package was developed at the University of Florida, and named Gatorade® for their Gator mascot. The drink was originally used to replace fluids and carbohydrate energy during long exercise bouts in the heat. Now a variety of sport drinks in many different formulas are available for a variety of uses.

What Do Sport Drinks Do That Plain Water Doesn't?

Studies of exercise in the heat show that people prefer the taste of a salty drink, so they drink more. The bit of salt in these drinks stimulates thirst, then makes you retain the water you drink. The sugar content in sport drinks allows more water absorption through the intestine than from a solution of only salts. In other words, the sugar aids water absorption, helping replace needed water into your bloodstream. The sugar also supplies calories for exercise. Specially formulated "replacement drinks" have high carbohydrate amounts specifically for the purpose of restoring carbohydrates after exercise. The specifics on "carbo-loader" and "carbo-replacements" drinks are explained in Chapter 17, "Ergogenic Aids."

What Sport Drinks Do

- Increase palatability, compared to plain water, so you drink more.

- Replace needed water, then help absorb and retain water.

- Stimulate your thirst mechanism to keep you drinking.

- Provide carbohydrate during long exercise bouts to delay fatigue.

- Replace carbohydrate after exercise.

You Get Thirsty Two Ways

One way you get thirsty is when you are low on water, called hypovolemic thirst. If you replace only water, your body sees that you have more fluid relative to electrolytes, because you have also lost electrolytes. Your body helpfully responds by "peeing" out some water to balance things out. You may still be a bit low on water because of this, even after drinking water.

The second way you get thirsty is when you have a high electrolyte blood content, regardless of your body's total water volume. This is called osmotic thirst. That is why salty things make you thirsty, even when you are drinking (and why bars serve you salty finger food—to keep you drinking). Small amounts of sodium in electrolyte drinks stimulate your osmotic thirst, then help you retain what you drink. That is why people drink more of these beverages than plain water.

What Is an Electrolyte Anyway?

An electrolyte is a substance that, when you dissolve it in liquid, becomes electrically conductive. Why does your body need an electric current? To transmit every signal for all the thousands of functions that nerves control to keep you alive, moving, and thinking, and to maintain an electrical potential across the membrane of every cell in your body, so that the cells can do their jobs.

No current flows through pure water. Dissolving even a trace of electrolytes in water makes water conductive. Electrolytes that are put into a liquid break up into ions. Ions are atoms or molecules with at least one electron fewer or more than normal, giving them a positive or negative electric charge. Table salt, for example, becomes the positively charged sodium ion, and the negatively charged chloride ion. Both are principle ions in your body. In physiology, the ions themselves are called electrolytes. Salt itself is not an electrolyte, but in liquid it becomes the ions that are electrolytes.

> Flashlights run on current passed by electrons through wire.
> Your body runs on current passed by ions through nerves.

The difference between current in electronic equipment and in your body is that electronic signals race through wire, passed by electrons, at up to half the speed of light, while in your body, nerve signals move through ions, thousands of times more slowly. Current in electronics uses electrons to pass the charge. The electrons themselves don't move far, but pass the charge along from one electron to the next like toppling dominos. In your body, nerve signals move along dissolved ions. Like electrons, the ions themselves don't move far in the nerve, but propagate the signal by positive and negative ions switching places on either side of the nerve membrane. That makes neighboring positive and negative ions want to switch places too, in a continuing action called the action potential, until the signal is passed along the nerve. Then the nerve ending uses a transmitter chemical to jump to the next nerve to start the signal traveling again, until the message is delivered.

Why Replace Electrolytes?

Losing some electrolytes through sweat is a good thing, to an extent. If you lost only water, your blood would get far too concentrated with electrolytes. Even though you lose electrolytes, your body regulates the loss so you don't lose too much. So, when you sweat, you lose proportionately more water than minerals, leaving your blood slightly more concentrated than normal, or hypertonic. Even though your body does not want to be more concentrated with electrolytes, that does not mean you should avoid drinks containing electrolytes. You can lose a substantial amount of electrolytes with prolonged sweating, creating a real need for replacement. Without replacement, your electrolyte and fluid levels fall too low, and your ability to exercise decreases.

With extreme electrolyte loss during long exercise, and only water to drink, you may abnormally dilute your body fluids and cells, a condition called water intoxication. Effects range from weakness to convulsion and occasionally death. Water intoxication is also called hyponatremia (high-poe-nay-TREE'-me-uh), meaning low sodium in the blood. Cases are usually reported in hikers and distance runners who drink only large amounts of water and eat no food. Occasionally, serious cases of hyponatremia occur in infants swallowing pool water during parent-infant swimming lessons.

Your Body Regulates Electrolytes

You eat varying amounts of electrolytes in your food and drink, and lose varying amounts with exercise and daily activity. Your body ordinarily keeps levels of everything within narrow ranges, no matter how much you vary input and output.

Your body restricts electrolyte loss when your supply is low, and gets rid of excess when you eat or drink too much. When you are inactive, the major exit avenue for surplus electrolytes is urine and feces. When you are active and start sweating more, your body restricts the amount of electrolytes that exit with sweat, and secretes a hormone called aldosterone (al-DOHS'-tur-own) into your bloodstream to help your kidneys retain more sodium.

Most people in Western society eat many times more salt than their bodies require, sometimes in astounding quantities in fast foods, and that's before they even pick up the salt shaker. When you eat more salt than you need, your body retains water to dilute the salt, and aldosterone secretion drops, encouraging your kidneys to excrete the excess.

Some "salt-sensitive" people with high blood pressure need to restrict salt to allow them to lose the extra water that salt retains. For the rest of the population, salt seems to not matter much. Your kidneys tightly regulate your output to get rid of excess electrolytes and water, or hang on to them, depending on what you need at the time.

> Many people worry about limiting salt intake.
> A small portion of the population is "salt-sensitive," and needs to restrict salt. For most other people, however, the body takes care of eliminating excess.

When Should You Replace Electrolytes?

Except for extreme endurance activities, you usually eat and drink more than enough electrolytes with your regular meals to keep you going. Ordinary recreational exercise does not deplete electrolytes enough to affect athletic ability or health. For that reason, after a one-hour bout of exercise, you don't ordinarily need to replace electrolytes immediately. It is also unnecessary to take extra electrolytes ahead of time to offset any loss predicted during your short bout of exercise. You don't lose enough to affect performance or cause fatigue. Unless you are in endurance races, or work long hours in hot environments with limited chance to eat and drink fluids other than water, health problems from electrolyte loss are unlikely.

Do You Need Sport Drinks?

- If you do endurance events lasting more than an hour or so, like marathons and triathlons.

- If you exercise in the heat for long periods.

- If you like to drink semi-sweet beverages more than you like to drink water.

Why You Get Dehydrated From Drinking Seawater

Sea-going birds, such as penguins, seagulls, petrels, and albatross, can drink seawater. Special glands in their heads excrete excess salt. Humans have no salt-excreting glands, yet you have to get rid of the extra salt in seawater because the amount is just too much for your system. Your blood is not similar in composition to seawater (contrary to popular belief). Your blood is several times more dilute. If your blood were like seawater, you could safely drink seawater, which is not the case. In the process of excreting the excess salt in salt water, the human kidney draws water from the body's supply, a process so dehydrating that if seawater were the only fluid replacement available, you could die of thirst faster by drinking seawater than if you didn't. Human inability to drink seawater for fluid replacement is reflected in Samuel Taylor Coleridge's Rime of the Ancient Mariner—"Water, water everywhere, nor any drop to drink."

Preventing Dehydration

Your health benefits by good hydration. Bring plenty to drink on trips and hikes. Drink water throughout your day. What you choose to drink is a matter of personal taste. Try different drinks to determine which works best for you. Everyone's system differs in what it tolerates. Drink before you're thirsty.

Sport drinks are quick and simple fluid, electrolyte, and carbohydrate replacement, and live up to claims for endurance events where you can't stop to eat or drink. For the general exerciser, they are not a magic energy food, but a good and easy way to keep hydrated.

17

Ergogenic Aids—
Does Physical Enhancement
Await on Your Plate?

Fillet of a fenny snake,
In the cauldron boil and bake;
Eye of newt and toe of frog,
Wool of bat and tongue of dog,
Adder's fork and blind-worm's sting,
Lizard's leg and owlet's wing,
For a charm of powerful trouble,
Like a hell-broth boil and bubble.

– Second Witch: Macbeth, Act IV, Scene I

A miracle drug is any drug that will do what the label says it will do.

– Eric Hodgins

The search for a personal edge that you can eat is a common one. Hundreds of years ago, Aztec warriors ate the hearts of fearless enemies, believing it would increase their own bravery. To prepare for battle, the Inca Indians chewed coca leaves, and Berserkers ate mushrooms containing muscarine. Norsemen drank the milk of Arctic reindeer in heat. In the Middle Ages, Dervishes whirled longer using coffee. Sigmund Freud used cocaine. Today, South American Indians know chewing coca leaves reduces hunger and fatigue. In the Middle East, khat leaves are chewed for similar effect; while in Asia and the South Pacific Islands, it's betel nuts; and in the Sudan, the kola nut. Some people take diet pills, eat protein supplements, use steroids, drink coffee, or try preparations with labels promising everything from muscle growth to energetic hair.

What Is an Ergogenic Aid?

Products that help physical performance are called ergogenic aids. An *erg* is a unit of work. The word "energy" contains the erg root and means the ability to do work. The suffix *gen* means "producing" or "generating." Putting them together forms the word "ergogenic" and refers to things used and, not incidentally, believed to enhance physical performance. Not everything claiming to be ergogenic is really ergogenic.

Some ergogenic aids are psychological, such as mental rehearsal, confidence training, and good-luck charms. Some are physical, such as swimming and lifting weights. (Don't forget that to get better physically, you can also work for it with exercise, not just by eating something.) Nutritional ergogenic aids include an assortment of drugs, supplements, and food concoctions. The variety is ingenious, from broccoli pills to carbohydrate injections directly into muscle. Some are hokum—many products on the market claiming to be ergogenic have no ergogenic properties at all. Others work well enough to be banned by athletic associations and Olympic committees. A specific few present health hazards.

Why Do People Use Ergogenic Aids?

Would you pay to eat a product called "This Won't Work," or would you favor "Beautiful-Body-For-Certain"? Many people buy products sold through clever advertising and false hope. Product names are not required by law to do what they claim, allowing ads to combine suggestive words like *power, energy, natural, super,* and *mega* on their labels. Who could think a vitamin named Ener-B didn't have anything to do with feeling energetic? Ads targeting the serious bodybuilder market suggest anabolic steroid capability with names incorporating word segments like *ana, testo,* and *bolic.* Product promotions may include quotes from flawed studies in obscure or faux journals. The Food and Drug Administration (FDA) does not currently require testing these products for proof of efficacy. An athlete may work and slave, eat low fat, train diligently, but then attribute all gains to a capsule or pill, and go on to promote the product through testimonials.

People might use products instead of making healthy lifestyle changes. They could have energy, weight loss, and increased physical abilities by exercising more, eating better, and stopping smoking, but instead, hope a pill will do it for them.

Many stimulant preparations are sold as "natural" and "herbal." That does not mean they are harmless or nonaddictive. Cocaine and nicotine, for example, are naturally occurring plant substances. Many people buy stimulants thinking there will be no problems with them because they are labeled "natural."

"Natural" and "herbal" do not mean
harmless or nonaddictive.

Another reason people use certain substances is that some of the potions work to various degrees. Some stimulants boost speed and endurance by increasing muscle contractility and/or energy use. Cardiac relaxants can improve aim in target shooting. Other substances increase muscle mass for strength and speed contests, increase endurance for long events, or just give an edge in the gym. Still others not only work, but are addictive, like caffeine.

Stimulants

Stimulant drugs exert their effects directly on your nervous system. People use them because they inhibit fatigue and appetite. Overstimulation and addiction are common, resulting in various effects that are not healthy. Interestingly, products all over the health food stores have all kinds of stimulant compounds.

Coffee. "Black as hell, strong as death, sweet as love," according to a Turkish proverb. Few who drink tea, coffee, hot chocolate, or cola drinks consider themselves drug users. These drinks all contain caffeine, the most commonly used stimulant drug in the world. Other people shun caffeine, and instead take "natural" stimulant herbs (discussed later). Caffeine is no less "natural" than any health food herb.

Caffeine was probably discovered in the Stone Age, and has been widely used ever since. Caffeine can extend endurance, and is banned in high concentrations by the International Olympic Committee for that reason. A big rage for caffeine as an ergogenic aid may have begun in 1978 when exercise physiologist David Costil, Ph.D., told *Runner's World* magazine that caffeine could improve marathon times. According to Professor of Medicine Randy Eichner, M.D., "This led to long coffee lines at big marathons, followed by long potty lines."

How caffeine helps is still studied and debated. Caffeine is thought to help endurance by directly stimulating your central nervous system, decreasing your perception of effort, helping your body save some fuel called glycogen, and, possibly, improving your use of fat as fuel. More recently, caffeine is thought to help short-term activity (so short that your body has no time to use either glycogen or fat) possibly by increasing recruitment of more of your muscle fibers and/or directly increasing their resistance to fatigue.

Some people react strongly to caffeine; others don't. That may be genetically based, and may change throughout your lifetime. It depends, of course, on dose, as well as metabolism, prior diet, fitness, and other interactions. For most people, nervousness, increased urine production, and heartbeat irregularities begin in the two- to three-cup range, with increasing tendency to irregular heart rhythms from caffeine as you get older. Side effects increase with dosage. Many preparations claiming energy effects from herbs contain caffeine or caffeine-like substances, so carefully read labels of any product claiming energy boosts.

If you don't already drink coffee or other caffeine drinks, there are no grounds to start just for an endurance boost. If you are a regular drinker, you may find the withdrawal symptoms of headache and weariness are not worth the effort to give it up for a day or week. Try to keep your use low to moderate; cut back if you comfortably can, and drink extra water to help offset the diuretic effect.

Sympathomimetic Stimulants. Part of your nervous system increases heart rate and constricts blood vessels, getting you "ready to go." That part of your nervous system is called the sympathetic nervous system. Substances with properties that mimic your sympathetic nervous system are called sympathomimetic (sim-path-oh-my-MET'-ik). Three examples are amphetamines, cocaine, and ma huang. (Caffeine and nicotine are not sympathomimetic. Not everything that is a central nervous system stimulant is sympathomimetic.)

Amphetamines. More potent than coffee, amphetamines became popular as "pep pills" and diet pills because they mask tiredness and hunger. Amphetamines were given to soldiers during World War II to delay fatigue, and were widely used in medical practice until recently, when their dangers became widely known.

Amphetamine users may get abnormally high or irregular heart rates, raised blood pressure, and, sometimes, mental states resembling paranoid schizophrenia. Abdominal cramps, incoordination, dizziness, dry mouth, nausea, and vomiting may also go along with initial use. Some people experience unusual effects on their blood cells. Amphetamines constrict the arterioles of the skin (small, end branches of skin arteries), increasing risk of overheating. Deaths in endurance competitions in the heat have been connected to amphetamine use. Amphetamines usually addict their user physically and psychologically after about 12 weeks. Abusers can gradually increase their doses from 10 to 1,000 times to retain the initial effects they liked so much.

For weight control, diet pills are ineffective. They undermine sound nutrition and allow the user to ignore the requirement of exercise in fat reduction. Both the older amphetamine types and the newer diet pills require extreme caution and the care of a qualified physician. Moreover, after two to three weeks, diet pills begin losing effectiveness. Justifiable medical uses of amphetamines are treatment of narcolepsy and (arguably) attention deficit disorder in children. Packaged amphetamines come with a warning about decreased ability to do hazardous tasks like driving or operating machinery.

What's a good substitute for amphetamine drugs? Exercise. Exercise increases feelings of energy and offsets food calories for weight control.

Cocaine. Cocaine enhances physical performance, with an unhealthy price. Cocaine is sympathomimetic. Here's how it works: Your nerve endings release nerve transmission chemicals called catecholamines across a space, called a synapse, to the next nerve ending. After they have done their job to transmit their signal, you have to get the catecholamine back out of the synapse so it doesn't keep signaling and signaling. There are several normal mechanisms for that, including gathering the catecholamine back up into storage areas in the nerve endings, ready for more signaling at another time. Cocaine blocks this re-uptake, prolonging the effects of released catecholamines. That's why you get so much signaling with cocaine. Lots of it. Signaling in some areas of your brain feels good.

As with other central nervous system stimulants, the extra signaling increases heart rate and muscle contraction, allowing more physical work, and making you feel "geared up" to do that work. Signaling to your heart and blood vessels, from the catecholamine called norepinephrine, raises blood pressure and increases abnormal heartbeats. Too much of this can cause a sudden, sometimes fatal, heart attack. Surviving that, the problem with not taking up your catecholamines again for reuse means that you can run out. Running out of your catecholamine stores leads to severe depression (the cocaine crash).

> Many health foods and herbal remedies sold as "pick-me-ups," athletic enhancers, and weight-loss aids contain various central nervous system stimulants.

Ma Huang. Ma huang is an herb that has direct nervous system effects. Many potions sold over the counter claiming energy and weight loss contain ma huang: *HydroxyCut, Yellow Jackets, Xenadrine, Optidrene, Energel, Diet Pep,* and *Up Your Gas.* Some have Asian-sounding names to somehow lend authenticity, like *Chi Power* and *Jade Energy.* The products contain one or more of the several forms of ephedrine, a stimulant compound that comes from the ephedra plant.

Ma huang is sympathomimetic — it mimics activation of your sympathetic nervous system, mostly by urging your nervous system to release the chemicals noradrenaline and adrenaline from your nerve endings. One effect is to open airways and decrease secretions, so ephedrine is used in allergy and asthma medications. In doses common in over-the-counter "health" and diet products, ma huang affects your body like an amphetamine (to a smaller degree). It can have serious side effects of raised heart rate and blood pressure, erratic heart rhythms, and chest pain, plus any of several nervous system effects like insomnia, tremors, anxiety, or seizures, depending on dose.

An advisory panel of experts convened by the U.S. Food and Drug Administration in 1996 reviewed reports of more than 600 health problems thought to be associated with ephedrine since 1993, including 17 deaths from overstimulation of the heart. The panel generally concluded that the amount of ma huang in products should be far smaller. Investigators from New England Medical Center in Boston looked at 926 reports of problems associated with ephedrine. There were 14 sudden deaths, 13 strokes, two mini-strokes, nine heart attacks, and six cases of rapid heartbeats. Thirty-eight of the people had no history of heart trouble.

Many people take ma huang thinking it is somehow safer or more natural than caffeine, but caffeine is as naturally occurring as ma huang, as is the nicotine in tobacco. All have negative side effects in large doses. Ma huang is advertised as "used medicinally in China for over 5,000 years." That doesn't mean it is healthy or safe. Opium was used medicinally too. If you think you need stimulant drugs, look at your health habits and determine why you can't function without them. For weight loss or to increase energy, it is safer and quicker to just go out and exercise.

Theobromine. Chocolate, gotukola nut, and several other foodstuffs available in health food stores contain theobromine, among other substances. Theobromine stimulates the nervous system and increases heart rate, similar to caffeine, but less intensely. Theobromine is used in certain medicines and advertised in "health food" items promising "pep" for that reason.

Ginseng. Herbal energy potions claiming that they are caffeine-free does not necessarily mean they are free of side effects or are healthy for you. Ginseng is an example. Because of ginseng's stimulant effects, it is popularly used for a variety of health problems and for a general "pick-me-up." Ginseng is used in pills, teas, sodas, and all kinds of candies and drinks. Ginseng can affect glucose metabolism, and raise heart rate and blood pressure. If you overmedicate yourself with ginseng, you can wind up with diarrhea, nervousness, skin rashes, and insomnia. Most symptoms will disappear when use is reduced or discontinued. This doesn't mean ginseng is bad; just that it is not harmless. It has effects. That's why people take it.

Most of the biological effects of ginseng come from ginsenosides. Investigations have found that content varies greatly, with some ginseng preparations containing no ginsenosides at all. There is no law requiring uniformity, or even labeling to identify content.

As with other stimulant use, take a look at your health habits to find out why you want stimulants. Taking them can produce a vicious cycle of dependence and fatigue without them, and a cycle of being too stimulated to sleep well at night, creating daytime fatigue. Poor eating habits, too much simple sugar, not enough exercise, and too much time spent indoors contribute to general malaise. Don't use stimulants to combat poor habits. Use healthy ways to give you energy. Herb stimulants are drugs the same as any other potions and pills.

Steroids and Steroid Substitutes

Anabolic Steroids. The word "anabolic" means promoting tissue growth. Not all steroids are anabolic. The anti-inflammatories cortisone and prednisone are steroids and are not anabolic. They do not stimulate growth. Neither does Vitamin D, another steroid that is not an anabolic steroid.

Anabolic steroids are drugs that have anabolic and masculinizing or androgenic effects. Large muscle mass gains from oral and/or injectable forms don't routinely occur without intense strength training. Adverse physical and emotional side effects of anabolic steroids are common. Most are incompatible with physical and emotional health—high blood pressure, elevated "bad" cholesterol (LDL), liver and kidney damage, greater risk of heart and vascular disease, volatile aggressive "roid" rages, and reckless uncontrolled behaviors.

Growth Hormone. Growth hormone, abbreviated "GH," has recently begun replacing steroids in popularity, probably because it is currently undetectable in drug tests. The American College of Sports Medicine (ACSM) strongly advises against GH for athletic enhancement because of ethical and physical problems.

GH in adults may irreversibly increase growth of the jaw, forehead, hands, and feet, even in cases where it does not increase strength. It may also increase risk of diabetes, high blood pressure, and heart problems.

Compounds supposedly having GH-releasing potential sell briskly in health food stores and gyms. Ornithine and sapogenin are two growth hormone hopefuls that fall short. Ornithine is often packaged in 250 milligram (mg) capsules, although the effective dose is far higher. Sapogens are derived from plants found in desert regions. Your body will excrete them without making any GH. If you want results similar to taking growth hormone, but in a natural, safe, and inexpensive manner without side effects, vigorous exercise does exactly that.

Anabolic Activators, Multipacs, and Enhancers. These are usually packs of food elements, labeled with the suggestive name "anabolic." They have no magical muscle-building abilities, and contain nothing that is not available in regular food. They are not steroid substitutes, except by name, and there is currently no law to prevent anyone from selling you potions called steroid substitutes, even if they have no anabolic steroid effect. The name "steroid substitute" means only that advertisers would like you to buy their products instead of steroids, not necessarily that the product works like steroids do. The use of the word "anabolic" could technically mean that, since some of these supplements have so many calories, they do promote tissue growth—of fat—the same way any other high-calorie food does. It's just snappy advertising.

Food Supplements

Protein. The most common belief about protein supplementation is that eating more protein will build bigger muscles. It won't. Consider this: Protein enters into thousands of body functions besides muscle assembly. Eating more protein will not automatically increase all those functions. Protein builds skin, enters into the reactions that create the pigment in your skin, and is a building block for the smooth muscle in your blood vessels. Extra protein doesn't grow you more skin, make you turn brown, or make your blood vessels more muscular.

> Protein has many functions in your body besides growing muscles. Eating more protein does not increase any of those functions in speed or amount. For example, protein is involved in pigmenting your skin, but eating more protein does not darken your skin.

Do You Need More Protein When Active? Studies find that for a brief time after beginning an exercise program, your body's protein balance falls, then restores to previous levels. Your need to increase protein (over the recommended minimum) may be brief and mild. Most people routinely eat more protein than the required recommended daily allowance (RDA). Because of all they already eat, any increased intake in meals or supplements is unnecessary.

> A high-protein meat dinner can keep you from sleeping well. Get grain and vegetable-based protein meals throughout the day, and most of your protein at breakfast and lunch.

You can't store protein the way you can store fat and, to a lesser extent, carbohydrate. Whenever you eat more protein than you need on any given day, most will convert to fat, and you will excrete the rest, a process requiring water. In high amounts, dietary protein contributes to dehydration.

For the average inactive person, the minimum RDA for protein is 0.8 grams for every kilogram of body weight. A kilogram is about 2.2 pounds, making your minimum requirement less than half a gram of protein for every pound you weigh. Protein requirement for a 180-pound (82 kilogram) person varies around 65 grams per day. That's only about 2 ounces. A 130-pounder (59 kilograms) meets minimum requirements with less than 50 grams.

An active athlete may need at least 1 gram per kilogram of body weight. Muscle magazines often state that you need a gram of protein or more per pound of body weight. This does not seem to be the case, and has not been shown to have any effect on muscle building. In fact, strength athletes usually need less protein than endurance athletes. It is the endurance athletes that need a bit more protein, as they burn more calories. Muscle requires little protein for growth. For active people, carbohydrate supplementation seems to be more important and contributes more to muscle building. See Chapter 14, "Nutrition Myths," for a closer look at protein.

> You need a certain amount of protein every day. You may need more than that amount when you are active. Since the average person already eats more protein than the minimum required, there is usually no need to supplement.

Carbohydrates. Carbohydrates give you energy for all your activities. They are so important that your body stores them, mostly in your muscles and liver in a form called glycogen. The larger your stores, the longer you can exercise before you fatigue, depending on your physical fitness.

There are many energy bars, mixes, and drinks formulated to give you carbohydrates. They are not magic potions; they are food. You can also build and increase your normal carbohydrate stores when you exercise regularly and eat regular meals of at least 60% carbohydrate.

Because athletes exercising at high intensities for long periods can delay fatigue and therefore work longer and harder with carbohydrates, including carbohydrate drinks, misunderstandings result. Taking carbohydrate drinks and preparations will not transform you into a better athlete. Your ability to do submaximal exercise like recreational running, swimming, biking, dancing, walking, skating, and so on, does not improve from any particular food or drink.

Carbohydrate Loader Drinks. Carbohydrate loader drinks are one of several kinds of sport drinks. Carbohydrate loader drinks have a higher carbohydrate content than regular electrolyte replacer drinks. Loader drinks have three main applications:

- During intense, long-duration exercise, they provide fuel to delay fatigue.

- For athletes who work out so much that they can't maintain their weight with regular meals and snacks, the drinks add calories.

- For people unable to eat a regular meal before physical activity because of time restraints or jittery stomach, the drinks become a temporary meal substitute or adjunct.

Carbohydrate loader drinks are not magic energy elixirs or stimulants. They won't give you a performance edge if taken before or during exercise much shorter than an hour or so, like an aerobics class, a half hour to hour of cycling, skiing, or basketball, or even a 6- to 10-kilometer jog. Athletes generally have enough of their own stored carbohydrate, called glycogen, to last about an hour to 90 minutes. Carbohydrate drinks are most effective to delay fatigue when carbohydrate concentration is between 6 and 8% and when exercise is tough stuff lasting over an hour. The commercial drink Bodyfuel 450®, for example, is 4.5% carbohydrate; Gatorade® is 6.0%; and Exceed® is 7.0%.

Carbohydrate Replacement Drinks. Carbohydrate replacement drinks are another kind of sport drink useful for replacing carbohydrates after exercise. They have a higher carbohydrate content than the loader drinks. Long, intense exercise depletes glycogen, an important fuel. Replacement drinks help restock your muscle and liver glycogen after hard activity. You need to replace glycogen as soon as possible after exercise. If you don't, your body can't make enough glycogen to replace the loss. Your muscle and liver reserves remain low even days later, limiting further exercise ability.

The first 30 minutes after hard exercise are crucial to the major restocking. Your muscles can restore more total carbohydrate if you begin to eat or drink carbohydrates within 30 minutes after hard exercise. The next two hours are the second important stage. You benefit by eating high-carbohydrate food as soon after exercise as you can. Unfortunately, many people get changed, pack away their gear, and return home before eating anything. By then, a critical maximum restock window has passed. For this reason, high-carbohydrate replacement drinks were developed for right after exercise. Eating your ordinary meals and drinking extra water would do just as well. Replacement drinks serve the market for those who prefer to drink rather than eat right after exercise, or who just want something pre-packaged and ready to swallow.

Sport drinks provide calories for the work of exercise. Don't go overboard with these, or the extra calories will not store as glycogen, but fat. The simple sugar is quick fuel for exercise. Drinking these when you are not exercising loads your system with simple sugar. You would do better with a snack of complex carbohydrate.

Carbo and/or Protein Drinks With "Buzz." Many packaged "health" and "sport" drinks contain stimulants of all kinds—ginseng, ma huang, and caffeine among them. These are advertised as "energy" drinks and "vitality" enhancers. Check the label. Remember that they are stimulants with associated health risks.

> If coffee and cigarettes were discovered today,
> they'd probably be in stores advertised as
> "wonder energy enhancers" and "natural" diet aids.

Creatine

Chapter 4 explains how you use a molecule called ATP to fuel short, hard activity. As quickly as you use ATP, you rebuild it for more activity using creatine phosphate that you store, mostly in your muscles. You can't store much, only enough for 8 to 10 seconds of intense activity, like a 100-meter dash. When you run low, you shift to another energy system at lower intensity. The hope of more creatine fueling intense short efforts is behind sales of creatine as a supplement.

Creatine monohydrate is a synthetic of the creatine phosphate you make in your body. Not everyone can absorb it, which may be why some people find results using it and others don't. Advice to eat lots of steak and pork, which contain creatine, doesn't work (for you or the pig). Once you cook meat, the creatine denatures (changes permanently), so you can't use it. Clogging your arteries with cholesterol won't help athletic ability either. You don't need to eat creatine directly because your body makes what you need from balanced meals, including vegetarian meals. One thing known to work well is to get in better shape. Good aerobic ability increases your ability to store the creatine you make and use it to rebuild your energy stores.

The USDA issued an advisory statement saying more is unknown than known about creatine side effects over the long term, and that there may be adverse effects on your kidneys and liver. Consult your physician before use.

Androstenedione (Andro)

"Andro" is another expensive "health-food store" supplement. You make it in your own body out of DHEA. People buy it because androstenedione breaks down to testosterone, a male hormone. But another hormone that andro makes is estrogen. There is more to body chemistry than "andro makes muscles because it makes testosterone." Also, your body is smart. If it has too much of a substance, it will try to get rid of the excess. That's why andro supplements can increase urinary levels. Not because there is more hormone in your body, but because your body is getting rid of the extra. Sometimes your body will stop producing its own testosterone if it intakes too much, making you more deficient than when you started. Sometimes andro supplements have other elements not on the label that can cause a positive drug test for banned substances.

Reports from gyms and andro manufacturers state that andro always greatly helps athletic ability. Carefully done studies in real labs don't always find that andro increases lean body mass, strength, or testosterone levels in healthy adult men. Some studies show increased strength, but only the same amount of strength as a control group who also exercised hard but didn't supplement with andro. Great changes into a muscular athlete don't happen from pills alone. Although andro is available over the counter, its use is banned by athletic bodies because of harmful side effects and ethical issues.

Vitamins

Many people regard vitamins as ergogenic aids. No scientific evidence supports vitamin supplementation as ergogenic. Unless you have a nutritional deficiency, increasing your intake will not improve your physical abilities. There are plenty of important roles for vitamins, but study after study demonstrates that ergogenics is not one of them.

Vitamins have no calories, so furnish no energy, by definition. Vitamins are often advertised as giving energy, even labeled with suggestive names like "Ener-B." Unless your fatigue relates to a deficiency, they will not make you energetic.

> Vitamin B12 has been called the least likely vitamin to affect sport performance and the most likely to be abused for nonexistent ergogenic effects.

Taking too many vitamins can be unhealthy. Some vitamins are fat-soluble. With repeated overdosing they can accumulate in your body to toxic levels. Other vitamins are water-soluble and you excrete them, but can still have side effects with long-term overdose.

Minerals

Like vitamins, minerals have no calories and no known ergogenic effects. Deficiencies may result in weaknesses, but taking amounts above your needs will not improve your physical fitness. Even so, many have been advertised with claims of ergogenic effects.

Boron is one of several minerals misrepresented as an ergogenic aid. A widely misquoted study found low dietary boron decreased testosterone in postmenopausal women. Levels rose when the deficiency was corrected. From that came many claims of boron as helpful to athletes to increase their testosterone levels, with "studies" seeming to back up those claims. Although problems stem from nutrient deficiency, there is no evidence that extra boron elevates testosterone. Large doses are toxic. Boron is an ultra-trace mineral. You need only tiny amounts and can get them from fruits, vegetables, nuts, and legumes.

Chromium (including chromium picolinate) and vanadium are also ultra-trace minerals in the diet. If a deficiency exists, the benefit of supplementation is to correct the deficiency. There's no good evidence that they otherwise alter your body composition, or enhance athletic ability to any extent that it matters to most exercisers.

Carnitine

The excitement over carnitine began when the Italian soccer team won a title while taking carnitine. Obviously, the team did many other things besides taking carnitine, like train at high levels. There was no real evidence to show the carnitine had anything to do with their season outcome, yet such advertising sells many bottles of carnitine.

Your body makes its own carnitine and distributes it to many of your body's cells. Primarily, it works to carry unoxidized fatty acids. There is a D form and an L form. Those initials just tell how the molecule rotates—to the right (dextro-, or D-rotatory) or left (levo-rotatory, or L form.) Eating too much of the D form of carnitine in supplements can make you lose the L form. In this case, supplementation can be harmful.

It's difficult to become deficient in carnitine through training. There's no good evidence that taking carnitine, in any of its forms, does much that can be considered helpful, but there is also not enough evidence to reject it completely. Some studies do show minor gains. For the small gains and big price tag, the average exerciser can get just as much gain through regular exercise.

Carbohydrate Injection

Korean speed skaters are reported to have been experimenting with glycogen injections directly into thigh muscle. The unanswered question for elite athletes is, "can it do any good?" The answer for regular exercisers is that it is completely unnecessary in any case.

Fluid Retention

Fluid retention has been examined as an ergogenic aid. The theory is that muscle leverage favorably changes as the muscle swells with extra water. You can increase your total body water in several ways—carbohydrate loading increases the water your muscles can hold, eating salt retains more water, and anabolic steroids swell you with water, before they have a chance to exert any androgenic effect.

But should you count on fluid retention to help you in sports or exercise? Most people don't drink enough water, which is a common, and hidden, cause of fatigue. Getting enough water is a good idea and can make you feel better by itself. As far as dosing on extra water, the effect would be small, if any. Your body will usually regulate things so that any excess is quickly eliminated.

Water

The most overlooked athletic ability aid is water. You need to replace body water before and after activity, and during long activities, particularly in the heat. Water is a good, inexpensive, and easy fluid replacer for exercise and daily activities. Try to drink eight glasses of water throughout the day, more when exercising in the heat. Drinking good, clean water is healthy and can help control your appetite. Drinking too much will not help you be healthier. Even too much water is not good.

What Will Give You an Advantage?

Overwhelming evidence points to regular good nutrition, good hydration, and regular exercise, not supplements, for athletic advantage. What can you do?

- Eat breakfast.

- Eat frequent, healthy meals. Don't starve yourself.

- Trade high-protein, high-fat, low-carbohydrate burgers for moderate-protein, low-fat, high-complex-carbohydrate meals whenever you can.

- Know the difference between simple sugars and complex carbohydrates. Eat complex carbohydrates for the vitamins, nutrients, and energy-giving fuel you need for activity.

- Get enough protein early in the day. Don't have a coffee and Danish for breakfast and a salad for lunch. Get protein from vegetables and grains all day. You'll sleep better without a high-protein dinner at night.

- Rest is a greatly ignored ergogenic aid. Get enough sleep and enjoy your life.

- Exercise for fun and health.

- Drink water, but not an ocean.

- Cut back (or out) on stimulants. Vicious cycles of dependence build. Stop unhealthy food, drink, and life habits that sap energy.

- Get outdoors in the sunshine (or the rain) every day. Wear sunscreen and sunglasses, take an umbrella, but go outside.

- Add up all the money you save on supplements.

- Be good to yourself—possibly the most neglected of personal enhancing devices.

18

Healthy Eating

A food is not necessarily essential just because your child hates it.

– Katherine Whitehorn

Eating nutrition-poor food is common. Sometimes, unhealthy foods are the only offerings at restaurants, movies, ball games, theme parks, and public events. Unhealthy eating is so easy to do, and so well-accepted as normal, that it often goes unnoticed as a major factor in fatigue, extra pounds, and some of the most common Western diseases, such as cardiovascular disease, diverticulitis, and diabetes. Many people turn to vitamins and health food products, hoping these will fix their low energy or poor health, without ever looking at the unhealthy daily eating habits behind their problem.

This chapter looks at a few common eating habits that lead to weight gain, fatigue, and health problems. It explains what to do to eat healthier, some myths of healthy and unhealthy eating, and how simple, good-tasting choices can improve your health.

Eating Backwards in Quantity

Eating backwards is a common bad nutrition habit. People often eat backwards in two main ways. The first is quantity.

Healthy eaters have larger breakfasts and lunches, and smaller dinners. People who eat backwards in quantity do the opposite—they eat little or nothing for breakfast, rush off to work, have little for lunch, take candy and coffee breaks during the day, then eat a large supper at night, and a snack or two later on. The results are often fatigue during and after work, candy cravings, crankiness, and extra pounds.

You may feel fatigued when you don't eat enough food at the beginning and middle of the day. You need carbohydrate energy to work, do physical activity, and get around enough to enjoy life. Although many people hope their bodies will burn fat if they cut back on breakfast, your body first turns to its protein stores, not fat, when dietary carbohydrate is low. Low-carbohydrate breakfasts and lunches often lead to snacks of candy. Sugary snacks are high-calorie, and may contribute to mood swings in those people susceptible to low-blood-sugar-induced crankiness. Large high-protein and high-fat meals at night add more calories, protein, and fat when you need less. After eating too much, too late, you don't sleep well, and have to get up to go to the bathroom.

Eating Backwards in Quality

The second main way people eat backwards concerns what they eat. Sometimes people have good-sized breakfasts, but filled with sugar and fat. They may stuff themselves on eggs, sausage, bacon, and pastry. Backwards meals are 40 to 50% fat, up to 30% and more protein, and full of simple sugar, but have little of an important nutrient—complex carbohydrate. Eating backwards in quality, as with quantity, often results in fatigue. You haven't supplied your body with enough complex carbohydrates for energy. Nutrition surveys find that many people eat backwards in quality. Healthy meals have most of the calories, about 65%, as complex carbohydrate, less than 25% fat, and the rest protein, depending on your body weight.

Typical Backwards Meals

A typical day of backwards meals begins with no breakfast, or a breakfast of coffee or tea, pastry or donuts, or eggs and sausage. Then a sugary snack at a midmorning coffee break because of low energy. Lunch may be a burger and fries—high fat and high protein, but low complex carbohydrate. Another late afternoon sugary/fatty donut, Danish, or cookie snack because you are starving for sugar; a fast-food snack full of fat and simple sugar; a large, meat-based, high-fat dinner with high-fat ice cream, cake, or pie for dessert; and often a sugary snack (or two) of cookies, or maybe potato chips, later that night to calm rebounding low blood sugar from earlier candy snacks.

Why Do People Eat Backwards?

Why do people eat backwards this way? A big reason, unfortunately, is the U.S. Department of Agriculture's old four food groups, two of which are the high-fat meat and dairy groups. There is good evidence that humans did not evolve eating high amounts of meat. Dairy is also a relatively late evolutionary addition to the adult diet. Modern Western diets often include meat and dairy every day, sometimes every meal. The human body is not designed to handle it all. Meat is not only protein, as often thought. Bacon, for example, can have around 80% of its calories from fat. Many meats are over 50% fat. (See Chapter 15, "Calculating Food Fat.")

On April 9, 1991, the Physician's Committee for Responsible Medicine released a statement that a diet based on the old four food groups will not ensure adequate nutrition, and promotes disease. This is not new information. A 1978 study showed that only 9 of 17 minimum daily required amounts of needed nutrients were met by meals based on the old four food groups. The 1977-78 Nationwide Food Consumption Survey stated, "Americans who eat diets based on the four food groups consume an excessive amount of fat."

Another reason for backwards eating habits is that many people remember when complex carbohydrates were called starches. They mistakenly regard complex carbohydrate as fattening food to avoid. They also confuse complex carbohydrates with simple sugars and eat sugar thinking it is energy food.

A third reason is that often the only food available at restaurants, office buildings, ballparks, picnics, and drive-throughs is nutritionally backwards packaged foods and popular fast foods, all high fat and simple sugar, and low complex carbohydrate.

Yet another reason is habit. The most popular snacks of packaged chips and lunch meats are backwards, but become habits at early ages. People eat these foods because they are part of their daily routines. People even spoon-feed cake and ice cream to babies in arms! Eating such seriously unhealthy foods will become seriously unhealthy habits throughout their lives. To rationalize it by saying that babies need some fun too would be like giving them cigarettes or street drugs. Automobile anti-freeze tastes sweet, too, but is still poison.

Food preparation can add fat to previously not-so-bad foods; for example, adding sour cream, butter, and cheese to a baked potato, and removing the skin. The skin is important for fiber, which helps keep blood sugar even and contains good nutrients. This turns a fairly healthy vegetable into a high-blood-sugar dish with lumps of fat.

> Eating candied yams, glazed vegetables, and buttered lima beans isn't "eating healthy vegetables"; it's eating a lot of fat and sugar—bad for your teeth, bad for your heart, and bad for the rest of your body in general.

Then there are honest mistakes. Food is often labeled as health food to make it sell when it is high fat, for example, granola bars.

Is It Natural?

Eating high fat is a common bad nutrition habit. It is easy to do and becomes natural. The taste perception of people accustomed to fat changes to the point where food that isn't fatty doesn't taste as good to them. People who switch from whole-fat milk to non- or low-fat milk say that the lower-fat product tastes watery at first. After an adjustment period, the same people tasting whole-fat milk again often protest that the high-fat item tastes too fatty, like drinking butter, which is not all that far from truth. Whole milk, though labeled 3% fat, is in truth close to 50% fat by calories. (See Chapter 15, "Calculating Food Fat.")

Children regularly fed high-fat and highly sugared foods develop the habit of eating them. When visiting anthropologists gave South American Indian children candy, the children spit it out as bad tasting. Although our bodies have an evolutionary survival tendency to prefer sugar and fat foods, foods as high in fat and sugar as we now eat didn't exist until recently. Many modern food preferences are just habit.

How to Make Bad Food Habits into Good Ones

Eating healthy should not be some hateful thing you do at certain meals because you have to, then discard the rest of the time to go back to your "real" foods. Like exercise, healthy eating can gradually become a good-tasting, normal way of life. Good eating habits are something that you can make a part of ordinary daily living.

Don't Eat Backwards. Healthy eaters have larger breakfasts and lunches, and smaller dinners. Healthy meals have most of the calories, about 60%, as complex carbohydrate; have less than 30% fat; and about 12 to 16% protein, depending on your body weight.

New Food Groups. The old four food groups have been replaced by a seven-group food pyramid. The large, solid, two-level base of the pyramid indicates foods to eat primarily and most often—grains, fruits, and vegetables. The smallest section is a sugar and fat group, to be eaten sparingly. The middle protein group includes dry beans and nuts. The new recommendations agree on vegetables as main dishes, with meat as side dishes if you eat meat, not the other way around. The new food pyramid isn't perfected yet, and has been criticized for including meat in the larger protein section of beans and having an entire equally sized section just for dairy. It is often argued that meat and dairy combined should be a smaller section than the others. But the pyramid recommendations for making vegetables, fruit, and grains solid main foods is an important concept for changing to healthy food habits.

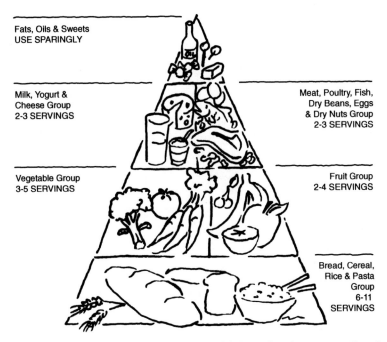

Fats, Oils & Sweets
USE SPARINGLY

Milk, Yogurt &
Cheese Group
2-3 SERVINGS

Meat, Poultry, Fish,
Dry Beans, Eggs
& Dry Nuts Group
2-3 SERVINGS

Vegetable Group
3-5 SERVINGS

Fruit Group
2-4 SERVINGS

Bread, Cereal,
Rice & Pasta
Group
6-11
SERVINGS

Figure 18.1. The food pyramid replaces the old four food groups. The food pyramid emphasizes that fat and sugar should be used only to a small extent, shown by putting it at the small end of the pyramid. Main meals of whole grains, oatmeal, vegetables, and fruits form the large, supporting base. Proteins come from legumes (foods like beans, lentils, and peas) and nuts.

Serving Sizes. Eating good food is one of life's great pleasures. Getting into shape and losing weight does not mean giving up that pleasure. It means learning a little portion control.

The food pyramid talks about "serving size," but what is that? In theory, it is one thing, but in practice, people eat far more than they think. A food label may say that snack crackers have 150 calories per serving, but that is only a few crackers. Eat the whole box and you eat over 1,000 calories. Too much of any food, however healthy, adds up. A few nuts are healthy. A one-pound can will be over 1,000 calories.

	Official USDA Serving	Typical Restaurant Serving
Ice cream	1/2 cup	1 cup+
Meat	3 oz	6–16 oz (and up)
Salad dressing	2 tbsp	4 tbsp
Slice of pizza	5 oz	9 oz+
Muffin	2 oz	4–6 oz
French fries	3 oz	6–8 oz+

Eat Breakfast. A healthy habit is to eat breakfasts with high complex carbohydrate, some fat, and moderate protein to fuel the day's work and exercise.

Eat Snacks. Animals like snakes and lions go long periods between meals. Humans seem to be natural snackers. Done right, snacking can help keep weight and food cravings down, and energy up. Frequent, low-volume eating is sometimes called grazing. The human body may have evolved to favor grazing between meals. If you graze on healthy foods, the body seems to adjust to more total calories without as much weight gain, compared to eating the same number of calories in one or two daily meals. Two important things happen, among many, when time interval increases between meals. In the short term, blood sugar goes down, signaling hunger. In the long term, your body learns that it must hold tightly to the fat it gets in order to survive. When meals are frequent, the body learns there will always be more coming down the tube. There is less survival-based need to hold on to each incoming calorie.

Try snacks like fruit, vegetables, whole grain breads, and air-popped popcorn for energy during the day. Make complex carbohydrates the majority of your calories, about 60%, in your regular meals.

Eat Before Activity. You need fuel to work hard enough to get a good workout. Some people can eat just about anything before exercising. Others can't stomach meals before activity, particularly not before strenuous activity. If you don't tolerate a regular meal before exercise, try small snacks of fruit or sport bars, liquid meals, and sport drinks. Experiment to find a balance that is right for you.

Eat Smaller Dinners. Food fuels your activities, so eat the bulk of your calories earlier in the day when you need energy to get things done. Large dinners often create trouble sleeping.

Choosing What to Eat

Protein. The amount of protein you need depends on your body weight. Most people in the Western nations get more protein than they need. The extra protein does not automatically convert into muscle, even with exercise. If you stop exercising, eating extra protein will not make you keep the muscles you have. Without exercise, your muscles will shrink in size. They don't turn into fat. The cells will still stay muscle cells, just smaller ones.

Grains and vegetables are important, healthy protein sources. You don't have to carefully mix them in every dish to get the right proportions of proteins, as once thought. Have a variety, often, as you should anyway, and everything will mix itself in your system. Make grains and vegetables your main dishes. You will have low-fat, high-fiber, healthy meals with plenty of protein. Choose from any combination of lentils, brown rice, barley, couscous, or bulgar wheat, for example. It takes about 30 minutes to cook. In the last five minutes, throw in a can of unsalted peas (or fresh peas), or any favorite vegetable, such as broccoli, spinach, mushrooms, or squash; add chopped raw carrots or apples to sweeten, or even a few raisins or chopped dried apricots. Add onion, scallions, chives, and/or leeks. Season with any variety of cloves, curries, lemon pepper, ginger, or whatever you like. Add sensible sprinkles of unsalted sunflower seeds, peanuts, or almonds. There are enough combinations in this one example alone for years of delicious low-fat vegetable dishes full of healthy "complete" protein. With any leftovers, you can make delicious sandwich fillings for lunch the next day. For example, mix with tomato sauce and spoon onto whole grain bread. Delicious. Cheaper, quicker, lower-calorie, and healthier than meat.

As a minimum, eat about 0.8 to 1.0 grams of protein for every kilogram you weigh. If you weigh 130 pounds (59 kg), get at least 47 grams of protein every day. If you weigh 150 pounds (68 kg), get at least 54 grams of protein. If you weigh 170 pounds (77 kg), get a minimum of 61 grams. If you weigh 200 pounds (90 kg), get 73 grams of protein. You can find the gram content of protein on the food labels. You don't need much more protein with heavy exercise, but you do need more carbohydrate to fuel that exercise. In fact, weightlifters need less protein than distance runners, for example, because the runners need more calories overall. Find out more about protein and protein myths in Chapter 14, "Nutrition Myths."

> Grains and vegetables are important, healthy protein sources. There is no need to carefully mix certain ones to get complete protein.
>
> There is a large variety of nutritious grains. They are quick to prepare, store easily in the cupboard in bulk, can be made delicious without adding butter or sauce, and are low cost compared to meat.

What is Texturized Vegetable Protein? Texturized Vegetable Protein (TVP) is defatted soy flour used as a meat replacement. It is very low in fat (3%), but check labels since commercial products sometimes add a lot of other fats to TVP foods. A 60-calorie portion has about 11 grams of protein.

TVP is not the same as HVP, hydrolyzed vegetable protein. HVP is a food additive, often with monosodium glutamate added (MSG).

What is Seitan? Seitan is an almost all-protein food made from wheat gluten. It has almost no fat.

Position of the American Dietetic Association:

Vegetarian Diets

A considerable body of scientific data suggests positive relationships between vegetarian diets and risk reduction for several chronic degenerative diseases and conditions, including obesity, coronary artery disease, hypertension, diabetes mellitus, and some types of cancer.

Position Statement

It is the position of the American Dietetic Association that vegetarian diets are healthful and nutritionally adequate when appropriately planned.

Fat. High-fat diets contribute to clogging up your blood vessels. In the short run, high blood fat generally impedes circulation. The American Heart Association calls for keeping dietary fat under 20 to 30% at most, with the majority of that as nonsaturated vegetable fat. Extremely low-fat diets, those of about 10% fat, have been found to not only stop advancing heart disease, but help reverse it.

What about cutting out fat entirely? Most natural foods have some fat. Even if you ate only beans, vegetables, grains, and fruits, with no oil or high-fat ingredients at all, you would get about six to 10% fat. Few people are this strict and most low-fat diets run about 10 to 20% fat. You'd have to eat only sugary junk foods to exclude all food fat, which wouldn't be healthy for several reasons.

A little fat is important to healthy eating. A small amount of fat helps absorb fat soluble vitamins like vitamin A, and supplies two essential fatty acids (EFAs): n-6 fatty acids and n-3 fatty acids (omega-3 fatty acids). Essential fatty acids seem to be good for your heart, nervous system, and joints. They are called "essential" because your body can't make them. You have to eat them.

Get n-6 acids (linolenic acid) from plant foods: oats, corn, leafy greens, wheat, flaxseeds, walnuts, soybeans, and other seeds and nuts. Omega-3 is found in most plant foods. Highest amounts are in green leafy vegetables, nuts, canola oil, soybean oil, and tofu. Don't eat bacon and cream and call it health food because you "need a little fat." How much fat is "a little"? Estimates vary from five to 15% of fat by calories as a minimum amount.

> Don't eat ice cream and cream sauce and call it "heath food"
> because you heard "you need a little fat in your diet."
> You need oil in your car, too, but too much and the wrong kind
> will kill your engine.

Complex Carbohydrates. They used to be called starches. It's a myth that starch, in itself, is fattening. Too many calories from any source is fattening, but complex carbohydrates are healthy eating and, like fiber, found only in plants. Make them around 60% or so of your calories. More before strenuous activities.

Eat more baked, boiled, and steamed sweet potatoes, brown rice, lentils, beans, soybeans, broccoli, whole grain bread, fruit, whole grain cereals, salads, and whole grains in general. Besides the complex carbohydrates that fuel your energy needs, many healthy vitamins and nutrients are only found in plant food.

What Are Phytochemicals? The word "phytochemicals" means "plant chemicals." They are simple compounds found only in plants that are increasingly studied as disease fighters. Find them in yellow-orange and dark green vegetables, such as broccoli, spinach, tomatoes, and carrots; fruits like apricots and cantaloupe, and nuts and seeds.

> People confuse carbohydrate (rich complex ones of whole
> grains) with simple sugar, so eat white bread thinking it is
> good, and shun grains as fattening.

Can Carbs Make You Fat? What about all the "carbo-bashing" starting with a *New York Times* article, "Eating Pasta Makes You Fat," and the wide media coverage that followed? The concern was that emphasizing carbohydrates would exacerbate "Syndrome X" in "insulin-resistant" people, an estimated 10 to 25% of Americans.

"Syndrome X" is a collection of risk factors for heart disease, including high blood pressure, low "good cholesterol," high triglycerides, and obesity. "Insulin resistance" is a topic with a lot of unknowns. It seems to involve a reduced number of insulin receptors. Body cells don't know how much insulin they already have had delivered. The pancreas secretes more and more insulin, not knowing when to stop. In theory, this insulin oversecretion causes the carbohydrates to be better stored as fat.

At the heart of the public's confusion were missing facts:

- Carbohydrate will store as fat only if you eat too much of it, the same as any other food.

- Even "insulin-resistant" people must eat excess carbohydrate calories before the carbohydrates are stored as fat.

- Losing excess weight and increasing physical activity are far more important in controlling insulin resistance than restricting carbohydrates.

- In most cases, insulin resistance seems to be caused by excess weight and inactivity, not the other way around.

What about the now-famous attack on pasta when fettuccine Alfredo was named "heart attack on a plate"? That was the high-fat, artery-clogging sauce. Obviously if you eat too much pasta you'll gain weight. Just like eating too much of anything.

What About Low-Carbohydrate Diets? Some weight loss diets claim that you gain more weight eating carbohydrate than fat or protein, and limiting carbohydrate will make you burn more fat. Neither seems to be the case. Several low-carbohydrate diets limit carbohydrates by lowering the carbohydrate percentage of your total intake, and raising the fat and/or protein percentage. All have the problem of being low in the one fuel your body needs to exercise well—carbohydrate. Without carbohydrate, you won't have energy to do the exercise to lose weight. For athletic or recreational events, you won't have the fuel you need for high performance.

> Remember that "carbohydrate" should mean the healthy, complex carbohydrates of vegetables, fruits, and whole grains, not the simple sugars of candy, cake, and fast foods. It's healthy to have a "low simple-sugar diet" but not a "low-carbohydrate" diet.

Low-carbohydrate and high-protein or high-fat diets create health problems. There is more to a diet than losing weight. If your long-term health is affected, the diet is not smart. Too much protein dehydrates you, is hard on your kidneys, and increases your risk of osteoporosis (see Chapter 14, "Nutrition Myths," and Chapter 22 on osteoporosis). Too much fat is well-known to promote many serious diseases. Many vitamins, minerals, anti-oxidants, and disease-fighting nutrients are found only in complex carbohydrates. Low-carbohydrate diets limit them and discourage healthy eating.

A healthy proportion of carbohydrates seems to be at least 60% for daily life and more for exercise. Keep most of this as complex carbohydrate, not sugar. Keep protein 12 to 15% or so, and fat under 20 to 25%, lower if you can. Claims of needing more fat or protein to put you into particular "zones" don't allow you enough carbohydrate to do enough exercise, and limit important nutrients from whole foods. Keep total calories to the amount you need for your healthy weight. More calories mean more weight, whether they come from fat, protein, or carbohydrate. See Chapter 14, "Nutrition Myths," for more.

White Processed Flour and White Rice. Most pastas, like many breads and other common foods, are made with refined white flour. The full-of-fiber and good-tasting hulls were removed in processing. Look for whole grains instead. Refined white flour lacks fiber and makes problems with your blood sugar. Learn about whole grains that are healthy and delicious.

Instead of white rice, there is brown rice and wild rice, of course, but try delicious, meaty lentils, and nutty barley, bulgar wheat (cracked wheat grains) and quinoa (keen-wah). Cook these in a little water or healthy soup stock. Add chopped green vegetables, onions, scallions, chives, leeks, and spices. You'll have a meaty casserole for a main dish. With many grains and greens, you can make dozens of interesting, healthy meals, different every day.

Whole Grain Alternatives. Instead of packaged cereal full of refined sugar and white flour, try quick oats, millet, quinoa or other good-tasting breakfast grains. Just cook in water (or soy milk) the way you do oatmeal. Spice with cinnamon, nutmeg, and fruit, not butter, milk, and sugar.

Instead of baking with refined white wheat flour, there is whole wheat flour, rye flour, spelt, teff, barley flour, soy flour, buckwheat, triticale, and quinoa flour, among many. Use whole grains instead of white flours. Try non-wheat flours. Not everyone feels well after eating wheat.

Don't miss flax seeds. Delicious, healthy, full of healthy oil and nutrients. Add them to your baking, casseroles, and morning hot cereal. Put them in your blender to mill them if you don't like the crunch. Use them as a butter substitute in baking. In health food stores, flax seeds and other things now recognized as healthy are usually expensive. Try a nut store or large supermarket where dry goods are sold in self-measuring bulk. Bring home a bag and experiment. You don't need to go to any specialty stores. Most large supermarkets now carry these items that are so common in many other parts of the world.

Eat chewy, healthful grains. Your gums and jaws need exercise to keep them strong and to support your teeth. Tooth loss is an early sign of thinning bones. Fluffy, refined white flour, soft white rice, and skinned vegetables are far from the healthy, fibrous foods that keep your entire body in shape.

Fiber. Fiber used to be called roughage. Fiber is the most complex of complex carbohydrates—so complex that your digestive system can't digest it. That's why fiber passes through your system, with healthy effects on your lower intestinal tract. Fiber is found only in plants, not in meat, poultry, fish, eggs, or dairy. Get lots of water-soluble fiber in oats, fruit, barley, and beans. Get insoluble fiber in vegetables and wheat. Keep the pulp in juice. The skins of many vegetables, like potatoes, are healthy and delicious when prepared well. Look for brown rice, whole wheat bread and pasta, and whole foods. Eat apple and potato skins too (after good washing). The fiber in whole grains, brown rice, and fruit with the pulp keeps your blood sugar even. Without it, previously healthy food becomes more of a sugar than a carbohydrate, and loses many important nutrients.

> White rice and white flour noodles are part of the "an hour later you're hungry again" phenomenon—stripped of fiber and complex carbohydrate to keep your blood sugar even. Look for brown rice and whole grains instead.

Simple Sugars. Don't confuse complex carbohydrates with refined sugars. Save sugar for occasional, not daily, use. You'll be surprised that you crave it less as you consume less. Eating simple refined sugar, so common in processed foods, can make you hungry. Eating more simple sugar feeds the vicious cycle.

Alcohol. Alcohol has no nutritional benefit, but lots of calories. When figuring how many calories you consume, remember that alcohol adds plenty. Each 12-ounce beer is about 150 calories (light beer closer to 100). A two-ounce margarita is about 150 calories. Half a cup of hot buttered rum has 250 calories. A glass of dessert wine can go up to 350 calories. Then there are the beer nuts, pretzels, fried chips, and other bar and party foods. A cocktail hour can run up an astounding number of forgotten calories. Alcohol is not metabolized as a carbohydrate, even though it is one. So it can't be rationalized as a "sports fuel." Remember, it's not a joke. Alcohol is a drug.

Handy Tips

If you are a beef-and-ale kind of eater, you don't want to be told to give that up and eat raw alfalfa. You won't do it anyway. The good news is you don't have to. Some simple, easy suggestions follow for making healthy eating a regular habit, not a hateful, poor-tasting thing you do because you're told you should. You don't have to choose between being happy and being healthy. Be both. Happiness is part of good health.

For new healthy eating habits, start with a few of the following suggestions. Then add others as you can and want.

- Eat breakfast.

- Tea and toast, or coffee and Danish for breakfast won't fuel you and can leave you irritable, low energy, and craving sugar hours later. Eat complex carbohydrates and protein for breakfast. Good examples are oatmeal, hot and cold grain cereals, and fresh fruit. Eat the skins of most foods, like apples and potatoes. The fiber makes them more nutritious and keeps blood sugar more even.

- Try eating larger meals in the morning and afternoon, and smaller meals in the evening. Most people eat backwards, eating little during the day and much at night. Large evening meals can disturb your sleep and make you have to get up to go to the bathroom. If you can't sleep through the night, try eating earlier and less at night.

- Keep healthy snacks, like fruit, small amounts of raisins and almonds mixed together, whole wheat breads, whole grains, whole wheat pastas, and others, handy.

- Learn about the new food pyramid.

- Avoid fad diets that omit major food categories. They are nutritionally unsound and don't work in the long run. You don't lose fat that way, but you will lose important nutrients, energy, water, muscle, bone, and other things you need.

- Try air-popped popcorn. Don't pour butter on it.

- Eat lightly before exercise—don't go hungry. Experiment to find foods and time schedules that agree with you if you have a tender tummy.

- Drink water with meals. Drink extra water when exercising, particularly in the heat. Don't overdo water so much that you float away.

- Have vegetables as main dishes and meat, if you eat meat, as side dishes, not the other way around. Combine different grains with vegetables for variety, nutrition, and great taste.

- Make your involvement with healthy eating a stress-free one. It makes no sense for your body and mind to be miserable in the name of health. Take a happy approach. Make sure your new program is one that suits you.

- Use seasonings rather than butter or sour cream dressings. Use nonstick sprays instead of thick layers of butter and oil in the pan.

- If you make your own juice, keep the fruit pulp in the juice, rather than throwing it out. In blender drinks, throw in apple slices (for example) with the skins (washed). The complex carbohydrates, vitamins, and fiber in the pulp and skin help keep blood sugar stable. Without the fruit pulp, juices are little more than flavored sugar water.

- Find healthy foods you love. Don't be miserable with your new plan to eat right. Find ways that make your stomach happy as well as your conscience.

- Good-tasting, healthier recipes are available for old favorite, but unhealthy, foods. Take a walk to the bookstore or library for a few fun books.

- Be good to yourself—possibly the most neglected healthy habit.

> Refined sugar and white flour lack nutrients and fiber and create problems with your blood sugar. Learn about whole grains that are healthy and delicious.

A Major Part of Healthy Living

Make healthy eating an enjoyable lifestyle, not just something to try for a day then stop because you've done it (and hate it). There's more to health and energy than eating right. It helps to surround yourself with favorable environmental factors, like exercise, clean water, clean air, good friends, good family, and happiness; and to avoid smoking, nonmedicinal drugs, perpetually stressful situations, and too much alcohol. Healthy eating is a major foundation of good health. Summing it up, that's nature, nurture, and nutrition. Or genes, means, and beans.

Resources for More Information

American Dietetic Association   (www.eatright.org)
216 W. Jackson Blvd.
Chicago, IL 60606-6995
(800) 877-1600

Physicians for Responsible Medicine   (www.pcrm.org)
P.O. Box 6322
Washington, DC 20015
(202) 686-2210

19

How to Lose Weight Without Dieting

*Eat less than you think you want, eat with your intelligence, not your stomach.
Never get up from the table with an inward, silent apology for being a pig.*

— Coco Chanel

Never eat more than you can lift.

— Miss Piggy

Having a little extra body fat is helpful for warmth, cushioning, and buoyancy in the water. Losing extra weight can benefit your joints, cardiovascular system, general health, and well-being. Sometimes it is even crucial. But severe calorie restriction and fad diets can be unhealthy, and they rarely work to maintain weight loss on a long-term basis.

There is no need to choose between the problems of being too heavy and the misery of dieting. You can do many things to lose weight without starving yourself or eating foods you hate. Good exercise and nutrition habits can become an easy, fun part of your lifestyle with attention and repetition.

Don't go at it without a plan. Aimlessly trying "diets" or vowing to "lose weight" does not work. It's not enough to say, "I'll lose ten pounds by next month." You need definite goals, methods to carry them out, and a schedule. Most important, you first need to take a good, hard look at the way you eat now, and how much activity you get.

Cut Back Fats

Reducing fat in your diet can help you lose weight. Eating less saturated fat also may reduce your risk of heart disease and some cancers.

According to some studies, cutting back fat is a better way to lose weight than cutting only calories. Some of the reasoning for this idea is that your body uses fewer calories to digest fat than it does to digest carbohydrate. High-fat meals end up as fat on your body more readily than high-carbohydrate meals with the same number of calories. The human body is designed to store fat, and more easily stores it when provided directly. That doesn't mean you can eat high-calorie meals every day as long as they are low fat. The extra calories will just turn into fat in your body.

Many of your food choices may be high fat without you knowing it, like muffins and granola bars. Other foods that you know are high fat may be higher than you realized, like most meat, including bacon, which can be around 80% fat. Not eating meat is also far cheaper than eating meat.

Many foods may be full of fat, but because they also have so much sugar, the overall percentage of fat on the label seems low. Don't be fooled. Lots of fat is still lots of fat. See Chapter 15, "Calculating Food Fat," to find out just how much fat many popular foods have. Take a good, hard look at what you eat and where all the extra calories are coming from.

> A low-fat percentage on the food label doesn't always mean the item is low-fat. It may be full of fat, but have so many calories from sugar that the proportion is low by comparison.

Make Your Own

Many common prepared "convenience" foods are just not healthy. They also cost more than making your own healthy foods. Making your own doesn't have to take time—often it's quicker than stopping for "convenience" foods.

- For a quick breakfast, instead of sugared cereal and milk, throw quick oats in a bowl. Add some sunflower seeds, walnuts, almonds, or pumpkin seeds, and cinnamon. Pour in boiling water and stir. There are dozens of other healthy things to add, from soy milk, to apples and bananas, to other quick grains like millet.

- For quick complete meals in a glass, throw soy milk in a blender (or unsweetened pineapple juice, water, or other healthy drink), and add any combination of hundreds of healthy foods. Add quick oats (uncooked), raw nuts, apple slices (with the skin) or unsweetened applesauce, peeled orange slices, apricots, flax seeds (the blender will mill them), sesame seeds, pumpkin seeds, grapes, carrots, or blueberries. Other flavor possibilities are unsweetened vanilla bean or unsweetened chocolate. Make as thick or thin as you like. Drink and go.

- Replace commercial soda with your own. Add lime to a glass of carbonated water. "Pure, natural" apple and citrus juices are high in simple sugar calories. Dilute them by a half or third with soda water. This is common in Europe.

Substitute

Don't deny yourself food—substitute a lower-calorie for a higher-calorie food, and healthy food for junk. When you are about to eat foods full of sugar and fat, eat something better instead—grains, fruits, and vegetables. Complex carbohydrates used to be called starches and were avoided. Now we understand that eating sensible amounts of complex carbohydrates, rather than too much fat and simple sugar, is a key to healthier eating. Be creative and find things you like.

For Snacks

- Raisins and grapes instead of candy. Not too much of these though, they are sugary. Brush your teeth after eating raisins. The sugar sticks to your teeth.

- Bananas instead of banana cake.

- Whole grain rolls instead of donuts.

- Many brands of fruit-flavored yogurts contain fruit-jam, adding the equivalent of eight or nine teaspoons of sugar per cup. If you eat dairy, get plain yogurt and add your own fresh fruit.

- Try chili powder and other seasonings instead of butter on air-popped popcorn.

- Have dry-roasted and raw nuts instead of roasted, honey-roasted, or salted nuts. Remember not to sit watching television eating a can of honey-roasted nuts, which can total over 1,000 calories. Don't be lulled by dry-roasted and raw nuts; they are not low calorie either, just a healthier food than processed snack food.

- Drink juice with the pulp. Processed grape juice, for example, is a common sweetener put in factory foods to masquerade as "healthy." It is little more than sugar water.

- Instead of chips and dip at your next party, serve cut sweet peppers; grapes, strawberries, and other easy finger fruit; nuts (not honeyed); and cubed, baked sweet potato and zucchini. Use chopped hot pepper salsa and unsweetened applesauce for dip.

For Cooking

- Bake, boil, and steam instead of fry.

- Use nonstick spray instead of butter, margarine, or oil. Use a quick squirt, not a layer—it is still oil and adds up. If you don't like aerosols, put flax seed or olive oil in a misting bottle and make your own non-stick spray. Or dribble half a teaspoon of oil on a paper towel and wipe it on the pan.

- If you must use oil, use less, and choose unsaturated oils, like olive oil, instead of butter or lard.

- If you must have butter, use less and choose whipped butter—it has more air and a bit fewer calories. Or try "light" butter. But don't be fooled—it's still a lump of flavored fat. Try seasonings instead of butter.

- Steam sauté in soup stock instead of oil, roast in seasonings, or braise in balsamic vinegar.

- Use aromatic foods to flavor sauces instead of butter, cream, or cheese. Aromatic foods include tomatoes, onions, garlic, mushrooms, leeks, fresh parsley, thyme, and basil.

- Refrigerate soups and stocks to separate and congeal the fat, skim it off, and use the skimmed product instead.

- Use whole grains, not white flour pastas. Use brown and wild rice, not white rice. Learn about the surprising variety of other delicious grains out there.

For Meals

- Make yolkless omelets. A three-egg-white omelet, prepared with nonstick spray and seasonings, has less than 50 calories and no fat. A three-egg omelet has 225 calories and 15 grams of fat.

- Roasting vegetables caramelizes the natural sugar. Roast sweet peppers with onions, mushrooms, and green vegetables. Brush with vinegar marinade or tomato sauce. Season with any number of healthy seasonings.

- Instead of pouring oil on your salad, try balsamic vinegar, pureed cucumbers, seasonings, low-fat yogurt, even hot sauce. Seasoned Japanese rice wine vinegar has some sugar in it, but often tastes rich enough to seem like there is oil in it. Make a vinaigrette with healthy flax seed oil or grape seed oil.

- Instead of cream on your potato, try lemon pepper seasoning, soy sauce, hot pepper, horseradish, or wasabi. Prepare it so you can eat the skin, too.

- Have a healthy sandwich instead of a Danish.

- When you cook vegetables, don't use sugar, butter, cream, or sauce. Throw in onion, scallions, chives, shallots, nuts like sunflower seeds and almonds, and hot peppers; and season with ginger, tamari, garlic, or curry.

- Make brown rice with lentils, peanuts, barley, green beans, peas, onions, or leeks, and hot sauce. Cook rice in fresh peaches with ginger. Cook in unsweetened pineapple and curry. Try tofu and tamari sauce. It's different every time.

- You can put soft, cooked sweet potato in just about anything—your morning hot cereal, the morning blender drink, afternoon sandwiches, pies, baked goods, rice, or lentils; make it sweet with apples or spicy with onions. Don't go overboard, of course. Sweet potato still has calories. Don't add sugar glaze or butter.

- You'd be surprised how good onions cooked with a sweet vegetable can taste.

- You can do a lot with mangoes. They can sweeten up vegetables, both cooked and raw. Mix chili peppers and mango into a sweet and tangy sauce. It's easy and fast.

- Instead of dairy, substitute mashed tofu, which is high-protein, high-calcium, and has no cholesterol.

- Substitute grain and vegetable dinners for meat. With all the fruit, vegetables, and grains out there, you can eat a different meal every day; then combine different things and you'll never repeat.

For Baking

Many favorite recipes, particularly baked goods, use large amounts of fat to retain moisture during cooking. With substitutions, your baking can be sweet and moist without the fat, sugar, or eggs.

- Substitute unsweetened applesauce, pureed bananas, apples, or prunes for most—or even better, all—of the oil and sugar. Substitute 1:1 by volume.

- Use flax seeds milled in your blender instead of oil and eggs.

- Add a sweet potato instead of oil or sugar for creamy, moist, good taste.

For Desserts

- For sweet desserts, try fruit and frozen juice popsicles, instead of pie and ice cream.

- Strain plain yogurt to make a creamy, cream cheese substitute.

- Get applesauce without added sugar or syrup. It is plenty sweet. Add cinnamon or nutmeg. Use over oatmeal instead of sugar, and over fruit for dessert and snacks.

- Make baked apple with cinnamon instead of sugar or honey. It will be plenty sweet.

- You can buy nonfat sour cream, nonfat cheese, and nonfat ice cream as easily as high-fat brands. There are also plenty of non-dairy (and non-chemical) desserts.

- Substitute talking with your friends or stretching for eating dessert.

- Dessert does not have to be simple sugar, and fat, and bad for you. Something can be good for you and still be a treat.

If all else fails, and you are eating when you are not hungry, drink a large glass of water, then brush your teeth or use a strong mouthwash instead of snacking. The water will fill your stomach, and it's hard to eat with the fresh taste of mouthwash in your mouth. More ideas for healthy substitutes are in Chapter 18, "Healthy Eating."

Don't Go Hungry

Fasting and semi-starvation diets make your body hang on to its fat stores. They also make you hungry and unhappy. Starving yourself, then snitching candy, can make you moody and craving to eat everything you see, usually in the late afternoons, then again at night.

Don't skip meals. Eat a low-fat, complex carbohydrate breakfast and snacks in midmorning and late afternoon. Eat complex carbohydrates often to help maintain steady blood sugar levels. Don't just eat "low-fat" cakes, cookies, and sweets. They are full of simple sugar, which will make you hungry within a few hours—usually sooner. Get protein from grains and legumes like lentils.

Eat Less Simple Sugar

"Simple" or "refined" sugar is just about everywhere in prepared foods. The label may say "no sugar," but don't be fooled. They can be full of other refined "empty-calorie" sweeteners, like dextrose, high-fructose corn syrup, maltose, grape juice, rice syrup, galactose, and others.

Eat complex carbohydrates like fruit and grains for snacks instead of candy, and high-protein, high-complex-carbohydrate oatmeal instead of donuts and Danish for breakfast. When you eat less sugar, a magic thing happens—you crave less. Keep a list if you have to, to see what you eat every day. Find out where all the extra sugar you eat is coming from. You'll save a lot of money and your health by not buying prepared snack foods. They're not good for you, and are worth cutting down.

Be Prepared

You may have created a healthy cupboard and refrigerator for yourself at home, but most offerings away from home at fast-food places, restaurants, the workplace, public events, and snack machines are high fat, high sugar, and low complex carbohydrate. Go prepared. Pack fruit, sliced sweet peppers, and nuts to snack on, so you don't wind up with fries, shakes, and candy. Or pack a brown rice and lentil lunch (cooked without oil or cream sauces) or other mixed grains with seasonings rather than oil.

Other options are the many commercial sport nutrition bars and drinks. Some are no more than candy with a sporty name; others are fairly good food. Sport bars and drinks are not magic energy potions; they are regular food in a wrapper. Read labels critically to find those that are low-fat. They usually come in at least a few flavors, are easy to throw in a briefcase or bag, and make a quick, easy snack, a small meal in emergencies, or meal adjunct.

Make It Easy

It's easier to reach into the refrigerator or cupboard and pull out a cookie or cake than take the time to fix a healthy meal. Have healthy food ready and easy to get to. Keep a bowl of fruit handy. Keep a container of cut vegetables within easy reach. Get and make healthy snacks ahead of time for when you know you will eat impulsively, and put them on the top shelf of the refrigerator and in the front of your cupboards.

Take Your Time

Lose weight the way you gained it—slowly. It will pay. Think long term. Food items are not worked off in single death bouts. Don't get discouraged if your body is not remade by the end of a week, or a month. Small daily calorie expenditures multiply over time. An easy 150-calorie-a-day walk translates into about 15 pounds a year. It works both ways—one extra 150-calorie-a-day piece of candy can mean you weigh 15 pounds more in one year. Make that work for you with slow, steady reduction that does not tax your system. Slow weight loss is more likely to stay off, is easier on your heart, and spares bone and muscle.

Check for Extra Calories You Don't Need

- You can cut many calories by not tasting foods as often when you cook, not licking icing from spoons, or not "just" breaking off halves of cookies to snack throughout the day. It can add up to hundreds of calories each day.

- Alcoholic drinks can add several hundred calories, plus hundreds more from the bar snacks and fried chips.

- Remember soda when you tally calories.

- Gum, mints, and small candies can have 10 to 15 calories each. It doesn't sound like much until you remember you eat a few dozen a day.

- Eighteen calories for a teaspoon of sugar doesn't sound like much until you count up all the two-packs in several coffees and teas a day. Milk, honey, and creamers add hundreds more.

- A big bag of chips, caramel corn, snack crackers, or cheese curls has over 1,000 calories, as does a can of roasted nuts.

- Trail mix and granolas are deliberately made to be high-calorie to sustain extended efforts in difficult terrain. They are not a low-calorie food. Half a cup of granola usually has around 200 calories. A big bowlful can have three to four times that. Add milk or soymilk and you have up to a 1,000-calorie snack.

- Many salad bars have vegetables with huge amounts of gloppy dressing and mayonnaise. Add cheese, croutons, nuts, olives, bacon bits, meats, etc., and you can easily eat up to 3,000 calories.

- Sports bars average 200 to 300 calories. They don't make you healthy just by eating them. Eating several is more than you need for exercise.

- Don't talk yourself into unhealthy foods because they contain a little fruit or vegetables in them. Packaged fruit cups are full of sugar and syrup. Don't think French fries are good for you because they are made from potatoes.

- Stop snacking while watching television.

- Sometimes all it takes to lose the 10 or 20 pounds you want is to cut out one regular bedtime snack. Stopping just one 300- to 400-calorie-a-night snack will make quite a difference.

Remember That "Diet Food" Is Food

Foods labeled as "diet food" are not magic potions that remove fat and calories from your body. They do not make you thinner by the action of eating them. They are food. Regular food. They have calories. Many are loaded with sugar and fat. They can make you fat if you eat too much of them.

What about meal replacement drinks? They also do not remove fat from your body just by drinking them. They are called "meal replacers" because you have one instead of anything else. You eat nothing else at all for that meal. Then you don't snack or sneak food before the next meal. It is better to learn healthy eating habits so you can have real meals that have fiber in them. Use a meal replacer when you are rushing somewhere and are really missing a meal. Don't have it in addition to your other meals as a snack. The extra calories will store as fat.

Do More Physical Activity

The major factor in overweight is a sedentary lifestyle. If you reduce your activity enough to gain only one pound per year, think how much heavier you will be in 20 years. Now think about only two pounds per year. These are pounds you will probably not notice on a day-to-day basis. Small things add up. Responsible plans for long-term weight loss include exercise. Exercise, in almost all cases, is a healthier, more effective weight loss method than starving yourself. A University of California study found that most of those people able to remain slimmed down were those who started exercising regularly.

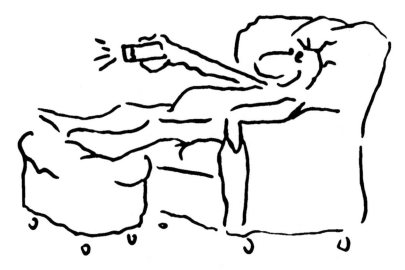

Figure 19.1. The major cause of overweight is inactivity.

Some people prefer organized exercise classes. They will drive to a gym and take the elevator to an exercise class, but hate to go out for a walk. Others haven't access or time to go to a gym, or they just hate the idea. Fortunately for them, getting in shape doesn't automatically mean three punishing sieges per week, pulse checks, group humiliation, and regimentation. Find an activity you like anyway, such as going to a dance club, bicycling, or walking. Then you don't have to go to a gym just to get activity. Make your life active. Try all kinds of things until you find something you love to do.

> The modern inactive life goes against the evolutionary history and design of the human body to be active. Going to a gym today is only a substitute for a natural active life.

How to Lose Weight Without Killing Yourself

Cut Back Fats. There are obvious ways you get too much fat, like fried food, rich desserts, and high-fat dairy products. Then there are ways you don't realize—creams and oils in sauces, salads, and snacks, and sloshed all over vegetables.

Make Your Own. Homemade food is healthier and cheaper than "convenience" foods.

Substitute. Substitute good-tasting, healthy foods for unhealthy ones. Be creative and find foods you like.

Don't Go Hungry. Starving yourself makes you hungry and unhappy, and makes your body hang on to its fat stores. Eat healthy snacks, not candy or cakes, to help maintain steady blood sugar levels.

Eat Less Simple Sugar. When you eat less sugar, you crave less.

Be Prepared. Pack healthy food to take with you to places that have only unhealthy food.

Make It Easy. Have healthy food ready and easier to get to than junk food when you know you will eat impulsively.

Take Your Time. Slow weight loss is more likely to stay off, is easier on your heart, and spares bone and muscle.

Want to burn more calories, even at work? The day is loaded with opportunities. If you drive to work, park farther away and walk the rest. Or commute by bicycle where feasible. Why wait for an elevator when you can improve your legs on the stairs? You may beat the elevator. If you work on an upper floor, take the elevator a few flights and walk the rest. Hand-deliver interoffice mail any chance you have. Instead of a smoke break, or donut-and-Danish break, take a walk-and-stretch break and have an orange.

Bend properly all day. You probably bend hundreds of times daily for the water fountain, the files, the trash can, to jot a message while standing, to pick up mail, or any number of other things. Bending over right at the waist is terrible on your back. Use your legs, keep your torso upright, and burn calories with every bend. Even people so heavy or injured that any activity is difficult can find something they can do. See Chapter 13, "How to Get Started Getting In Shape," and Chapter 26, "What to Do About the Shape You're In," for more on exercise ideas for weight control.

Check for Extra Calories You Don't Need. Sometimes all it takes to lose the 10 or 20 pounds you want is to cut out idle snacking, foods that are terrible for you anyway, and late-night extra meals.

Remember that "Diet Food" Is Food. It does not make you thinner by eating it. It makes you fat if you eat too much of it.

Do More Physical Activity. The major factor in overweight is a sedentary lifestyle.

Make It Fun. Make your new, healthy lifestyle a fun one so you stay with it, and enjoy it.

Eat More Slowly. Put your fork down between bites. You'll eat less.

Turn Off the TV, and talk to your friends and loved ones over dinner.

Bend and Lift Properly. People kill their backs all day every day when they could instead burn hundreds of calories and exercise their legs by lifting properly with torso upright and knees bent. Examples include getting things out of the refrigerator, desks, low shelves, and closets; tying shoes; picking up mail, babies, papers, and laundry; vacuuming; making beds; leashing pets; and countless more.

When you think about it, the human body was designed for activity, and was active through the eons. Today in much of the "developing world," people commute by bicycle, regularly lift and carry loads, and sit and rise from the floor often. Modern life became inactive, bringing diseases of inactivity with it. Going to the gym is just a substitute for having an activity level that seems to be programmed into the human body for health. With practice, you can find activities that are fun and do them often until they become a natural, healthy part of your life.

> Being more active is the key to weight control. Find ways to be more active as part of your everyday life.

Make It Fun

All the ways to control your weight without diets can become easy, safe, good-tasting, and fun lifetime habits that work. Eat healthfully and increase your daily activity level by making common lifetime activities part of your exercise. It will pay off in a lifetime of better health and enjoyment.

Resources for Low-Fat Cooking

The (Almost) No Fat Holiday Cookbook: Festive Vegetarian Recipes. Bryanna Clark Grogan. Book Publishing Company, 1995. ISBN: 1-57067-009-9. Over 100 vegan holiday recipes for 17 festivals from a variety of cultures (from the Fourth of July to Kwanzaa to Eid-Ul-Fitr, the end of Ramadan).

The Lighthearted Vegetarian Gourmet Cookbook. Steve Victor. Pacific Press Publishing, 1988. ISBN: 0-8163-0718-0. Fifty extremely low-fat, vegan recipes with no concentrated sugars from any source, and no high-fat vegetable ingredients. One hundred humorous and densely written pages.

Part III

HEALTH

A person ought to handle his body like the sail of a ship, and neither lower and reduce it much when no cloud is in sight, nor be slack and careless in managing it when he comes to suspect something is wrong.

— Plutarch

20. Back and Neck Pain—Why?
21. Back and Neck Pain—Prevention and Treatment
22. Calcium, Protein, Space Flight, Exercise, and Your Bones—A Detective Story
23. Body Fat—It's Not All Bad
24. Problems of Being Overweight
25. Body Fat—How to Tell How Much You've Got
26. What to Do About the Shape You're In
27. Cardiovascular Disease
28. Good and Bad Cholesterol Explained
29. Headaches
30. Leg Cramps and What to Do About Them
31. Funny Physical Facts and Foibles

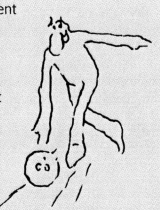

20

Back and Neck Pain—Why?

We sit at breakfast, we sit on the train on the way to work, we sit at lunch, we sit all afternoon...a hodgepodge of sagging livers, sinking gallbladders, drooping stomachs, compressed intestines, and squashed pelvic organs.

– John Button, Jr.

Sitting is very tough on your back and neck. Back and neck pain are common, and can be very painful. Although often mistaken for a mysterious, permanent, unavoidable condition, back and neck pain are almost always easily treated, and more easily prevented.

Why read this if your back or neck doesn't hurt? Odds are they will one day. Statistically, eight out of 10 backs and necks over the age of 18 will hurt a little, a lot, or an awful lot sometime in their lives. Only the common cold beats back pain as the top cause of work absenteeism in the United States. Americans lose an estimated 90 million production days annually due to back pain. Back injuries are the work industry's single greatest medical expense, estimated at $100 billion in the United States alone in medical costs, compensation, and lost productivity and wages—every year.

An Injury, Not a Condition

The real cause of most back and neck pain may surprise you. Just like heart disease and lung cancer, back and neck pain usually develop slowly over time without your knowing it. Back and neck pain are almost always a repetitive strain-type injury, not an unavoidable, sudden "condition," or evolutionary punishment for walking on two legs. This is an important distinction. Your chronic backache, your killer back-of-the-neck pain, or the back that just "goes out" once in a while are injuries that usually develop slowly from harmful patterns—things that you do every day. Even if you have structural problems of arthritis, or things breaking down or not being where they should, your daily habits can be causing or worsening the condition.

> Someone who breaks their leg would not go around year after year saying they have a "leg condition." Back pain is an injury that can be treated, not a "condition" that cannot be changed.

Just as you heal after a sprained ankle or broken arm, you can heal from back pain and resume your normal life. The key is to identify and modify abusive patterns, detailed in the next chapter on treating and preventing back and neck pain. First, a quick look at your interesting anatomy, so you can see why the things you do can hurt so much.

> Just like heart disease and lung cancer, back and neck pain are usually developed slowly over time, from small, repetitive bad habits that cause injury. That means you can do something about it before it happens, and change things to reverse the course once started.

Your Interesting Parts

Your Spine Bones. The bones of your spine are called vertebrae. The top seven vertebrae are your neck bones, called cervical vertebrae. Their names are C1 (from the top) down to C7. If you tip your head forward and feel the back of your neck, the bump at the bottom of your neck is usually C7. Your next 12 vertebrae are thoracic vertebrae (T1–T12). Your rib bones attach to these vertebrae, 12 on each side. (Both men and women have 12 paired ribs, 24 total. Men do not have one fewer rib, contrary to biblical speculation.) The next five vertebrae do not have ribs attached. These are your lower back bones, the lumbar vertebrae (L1–L5). This is where a lot of back pain occurs. More on why in a bit. Below them are your five sacral vertebrae (S1–S5), fused into a single bone, the sacrum. The sacrum forms the bony back wall of your hips. Attached to the bottom of your sacrum is the coccyx, your tailbone.

Your Discs. Discs are flat, fibrocartilage cushions that sit like washers between bones in several areas of your body. The discs you hear about most often sit between each of your vertebrae. These intervertebral discs cushion shocks transmitted through your spine with your every step and prevent your vertebrae from rubbing directly against each other.

There are also discs in other areas of your body. Tiny little discs cushion the joint between your head bone, called the temporal bone, and your lower jawbone, called the mandible. Sometimes, these little discs wear out, causing pain at the joint between them, the temporomandibular joint (TMJ). You have two larger discs, called menisci (singular is meniscus), in each knee. Injuring a meniscus is one cause of knee pain.

The discs most often involved in low back pain are your vertebral discs between L4 and L5 and, particularly, between L5 and S1. That is where most people give the most punishment to their backs.

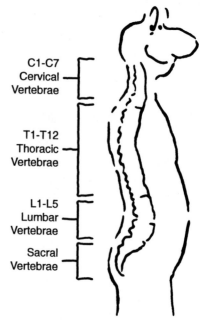

C1-C7
Cervical
Vertebrae

T1-T12
Thoracic
Vertebrae

L1-L5
Lumbar
Vertebrae

Sacral
Vertebrae

Figure 20.1. You normally have seven neck vertebrae (cervical); 12 upper back vertebrae (thoracic); five low back vertebrae (lumbar); five sacral vertebrae, fused into the bony back wall of your pelvis; and your small tailbone or coccyx, made of several fused rudimentary vertebrae.

The Quick Way and the Slow Way to Get Back and Neck Pain

There are two main ways to hurt your back and neck: the quick way and the slow way.

The Quick Way. The most classic onset of back pain is after you lean over, twist to the side, and lift something. Why is this?

If you do nothing more than stand still and bend over with straight legs, you put hundreds of pounds of force on each vertebral disc, the most on L5–S1. Twisting when you lean is worse. Yanking a weight is often the death blow. There are many opportunities to do exactly those three things: picking up packages and children, lifting things out of cars and trunks, making beds, taking out the trash, doing laundry, and grabbing your bags at the airport baggage claim.

It's not that lifting by itself is bad for you. Lifting properly is no problem and is good for you. Lifting improperly is what injures, eventually. Many people lift dangerously for years without outward sign of injury—until one day....

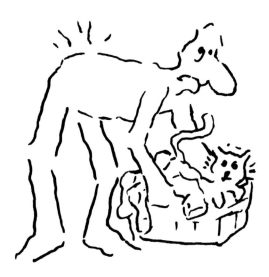

Figure 20.2. The "quick way" to ruin your back—lean over, twist, and lift.

The Slow Way. Years of wear and tear add up. Chronic slouching can injure your back and neck over several years as badly as a single accident can. Your body weight alone is enough to injure your muscles and discs through poor sitting, standing, and bending habits.

The small of your back is supposed to curve inward to a certain extent. One of several ways to slowly hurt your low back involves reversing your normal slight inward curve so that you curve forward instead, like the letter "C." This bad posture involves a motion called lumbar flexion.

> The pressure of your own body weight on your muscles and discs over several years of poor posture is enough to injure your back as badly as a single accident.

Flexion is when you bend a joint to make it smaller. Bending your elbow is elbow flexion. Putting your chin on your chest is neck flexion. You do hip flexion when you bend forward at the hip or raise your leg. Genuflection (*genu* is the Latin word for "knee") is when you bend your knee in church; but it's just plain knee flexion any other time. Sitting, standing, and lifting with a round back instead of maintaining the normal inward curve of your lower back is lumbar flexion. Too much lumbar flexion squeezes and pushes your discs outward toward the back. The disc may eventually fray and give out like a worn tire. Continuous back flexion also overstretches the long ligament down the back of your spine, weakening the back and allowing discs more room to protrude. On top of that, chronically holding back muscles, or any muscles for that matter, in a stretched position weakens them.

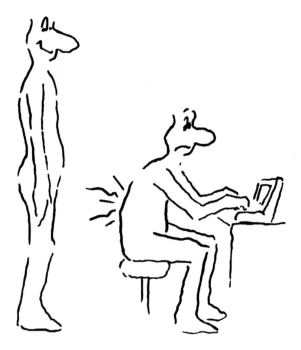

Figure 20.3. Normal good back posture has a small inward curve in your low back. Chronically reversing your normal curve or exaggerating it with poor posture can lead to back problems.

Habitually standing with your head forward overstretches and "uncurves" the back of your neck with similar results. A forward head contributes to upper back pain, usually between the shoulders, just under the lower point of the shoulder blade, and may also radiate to other areas.

> One of several ways to slowly hurt your back is sitting and bending so that the normal inward curve of your lower back curves outward. This eventually pushes discs outward and overstretches the long ligament down the back of the spine, weakening your back and allowing discs more room to protrude.

The second main bad posture is caused by not using your abdominal muscles so that you allow your low back to sway, exaggerating the normal inward curve. This does not cancel out problems from excess flexion, but creates back pain and injury of its own. Often, people who sit and bend with too much back flexion also stand excessively arched. Too much arching can cause the same wear-and-tear problems as too much flexion. Occasionally, too much arching irritates the joints, called vertebral facets, where each vertebra attaches to the one above and below it.

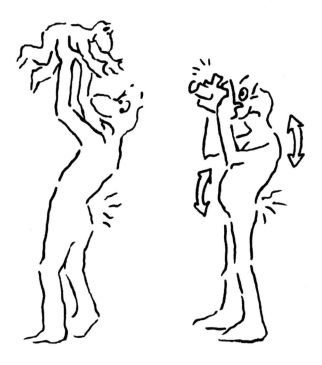

Figure 20.4. Chronically exaggerating and forcing the normal inward curve of your low back is a poor posture that can lead to back pain.

According to some estimates, men suffer back pain two to three times more often than women. One reason is the load of carrying around their larger shoulders, bigger backs, and longer, larger torsos relative to their bodies. Women usually keep more of their weight lower and biomechanically safer.

Most people unknowingly abuse their backs all the time in their daily activities. Just as smoking one cigarette at a time eventually can cause much trouble, you can gradually accumulate a back injury that may not become apparent for years.

In an average day, most people repeatedly abuse their backs unknowingly. In this way they are brewing a back injury that may not become apparent for years. Ironically, once their backs finally begin to hurt, they give up active exercise that helps backs, and they continue sitting and lifting with a rounded back, and standing with too much arch—both major back-injury-producing actions. A particularly ironic sight is back pain patients in physicians' and physical therapy waiting rooms, sitting in lumbar flexion and bad neck posture and worsening their condition while they sit. What follows is a series of seemingly harmless daily habits that are continuous, major back and neck pain producers.

An Average Day of Ruining Your Back and Neck. You wake up and sit at the edge of the bed, curled in back and neck flexion. Then you slouch over to the sink and bend over the sink to splash your face awake. Bend over, twist, and lift to make the bed. Get dressed, bending over while sitting to pull on shoes and socks. Put a wallet in your back pocket that makes you sit crooked. Sit curled forward in lumbar and neck flexion in a kitchen chair for breakfast, then again in the car or public transit to work. Commuting healthy by bicycle? Back flexion there too if you curl over the handlebars in poor form, worse with racing handlebars. You add to your neck troubles when you crane your neck forward for the ride. Sit in flexion at work, including lunch. From your chair, lean over, twist, and yank open file cabinets. Crane your neck forward at your desk to view the computer monitor. If your computer monitor is in the usual low position on your desk, you hold your head both forward and down to get your work done. Stand and walk with excess back arching (and also a forward head, often carrying packages, which compounds the strain). Reach overhead for shelves by arching your back. Lift boxes by bending right over at the waist, then lift them by arching your back. Commute home, sitting in flexion. Then flexion at dinner, in front of the sink, and in a rounded chair or couch in front of the TV with your head craned forward. Have young kids? Bend over incorrectly to pick them up. Hold them while standing arched. Flexion to tuck them in. Add chronic bad lifting mechanics during house and yard work.

Do you go to the gym? Several popular exercises do more to weaken your back than strengthen it: weightlifting while leaning over unsupported; straight-leg dead lifting; forced repetitive back bending, like touching toes from a stand, or swinging elbows down to opposite knees; and forced repetitive back arching, like "donkey kicks" that swing the leg overhead from a hands-and-knees position. Other damaging exercises include: lifting weights overhead while arching your back; doing sit-ups and crunches that hunch you forward in poor posture; and curling over stationary bicycle handlebars with head forward and back rounded.

Well-meaning exercisers often start their routine with back abuse—they bend over straight-legged to touch toes, and make it worse with bouncing and without warm-up. Although it often feels good on tight muscles, it's tough on your back in the long run. Moreover, stretching is not a warm-up, and should not be done until you warm yourself by muscular activity like jogging or bicycling. Necks get yanked forward during sit-ups, crunches, and several other exercises involving the hands behind the head and pulling the upper body forward. Chest exercises shorten and strengthen the upper chest muscles, while upper back muscles are ignored, furthering the rounded shoulder-forward head posture problem. Healthy alternatives are in Chapter 6 on stretching, Chapter 7 on abs, Chapter 8, "What Exercises Do You Need to Be Fit?" and Chapter 9, "Good and Bad Exercises."

Do you use rowing machines or go rowing? Rowing can be terrific exercise when done correctly, but problematic when done incorrectly with a rounded back. Sit upright, keeping the lower natural inward curve of your low back. Push off your heels, rather than your toes, to get better exercise for your legs, and keep the effort on your muscles, not your knee joints.

Still doing sit-ups? Still doing leg-raises? Those two do little for your abdominal muscles and are tough on your lower back, specifically where the muscles you use for sit-ups and leg lifts connect. Crunches can be terrible for your posture and don't train your abs the way you need them for real life. See Chapter 7 on abdominal muscles for a detailed explanation of why sit-ups and leg lifts benefit other muscles more than your abs, and what to do instead.

Finished your workout? Do you bend over and twist to pick up your gym bag? A paper on "Asymmetrical Loads and Lateral Bending of the Human Spine" in the July 1993 *Medical & Biological Engineering and Computing* reported that bags worn over one shoulder curl your spine slightly. The researchers concluded that such unequal forces might contribute to the high percentage of school children turning up with scoliosis. They suggested switching to knapsacks to distribute the load. In adults, shoulder bags can contribute to muscular pain. But it's not because of the bag; it's because of letting your posture sag. Not only do people let their posture slouch under their own body weight, they allow their body to sag under the weight of things they carry. You could burn calories, and get an ab and back workout, by simply holding

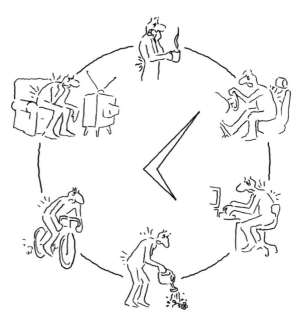

Figure 20.5. An average day of slowly ruining your back with poor posture starts in the morning and goes on all day, every day, for many people. Hurting your back is not caused by lifting wrong just once; it is from cumulative things you do all the time without realizing it. Like smoking, the ill effects take years to accumulate.

good posture against the pull of the bag, no matter where you wear it. Use packages, knapsacks, and bags as a free workout for your abs and back.

This overview just scratches the surface of what's behind back pain, but you get the idea. Like braces on your teeth, the continuous pull of bad posture habits on your back and neck will eventually reshape your body—but in unhealthy ways. Major factors in this process are weak muscles, lack of flexibility, and poor sitting, standing, and bending habits. It's not just lifting wrong one day. The effects are cumulative, like smoking. Then, one day you bend over to pick up a sock, and your back has had enough.

> The relentless pull of bad posture habits all day, every day on your back and neck will eventually reshape them, just like braces on your teeth. Only the result is not pretty or healthy.

How You Usually Get Back and Neck Pain

Although you may have specific back conditions like arthritis, osteoporosis, or scoliosis, the bad habits described here increase anyone's risk of pain and injury. For more on osteoporosis origins and prevention see Chapter 22, "Calcium, Protein, Space Flight, Exercise, and Your Bones—A Detective Story."

Muscles. Most back and neck pain is muscle-related. There are several ways you contribute to this:

- Ordinary daily bad habits, like chronic poor sitting, standing, and bending, eventually overstretch, strain, and contract your muscles into painful knots.

- Bad posture puts your head and torso into positions that put relentless pressure on discs, nerves, and muscles. Microtears, spasm, and inflammation result, creating more pain.

- Sometimes, muscles on one side of your spine or hip are stronger than the muscles on the other side. The weaker side can't counter the pull of stronger opposing muscles, furthering bad posture stress.

- Sometimes, muscles on one side of your spine or hip are too tight compared to the muscles on the other side, pulling your body into a continuing cycle of poor posture and joint stress.

- Tight muscles can strain instead of stretch during activity. Even a small range of motion can strain tight low back muscles, accounting for many painful backs at the end of a day.

Figure 20.6. Your hip flexor muscles cross your hip in the front and attach to the top of your leg. They work to bend (flex) your hip joint. One set of hip flexors starts on your spine, the others on the top of your hip. Tight hip flexors can change the way you stand and walk, and can contribute to back pain.

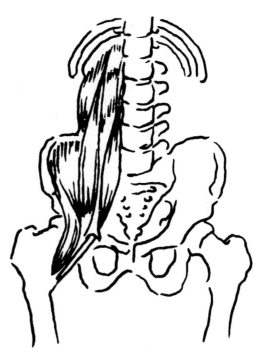

- Muscle strength and flexibility inequalities can occur even in people who work out regularly, if they don't work muscle groups evenly, a common practice.

- Muscles called hip flexors bend you forward at the hip. One set of hip flexor muscles begins on your lumbar vertebrae (lower back bones) and extends forward and down to a knob on your upper leg bone (the greater trochanter of your femur). When these muscles are tight, common in people who sit a lot, they sometimes pull enough on your lower back to increase its normal arch. This extra pulling and tilting can contribute to low back pain.

- Other sets of muscles pull on your hip bones from the back. Hamstrings are the triple set of muscles in the back of your thigh. They work to both bend your knee and swing your leg behind you. The three hamstrings of each leg start at the bottom of your hip bones, on the bony "bumps" you sit on, called ischial tuberosities. The hamstrings run down the back of each leg, and cross the back of your knee, where you can feel their stringy tendons on both sides. Tight hamstrings can pull on your hip bones and tip your pelvis rearward, reversing your normal arch and contributing to back pain.

- Muscles that are tight from inflexibility, and muscles that are tightly in spasm from bad posture habits, can compress nerves, mimicking the kind of pain produced by herniated discs pressing on nerves. One of several muscles that seems to like to do this is the piraformis muscle. The piraformis lies deep in your pelvis under your buttock muscles. In a small percentage of the population, the sciatic nerve goes through the piraformis. In most others, the sciatic nerve is not in the piraformis, but close by. In either case, if the piraformis is tight, it can compress your sciatic nerve, causing pain and sometimes weakness in the buttock and down your leg.

> Tight hip, back, and leg muscles can cause the poor postures that lead to back and neck pain.

Any of these various muscle problems are often enough to cause back pain by themselves. Worse, several of them frequently occur together. Add slinging weights and packages (and yourself) around in ways your back isn't designed to withstand, and back pain eventually afflicts the majority of people.

> Most back and neck pain comes from daily bad sitting, standing, and bending postures.

Poor neck posture often brings on pain, and sometimes numbness in back of your head, down the side of your neck, across the top of your shoulders, between the shoulders, under the shoulder blades, and sometimes down your arm. Poor neck posture is a common cause of headache.

The most common poor neck posture is standing and sitting with your neck sloped forward, which juts your head forward of the center line of your body. This bad posture is called a forward head. Many people have a forward head without knowing it. Think of a bowling ball. Now imagine continuously holding that heavy bowling ball out in front of your body. Soon, your back and neck muscles that hold it will fatigue, then hurt. That bowling ball is your head.

A forward head looks like E.T. sniffing a flower. Less comical is its effect to overstretch the ligament down the back of your neck, putting pressure on your discs. A forward head can eventually damage neck and upper back structures, when they begin to bend and rub at angles they were not built for. Your discs can degenerate or begin to protrude. Protruding (herniated) discs can press on nerves that go down your arms. Chronically holding your neck muscles, or any muscles, in an overstretched position weakens them. You wind up with shortened, contracted muscles down the front of your neck, and a stretched, weakened upper back. You may have seen this forward-head posture on older people and wondered how they got that way. The answer is practice.

The forward head can also contribute to shoulder trouble. The forward-head posture brings the top of the shoulder bone over the top of the arm bone, limiting overhead reaching, and, over time, contributing to shoulder impingement problems.

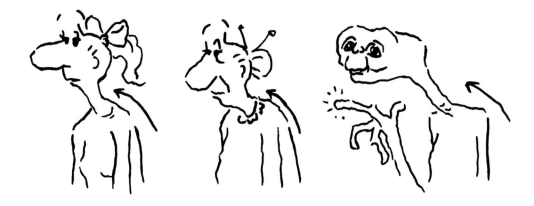

Figure 20.7. A forward head can cause a lot of neck, shoulder, and upper back pain. A forward head can make you look older. A forward head is so common that it looks normal, and is just about taken for granted in older people. But it is a posture that can be avoided.

An average day is filled with opportunities for the bad habit of the forward head:

- Sitting with your head craning forward in front of the computer screen.
- Hunching over your desk.
- Using your shoulder to cradle a phone receiver against your ear.
- Commuting in car, bus, or train seats.
- Bending over the kids.
- Walking.
- Doing household chores.
- Watching TV.
- Craning your head forward while exercising.

In short: All day, every day, at work and play, even at rest in a chair, and then all night if you sleep on your back with your head pushed forward with pillows. No wonder your neck and back are killing you.

> The average person does so many things every day to damage their back and neck that it is amazing they don't hurt more.

Discs. Disc protrusions, called herniations, can result from chronic outward pressure on discs. In your neck and lower back, this pressure occurs from the bad posture of slouching your torso forward into the shape of the letter "C" when sitting, bending, and lifting, rather than keeping the normal inward curves of the neck and lower back. Continually putting grinding, unequal pressures on your discs can cause them to break down (degenerate) over time. The curled posture also pushes discs out, out, out, over time. The edges begin to fray like a wearing tire. Eventually, one day, after even a small provocation, the disc finally protrudes far enough for a sudden onset of disc pain. Then you attribute the injury of the "slipped disc" to the one event that brought on the pain, never realizing it was brewing all along from the way you sat, stood, and lifted, day after day, year after year.

> Year after year of poor sitting and standing posture can wear out your discs. One day, a disc finally "goes," while you are doing nothing more than sneezing or reaching for something. The "slipped" disc wasn't caused by the one event; it was brewing all along.

Discs don't usually protrude straight back. Their path is blocked by a long, tough, vertically running ligament, called the posterior longitudinal ligament. That is good because your spinal cord lies behind the discs. But that also means that a disc herniation will usually push out sideways. The long nerves serving your legs also exit your lumbar vertebrae to the side. When a disc bulges against these nerves, pain extends down your leg. The most common nerve to be pushed on by bulging discs is the sciatic nerve. The sciatic nerve has both sensory and motor functions, meaning that if compressed, it will hurt and can reduce the function of your leg. In the most serious cases, discs can protrude directly backwards against your spine, disrupting your ability to move from that level down and to control your bowel and bladder.

Although "slipped" or herniated discs used to be thought of as a life sentence, we now know that is rarely so. Many disc protrusions heal if you let them, and you can go back to your life, as after any other injury. Chapter 21 covers treating and preventing muscle- and disc-related back and neck pain. It's not hard, and rarely requires surgery. Best of all, back and neck pain, whether from muscle or disc, is almost always avoidable.

> Most disc herniations will heal with proper exercises and stopping the bad habits that made them herniate in the first place.

Other Ways You Get Back and Neck Pain

Your Legs. A knee or ankle injury may throw off how you walk and stand. Poor posture of your legs causes you to distribute your weight unevenly across your legs and feet. This can affect how you walk, and adds to chronic wear and tear on your muscles and joints.

Unequal leg length can add to back pain. It is a myth that everyone has unequal leg length. For those who do have unequal leg lengths, the difference is not always in bone length. Muscle spasm can pull on your hip and lower body, making a "functional" leg length difference, rather than a true structural one. These spasms can be easily dealt with by a good physical therapist, orthopedist, physical medicine physician, osteopath, or massage therapist with appropriate training. Often, simply slouching more on one leg than the other or letting one ankle roll in more than the other results in dramatic leg length differences that are not "in the bone." If after ruling out these causes, your doctor finds you have a true leg length difference, wear a properly measured, padded shoe lift that fits well.

Your Feet. An often overlooked source of back pain is your feet. Your feet and legs have posture just like your neck and back. You may walk with your feet too flat (pronated) or too arched. Or turned in or turned out. Bad foot posture throws off how your legs distribute your weight. Another foot problem involves your big toe. When your big toe joint works as it should, it bends pliably, and your foot and leg pivot around it to walk normally. Sometimes, although it may not hurt or be obvious, it does not bend enough during the push-off phase of walking, throwing off foot position and gait, and pushing the posture of your head and trunk forward. Your lower back muscles and discs bear the brunt. For more on how important your feet can be in pain and injury prevention, and exercises to prevent problems, see Chapter 9, "Good and Bad Exercises."

Your Middle. The extra load and altered posture of beer guts and pregnancies are tough on your back. But it is not the pregnancy that hurts the back. It's allowing the back to arch backward to carry the load instead of using your ab muscles to prevent arching backward in bad posture. For more on how and why your abs control posture and can be used for pain and injury prevention, and for exercises to prevent problems, see Chapter 7 on abs.

Your Walk. Walking "hard" shocks your spine (and hip and other joints) and adds to early wear and tear. Some people come down so heavily on each step that the skin on their face jiggles. Think of your car. Without good shock absorption, your frame will wear out early. You have several ways to add to your necessary, natural shock absorption:

- Your major bodily shock absorbers are your thigh and backside muscles, the quadriceps and gluteal muscles. Exercise them for better back health.

- Strong back muscles are shock absorbers, much more so than weak back muscles, another good reason to do your back exercises.

- Wear a good, padded insole in your shoes every day. Two good brands of padded insoles are Spenco® and SecondWind®. When you buy new shoes, take your padded insoles with you and try them on in the shoe. If you have to buy a half size higher to fit the pad, it's worth it.

- More important than "external" shock absorption, like insoles, is to maintain good posture by keeping the normal inward curve of your lower back. Your spine is like a spring and absorbs shock through its normal curves. Straightening out the curve by slouching removes the normal spring action. Accentuating the normal curve through too much arching also reduces shock absorption.

- Walk softly all the time. Roll heel to toe, don't walk on tiptoe. Bend your knees when walking, descending stairs, and stepping off curbs.

> Your legs and feet have posture, too. How you stand and walk makes a big difference between getting healthy exercise, and putting extra pressures, shocks, and wear and tear on your joints.

Sitting Down Heavily. When you sit down, you should be using your leg muscles to decelerate so that you don't wham down onto your behind. The shock jolts you throughout your spinal column and wears out your discs. Watch people for this and check yourself. Do you need your arms to help you lower into a chair? Do your knees come together? Your leg muscles are critically weak. You need to strengthen them. Practice rising and lowering with good form. Don't lean forward. That puts weight on your knee joints. Push off your heels to use your leg muscles. Work up to several sets of 10 for a simple, free exercise that directly benefits your life.

> Do you let yourself flop down in your chair without using your leg muscles to decelerate? That jolts your spine and loads your discs. It may be just a bad habit, or your leg muscles may be too weak. Lower yourself with strength and ease.

Neck and Back Pain From Outside Your Body

Your Shoes. Shoes are often made with little or no shock absorption, particularly fashionable dress shoes. They are also frequently too tight for good walking dynamics, even if they do not feel too tight.

- If you have marks, bruises, roughness, or calluses on your feet or toes, chances are that your shoes are too tight.

- If your toes fit like puzzle pieces, tight shoes probably molded them that way. There is supposed to be space between your toes, and toes should be able to wiggle easily.

- Tight shoes aggravate and accelerate bunion formation in people predisposed to them. Bunions alter healthy walking mechanics.

- High heels are well-known as major contributors to foot injury and disruption of normal walking mechanics of the entire leg, transmitting problems to your back, and even to your neck.

- Worn-out shoes can create a vicious cycle. If you walk unevenly, your shoes wear unevenly. Turn your shoes over and look at the heels. See if they are much more worn down on one side than the other. This uneven sole will tilt you further to that side, making you walk even more unevenly.

- Walk straight, and keep the heels of your shoes in good repair. Don't wear old, worn-out shoes.

- Don't wear tight shoes for "support." You are supposed to use your own muscles to hold yourself up. Don't let your feet atrophy by never using them to hold yourself up properly. Don't let your feet and knees sag. Use good leg and foot posture—parallel feet, knees that face straight forward, not tilting inward or outward.

It's a myth that sneakers don't have "support" or are bad for your feet. Dress shoes are more often the culprit. With practically nothing between the soles of your feet and the hard pavement, and raised heels that alter normal walking dynamics of the foot, it's a marvel that your back and neck don't hurt more often.

> Good shock absorption is important to healthy backs
> and necks. Wear shoes with low or no heels,
> padded insoles, and soft soles.

Remember that your most important shock absorption should come from your own muscles and gait. Walk softly.

Hidden Causes of Back and Neck Pain

The major, usual causes of back and neck pain are tight, weak back and leg muscles, a forward-head posture, and poor standing and sitting postures. Some surprising and often overlooked contributors to pain are:

- Funny leg posture. Keep your knees facing straight ahead rather than letting them turn in or out. Keep them in line with your ankle joint rather than letting them bow out or sag inward.

- Funny foot posture. Stand with your weight distributed evenly so that you do not roll in or out on your arches. Check your shoes to see if they make you stand funny. Don't walk with your toes pointed in or out.

- "Stuck" big toe. Your big toe needs to bend with each step so that you can push off your toe, rather than lifting the entire foot stiffly. Keep your feet flexible, particularly your big toe joint.

- Beer guts.

- Walking "hard." It shocks your spine and adds to early wear and tear. Use your muscles to decelerate when you step, don't just stomp or flop your feet down.

- Not wearing sneakers often enough. Just like a car, you need good shock absorbers or your frame will show early wear.

- High heels. They alter just about everything natural about your foot, leg, and back posture, all the way to your neck.

- Old shoes that are unevenly worn, or new shoes that do not fit right so that your foot is allowed to, or made to, tilt to either side.

- Tight pants and belts.

- Mattresses that are too hard.

- Chairs that make you sit funny.

- Computer monitors at desk level, rather than head level.

- Smoking. It adds to disc degeneration.

Your Clothes. Tight pants and belts can make your back hurt.

Your Mattress. Too-hard mattresses are a common cause of tight, stiff morning backs. It is an "old husbands' tale" that back pain sufferers must sleep on a hard board. Try a foam "egg crate" on top of your hard mattress.

Your Chair. Check your car seat. Does it make you sit curled forward? Is it worn out on one side, making you sit with one hip hiked higher than the other? Check your chair at work. Do you sit crooked? Maybe your seat is not level. Put your computer monitor up on blocks so that you look at it straight on, not craning your neck down and forward to view it at desk level. Check your chair height at your desk.

Your Cigarettes. Smoking contributes to degeneration of your discs.

> People do things 23 hours a day to tighten, weaken, and wreck themselves. Then they spend an hour exercising and wonder why it doesn't "work."

21

Back and Neck Pain—
Prevention and Treatment

*We don't consider a patient cured when his sprain has healed or
he's restored to a minimal level of functioning. The patient is
cured when he can again do the things he loves to do.*

— Stanley A. Herring, M.D.

The previous chapter described some of the common ways to get back and neck pain. To review, back and neck pain often result from things you do every day without knowing it. Although back pain often comes on suddenly, the injury that causes pain is rarely a sudden event. It brews with years of abuse. Wear and tear from your body weight alone, from poor sitting, standing, and bending habits can injure your back over time as badly as might happen in a single accident. The main factors in back and neck pain are poor sitting, standing, and lifting postures that often result from inflexibility and weakness of muscles supporting your torso and back. This can happen even if you work out regularly.

Pain From Poor Function, Not Structure

Someone with back pain may go to a doctor and get an x-ray or other imaging. The pain is from all the poor body mechanics all day, not any organic problem. The scans show nothing. What they need is exercise and muscle and posture retraining, but they are told they are imagining everything or that it is stress. They continue all their poor habits and their pain continues, or worsens.

Or the scans may show arthritis, a bulging disc, or degenerating or slipping structures. Just like car tires that are mid-life but perfectly good, an exam may show some wear that is completely unrelated to performance or pain. The pain is falsely ascribed to the structure, even though the pain is from all the poor mechanics over the years. They may be told to give up activities or have surgery, when what they need is exercise and muscle and posture retraining.

Sometimes, the scans show a major structural problem. Poor mechanics may be contributing to the pain, or even causing the problem. But the person goes for surgery, sometimes major surgery. The pain persists because of uncorrected poor mechanics. The problem itself, such as a herniated disc, may return due to poor mechanics.

Most Back and Neck Pain Is Preventable

Almost all back pain is preventable. You can easily reduce your chance of back or neck pain and reduce pain you already have. You first need to identify and avoid things you do that chronically abuse your back and neck. Then do several easy exercises and good postural retraining to help you recover and make your back more injury-resistant.

Even with things you can't prevent, such as certain inherited back disorders or serious accidents, you can usually reduce or eliminate pain with good habits. Tendency toward arthritis, for example, increases with habits that contribute to wear and tear, and with lack of proper exercise. Scoliosis is aggravated by carrying shoulder bags without postural control, or skipping exercises to strengthen muscles that support the spine. There is much you can change.

> Almost all back pain is preventable.

Avoid Bad Standing, Sitting, and Lifting Habits

Your Back. Do you sit, stand, and bend with your lower back rounded outward rather than inward? That is the most common way to slowly ruin your back. The concave back of most chairs makes you sit with a rounded back and a forward head. Watch for bad chair engineering in office, bus, train, and plane seats. Other problem chairs are bench seats in restaurants and church pews. Plane and bus seats seem to be exceptionally bad. Boat benches are often hard, with no back at all. The stress to your back may be made worse when pounding over waves. When riding in trains, planes, and automobiles, bring a small cushion or use your jacket to roll in the small of your back, to sit keeping the normal inward curve of your lower back.

> Sitting stresses your discs more than standing.
> Poor sitting posture makes the strain far worse.

Do you stand with too much arch in your back? You need abdominal exercises to retrain the forward "guy wire" muscles that would prevent backward sway. See Chapter 7 on abs.

Do you pick things up by bending at the waist with your legs straight or nearly so? Don't do that. Keep your torso upright, not bent over, and bend your knees. A common complaint is that using the legs is difficult. Exercise your leg muscles, as discussed later in this chapter, to make it easier. Using your legs is free exercise and burns calories, so be glad. When you have one hand or elbow free, support your upper body weight with that hand or elbow on your knee or other support. Don't twist to one side during a lift or bend.

> As a child you were told, "If you make a funny face, it will stick like that." If you spend your daily activities with your head and shoulders hunched forward, your body will eventually tighten up and stick like that. "As bent the twig, so grows the tree."

Your Neck. Do you stand and sit with your head forward? That's a common source of upper back, neck, and head pain, particularly pain between and across the shoulders. A forward head is so common that it looks normal, but is a serious problem. Keep your ears over your shoulders, not in front of them. A common mistake is just lifting the chin up, which just compounds the pinching, rather than pulling it back and in. Put your computer monitor up on blocks, rather than sitting it on the desk, so that you can look at it straight on without looking down. Place your TV screen at head level. Reading and writing at a desk is no excuse to hunch over. Keep your body upright, and head pulled back while you look down, rather than tipping your head down and forward.

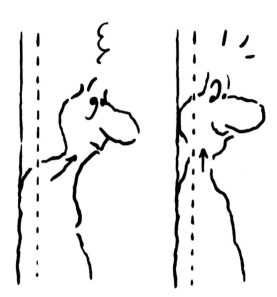

Figure 21.1. Correct a forward head by lifting back and in, bringing your ears over the center of your shoulders without looking up or down. Lift back without strain or tension. This is also a good exercise to relieve pain and tension in back of your neck and shoulders.

Relieving back and neck pain does not mean giving up
activities you love, or sitting and standing stiffly like a soldier.
You need physical activity and flexible posture.

Your "Guy Wires." Your back needs support from all sides. In brief, when you use the muscles running along your back, they pull on the back of your spine to keep you from slouching forward. Abdominal muscles run down your front from your ribs to your pelvic bones. When used, they pull to keep you from arching backward during normal standing and sitting. Weakness and poor use of your guy-wire muscles allow you to sit and stand in positions that slowly injure you without you being aware of it. The degree of strength and muscular endurance of your back muscles can make the difference between an uneventful day, and a tired, achy back that night. That's why back exercises are so important. Exercises won't automatically make your muscles hold you in the right position. You must consciously remember to *use* the muscles to stand and sit properly. Don't just let your body sag to wherever it sags.

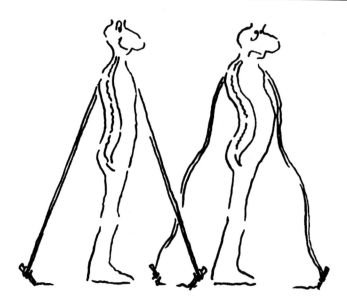

Figure 21.2. Your abdominal muscles are your "guy wires" that, when used, pull your spine from the front. Your back muscles are your "guy wires" in the back. Weak or unused guy-wire muscles allow you to sit, stand, and move in poor postures that can slowly cause back and neck pain.

Avoid Too Little Exercise

Without enough exercise, your back easily becomes weak. Weak muscles can't hold the good posture necessary for anatomic structures to fit together without strain and rubbing. This can happen even if you are in "good shape" or go to the gym. It is easy to underwork some muscles and overwork others so that they overpower the back and neck muscles.

> Don't let bad postural mechanics grind your back structure down to where it will be harder to fix later. Good muscle support around the joint comes from proper use and educating the muscles how to support the area, not by stopping your activities and "resting it."

Avoid Too Much Exercise of the Wrong Kind

Several exercises common at gyms and exercise studios can do your back more harm than good. A few bad exercises now and then usually do little damage, but give it a chance. Like smoking, the repeated damage of the exposure can harm at a rate faster than your body can repair.

Tough-on-the Back Exercises

- Straight-legged dead lifting and other continuous, weighted, forward bending. You hear all the time never to lean over and lift packages with straight legs. Why does it magically become all right to do that in a gym? Many lifters believe it strengthens the back, but straight-legged dead lifting and bent-over lifting can injure you.

- Standing toe touches. It is just more leaning over with straight legs.

> It's well-known that you should never lean over and lift packages with straight legs, so why does it magically become all right to do that in a gym? Straight-legged dead lifting can seriously injure your back.

- Sit-ups and leg lifts. (Unless you need them for activities requiring high hip-flexor strength, like ballet, placekicking, and martial arts.) Sit-ups and leg lifts use the hip flexor muscles that attach to your lower spine, far more than they use your abdominal muscles. They are tough on the back with little reward for the abs. Substitute ab exercises, described in Chapter 7 on abdominal muscles.

- Forced, repetitive back arching that, over the years, can irritate and grind your facet joints, where each vertebrae joins the next, and smash soft tissue. Examples are continuously swinging your leg backwards in the air in an exercise called "donkey kicks," and moving and standing with too much arch, particularly when lifting weights or reaching overhead.

Abs Are Not Enough. Many people mistakenly concentrate on abdominal exercises like crunches, thinking that these alone will keep their backs injury-free. Abs create an important support structure for your torso, but they are not the entire support. It is all too common for exercise classes to spend much time on abdominal exercises, and never turn over to do back exercises. Without also working the back muscles, the resulting forward slouch slowly injures. Crunches are the exercise usually thought of for ab exercise and back pain control; however, they create a hunched-over posture, encourage a forward head, and are not how you need your abs in daily life. They do not automatically make your abdominal muscle work properly while standing, so are not a good, functional exercise. Chapter 7 on abs explains this in detail and what to do instead. Back exercises are detailed later in this chapter.

Crunches are a common ab exercise; however, they do not train your torso muscles the way you need them for back pain control, and they encourage hunched-over posture.

To Avoid Back and Neck Pain, Avoid These

- Continuous incorrect lifting, sitting, and standing.
- Sitting with your back rounded.
- Standing with your back rounded or too arched.
- Standing with your upper back too rounded *and* your lower back too arched.
- Continually holding your head forward.
- Chronic bending at the waist and hip.
- Twisting during a lift or bend.
- Damaging exercises.
- Beer guts.
- High heels.
- Smoking.
- Lack of exercise.
- Poor flexibility of back, hip, and hamstrings.
- Doing ab exercises without turning over to counter them with back exercises.
- Not using your muscles to control torso posture. Good posture doesn't happen automatically just from doing exercises.

Posture Matters More Than You Think

Posture can make a difference between a pain-free back and neck, and chronic misery. People don't take posture seriously as the main contributor to back and neck pain. Think of it as mechanics. If your car had crooked parts, you'd know right away that would cause grinding and early wear. Think of posture as muscle retraining. Keep your ears over the center line of your shoulders. Keep your back from rounding, and stand without leaning backward or tilting forward from the hip. Don't let your legs turn in or out. Keep your toes facing straight forward.

Good posture doesn't mean standing stiffly for a moment, then stopping because it doesn't feel natural. It means getting the flexibility and strength so that you are able to move into the right position and hold it. Most people don't have the flexibility even to stand straight. They crane their necks. Their tight chests and shoulders feel more "natural" slumped. That is a signal that you have to stretch and strengthen, not slouch.

> Strengthening muscles through general exercises doesn't automatically "give" you good posture. Plenty of muscular people have terrible posture. Posture is a conscious muscular activity, so it burns calories and is good exercise by itself.

The fitness of your supporting musculature will determine whether you can maintain good posture, or slouch and crane into postures that eventually will be a pain in the neck or behind. How can you tell?

Posture Test. To identify how your body segments line up:

- Stand very near a wall, facing away from the wall, but not touching it.

- Assume a posture that you feel is normal.

- Slowly back up and contact the wall.

- Did your head, shoulders, back, behind, calves, and heels all touch at once? Good posture. Did your behind touch first? You probably slouch forward. You need to concentrate on the back muscles that support your posture upright by pulling toward the back. Did your shoulders touch first? You might be arching backwards and need extra abdominal muscle strengthening to keep your guy wires supporting you from the front. Did the back of your head never touch? You probably have a forward head.

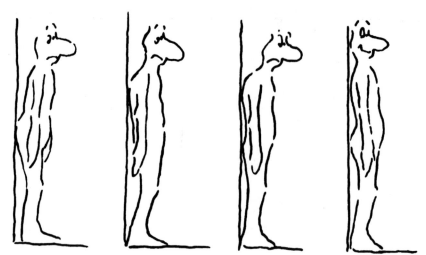

Figure 21.3. Try a posture test by slowly backing up against a wall. Did your behind touch first? Or your shoulders? Did the back of your head never touch? Touch all your segments to the wall comfortably. Keep that good posture all day. Posture can make a difference between a pain-free back and neck, and chronic deformity and misery.

If you habitually keep your head forward of your shoulders, you can learn to correct that by pulling your chin in. Don't tip your chin up or down. Slide your head back until it touches the wall with the rest of your body. Learn this as your daily posture.

Watch other people from the side as they stand, walk, and sit, so that you can identify a forward head. At home, spend time to learn about your own posture. Stand sideways in front of a mirror. Use a second, handheld mirror to look at your profile, or use a three-way mirror. See where your ears are relative to the middle of your shoulder. See where your shoulder is relative to your back and hips, and so on.

Notice how often poor posture is represented in popular magazines, not only by models who do it as an art form, but by people shown in athletic activities. Begin to see how the poor postures put strain on their joints during their activity.

In posture, don't forget your legs, ankles, and feet. Don't let them sag to wherever they sag. Use good leg and foot posture—parallel feet, knees that face straight forward, not tilting inward or outward. When bending your knees for good lifting and for exercise, keep the knee over the foot, not swaying inward. Keep the knee far back— over the heel, rather than leaning forward and allowing the knee to pass the toe.

Good knee posture puts weight on your muscles, rather than on the knee joint. You get free exercise and keep your knees from wearing out.

> Do you feel unnatural standing with good posture?
> When the postural muscles of your back and abdomen
> are so weak and tight that they cannot comfortably support
> you, that means you need to work them to be comfortable,
> not slouch to be comfortable.

Posture Exercise. Many people have such tight muscles in front, and such stretch-weakened muscles in back, that standing up straight feels uncomfortable, tiring, and unnatural. Being unable to maintain upright posture comfortably is a signal of the simple but important exercises that need to be done. The following "wall stand" posture exercise helps you identify and relearn good posture:

- Stand against a wall with your heels, behind, shoulders, and the back of your head all touching the wall at once.

- Look straight forward and hold. Don't force back or stand rigidly like a soldier. Just hold your body upright.

- Pull your shoulders back—not until they hurt, but until the midline of your shoulder is in line with the midline of your body, not in front of it. Your back may be touching the wall, but your shoulders may still be rounded forward.

- You may need to stretch your chest to allow your shoulders to line up with the midline of your body, rather than rounding forward.

- Get the feel of this correct posture, then do it as a habit.

- Do this every 15 minutes or so when you are spending time sitting in a chair or leaning over work on a table.

- An easy way to line up your posture is just to stand with your back against a wall, with your back, behind, and heels touching. Touch the back of your head without lifting or dropping your chin. Don't arch your back; just keep a small natural curve. Do this in the elevator, on the door jam when going into and out of meetings, and against the wall while waiting. When you walk away from the wall, keep the great new posture.

> But isn't it natural to slouch? As natural as wetting your pants.
> At first you make mistakes, but then you learn to "hold" it,
> even when you don't feel like it.

Healthy Sitting Posture

Healthy Sitting With a Lumbar Roll. When you sit in a chair or in the car, use a lumbar roll.

- To get the idea of what a lumbar roll does and what size is good, sit in your chair with your entire back against the back of the chair. Put your forearm behind you, between your low back and the chair. Nestle your arm in the natural space. Lift your upper back against the chair. Your forearm is usually just the right size to fill the space of your low back. It should feel comfortable.

- Try a small rolled towel or commercial lumbar roll between your lower back and the chair. Used properly, the roll will help you have healthy lumbar posture with normal inward curve.

- Don't force your body into an unnaturally straight or arched posture. Lift your upper back against the chair instead of pressing against the roll. Keep your head up, not tilted forward.

- If you find yourself without your lumbar roll at meetings or movies, use a small rolled towel, an article of clothing, or your arm. Inflatable pillows are inexpensive and pack flat and light.

- Commercially available rolls are sometimes too fat. An easy solution for those made of foam is to cut them in half lengthwise, making two long rolls, each round on one surface and flat on the opposite. Put the flat part against the chair and the rounded side to the small of your back. Keep one in the car and one at your desk.

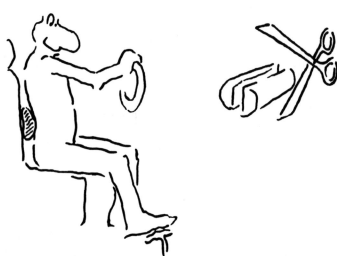

Figure 21.4. Use a lumbar roll when you sit, to maintain the normal inward curve of your low back. Make a lumbar roll from a small cushion or a rolled towel, or cut a cylindrical foam roll into two half-rolls for a custom fit.

Healthy Sitting in Chairs. Chairs often are shaped in a way that, if you sit conforming to them, makes you sit in terrible curved-forward posture. Airplane, bus, and train seats are most famous for this. People worsen the problem by putting a pillow behind their head, instead of low back. For airline seats, use two pillows, one in the natural curve of your low back, and a second behind your upper back. This will help you lean back in the chair, instead of forward. You have to sit upright to rest the back of your head against the headrest.

What about "ergonomic" chairs, "ball" chairs with no back, or kneeling chairs? You can sit poorly in any chair if you slouch and hold your neck tilted forward, no matter how expensive or engineered the chair. They cannot "make" you sit up properly.

Healthy Work Habits

You can do many healthy things for your back during the day:

- When working at your desk, remember to stand up every half hour or so and arch your back in the other direction.

- Chores are no excuse to slouch and reverse your lumbar curve. When cleaning, painting, or fixing, bend your knees rather than curl over the task. Keep your torso upright, and preserve the natural inward curve of your back. It's free exercise – burning calories, toning leg and back muscles—and keeps weight off your joints.

- After bicycling, gardening, cleaning floors, or any other activity where you lean forward for prolonged periods (even with bent knees and good posture), lie facedown, propped up on your elbows so that your back curves backwards.

- When stuck sitting for long periods, during movies or traveling, do small range of motion stretches. Alternately tense and release your leg, back, and torso muscles. Press your palms against your thighs while breathing in and out. Press your palms firmly against the back of your head, and push back with your neck. Make up fun ways to fidget. Keep breathing during all exercises.

- Any time you find yourself bending forward for long periods, counter it with leaning backward.

> Doing your back exercises a few times a week, but keeping the old, bad postures and habits that hurt your back in the first place is like eating cake and ice cream morning, noon, and night, and doing five minutes of aerobics a few times a week. You are not balancing out the harm done.

Healthy Lifting Habits

Exactly what is "lifting right"? Any time you bend over, whether for a drink of water, to jot a note, wash your face, tie your shoe, start the lawn mower, or lift anything, bend your knees and keep your torso as upright as possible. It's not wimpy. It will save your back from cumulative abuse that it was not built to withstand.

- Get close and face the weight.

- Keep your feet apart.

- Bend your knees, not letting your knees flop forward past your toes. Keep your weight back on your heels, not toes. This shifts your weight onto your leg muscles and off your knee joint.

- Keep your torso upright. Don't put your head down to your knees and claim it is healthy lifting because you are bending your knees.

- Take a deep breath and breathe out as you lift.

- Push off your heels, not toes, to keep weight on your muscles, not knee joint.

- Think, "I don't want to hurt my back," *before* you just lean over and yank.

- Lift slowly. Don't arch your back on the way up, or if you lift the weight overhead.

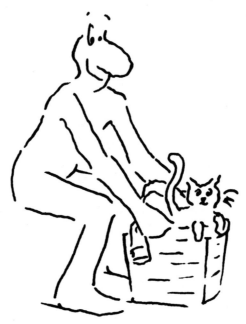

Figure 21.5. Safe lifting technique. Keep your torso upright, get close and face the weight, bend your knees keeping your feet apart, and lift slowly. Do this any time you lift anything—laundry, packages, or weights in the gym.

If you lift dumbbells for back strength, don't bend over and lift. Lie facedown on a flat or tilted bench. If you choose to stand, support your weight with one hand on a bench or your knee. You hear all the time not to bend over and lift anything because it's bad for your back, yet people go to a gym and magically forget this. They bend right over and lift weights, even thinking it will help their back.

Safe Lifting With Bad Knees. Many people use the excuse of bad knees to bend and lift straight-legged. Bad knees are no excuse to make your back bad, too. If your knees hurt, go to a good orthopedist to find out why. Many knee complaints result over time just like back and neck pain—from poor walking and standing habits that wear, tear, and unevenly load the knee joint, and from uneven muscle strength and flexibility. Get your knees properly diagnosed, then do the knee exercises your doctor or physical therapist prescribes to make your knees better. (Knees are for another book.)

Proper bending should not hurt your knees. Bending and strengthening your legs often is important to strengthening your knees to make them better again.

Use the "golfer's pickup" to bend over:

- Put one foot in back of the other.

- Put your hand on your thigh.

- Lean your weight on your hand.

- Bend your knees as much as comfortable, keeping the weight of your upper body supported.

- Keep your weight on the heel of the forward foot, not toe. Keep your weight on both legs, not only thrown forward onto the front knee.

Try it now for practice.

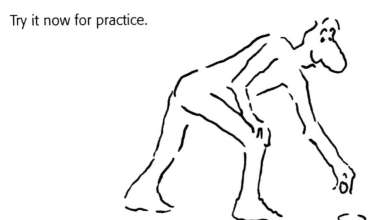

Figure 21.6. Use the "golfer's pickup" when picking up small things. You protect your back by supporting your upper body weight on your knee, and reduce stress on your knees by keeping a wide stance.

Healthy Standing Around

Whether standing in line, talking with people, or doing dishes, you can do several, easy, quick maneuvers to help your back.

- Check your back posture and correct it—are you arching too much? Use your abs to correct it as detailed in Chapter 7 on abs. Are you slouching so that you are rounding your back or removing the inward curve of your low back? Pull yourself up with your back muscles. Use your muscles all the time.

- Check your neck posture and correct it. Is your head forward? Chin out? Pull it back in without tensing your neck. Just like bending your arm, you don't tense it, you just move it to where you want it to go.

- Check your leg posture and correct it. Are your knees and toes facing straight ahead? Are they facing in or out, or swaying or bowing? Keep your knees slightly bent and your weight up on your muscles; don't "lock" your knee straight. Keep weight on the sole of your foot, not the arch.

- Stand with one foot supported. That's why bars have that rail at shin level. At the kitchen sink, you can open the under-sink door and rest your foot on the shelf.

- When stuck standing around for long periods, tuck your hips and pelvis in to stretch your back. Alternately tense and relax your ab, leg, and back muscles. Press your palms firmly against your thighs and release to work your torso muscles. Movement and muscle contraction keep blood from pooling in your legs.

> Being told to "stand up straight" is like being told, "When someone is a complete jerk to you, don't get angry." You know that is the healthy response, but how do you do it? You need to learn specific techniques and do it even when you don't feel like it.
>
> It's like saying, "To bowl a 300 game, throw a heavy ball against the pins and knock them all down every time." It's true, but you need motor control and practice.
>
> Good posture needs training, lots of practice, and doing it even when you don't feel like it.

Healthy Exercises

Unfortunately, back pain is sometimes regarded the way a heart attack was years ago—as a condition, not an injury. Sufferers of both were relegated to the "cardiac cripple" status of inactivity; they were told never to exercise or lift weights, and even to restrict activities of daily living. In that way a tragic cycle of disuse and declining ability perpetuates. Back muscles, like heart muscles, need exercise to develop in progressive sane ways until they meet your needs. Increased endurance of posture muscles of the back reduces back and knee pain over a long day. Increased strength reduces your chance of hurting your back, knees, and shoulders from lifting packages and weights. See Chapter 3, "Improving Your Fitness," for more on increasing muscle endurance and strength.

If you have back and/or neck pain, the exercises you need to do will be specific for the type of pain. There are many exercises that strengthen and stretch the hips, back, neck, abdominal muscles, and leg muscles, to reduce back and neck pain. See your physician or physical therapist before starting any exercise program, particularly if you have existing pain.

Neck Exercises. One exercise that corrects a forward head is called the "double-chin" exercise. Pull your head back into proper alignment in an exaggerated way, so that your chin becomes a "double chin." This exercise doesn't "fix" the problem, but helps you identify the muscles in back of your neck and how to pull your neck in. Hold for 10 counts, release, and repeat. Then remember to hold your head back in normal position all the time.

Abdominal Exercises. Abdominal exercises are covered in Chapter 7. Proper use of abdominal muscles is important to support your torso from swaying backward. Don't make abs your only exercise. Exercises that contract your back muscles are crucial to complete the support your back needs to keep from slouching forward. These important exercises are described next.

Upper Back Extension (also good for your neck)

Besides giving you a beautiful line down your back for evening gown wear, this exercise is a mainstay of most back-strengthening and pain-reduction programs.

- Lie facedown, hands at your sides, and off the floor. Slowly lift your upper body a few inches. This action is called back extension. Then lower back to the floor. Don't force. Don't tilt your head back. Keep your head in line with your body. If you feel any pinching, don't do this exercise, and see your doctor. If you feel muscles working, that is right. Start with one or two lifts. See how you feel the next day. If you feel no pain, gradually increase to 10 repetitions three times a week.

- To progress, do more repetitions, and move your arms from your sides to overhead.

- If you have a bench, lie on the bench facedown. Let your legs hang off the bench and your feet touch the floor. When you lift your torso, lift until your back is straight, rather than arched.

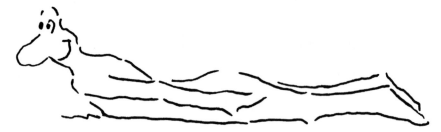

Figure 21.7. Upper back extension strengthens your upper back muscles, important for posture and back pain control. Don't yank or force upwards or tilt your head back. Lift your arms and upper body with control.

Lower Back Extension. Following are several ways to contract the muscles of your low back to work them:

- Lie facedown, chin on hands. Lift one leg off the floor, knee straight. Hold and lower. Easy does it. Then switch legs.

- To progress, lift both legs together. This exercise is great for your back and behind.

- If you have a low bench, lie on the bench facedown, and let your feet touch the floor. Lift your legs until your back is straight, rather than arched.

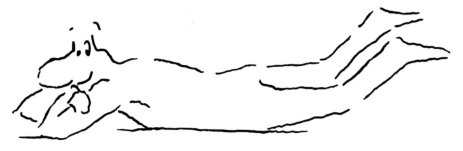

Figure 21.8. Lower back extension strengthens your lower back muscles, important for posture and back pain control. One way to do lower back extension is to lie facedown on the floor or over a bench and gently lift one or both legs.

- Lie on your back, both knees bent. Lift your behind off the floor and hold for 10 seconds, then lower. Work up to 10 repetitions. To progress to a harder variation, do this with only one leg. Cross one ankle over the opposite knee, or just hold one foot off the floor, and lift your hips. This works your back, abs, and hamstrings.

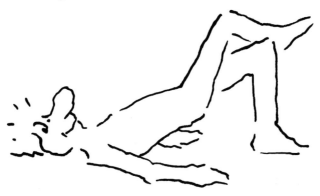

Figure 21.9. Supine lower back and gluteal extension strengthens your low back, lower abs, hamstrings, and gluteal muscles.

- If you go to a gym that has weight machines, look for the back machine. You sit with a pad against your back and curl it backward. It should be next to the abdominal machine (where you sit with a pad against your abdomen and curl it forward.) In a physical therapy setting, these machines will have special locks that limit how far you can push backwards. As your back gets better, the lock is moved to allow more range of motion. This limit to motion is important during physical therapy of injured backs. Check with your doctor before using machines if you have a back injury.

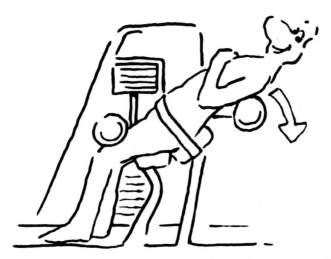

Figure 21.10. Exercise to contract your back muscles is crucial for back health, good posture, and pain control.

> Most back pain is a simple matter of muscle weakness, tightness, and non-use creating mechanical stress, segments slipping around, and wear and tear, so is retrainable and easily remedied.

Modifications for Special Populations. Some people with specific back disorders like facet pain and a slippage of vertebrae called spondylolisthesis (spon-di-lo-lis-THEE'-sis) should not actively arch their back to a high degree. However, contracting the back muscles is crucial to strengthening and necessary to retrain the muscles to support the area properly to prevent damage from the poor resulting postures. Exercises that contract the back muscles without arching past the neutral-straight position are effective and important for rehabilitation and pain control. Physical therapy centers and many gyms have back machines that allow active back extension while limiting the range to not exceed the straight position.

If you have been told that you shouldn't extend your back past the straight position, you can still exercise your back muscles in several ways.

- For your upper back, one easy exercise without arching your back is to lie facedown on the floor or over a bench, and lift only your arms, not your upper body.

- For your lower back, lean over a chair and lift one leg in back. If you have a bench, you can lie on the bench, so that the bench extends from your chin to your hips, with your legs hanging freely to the floor. Then lift one or both legs up from the floor until your body is straight.

- Kneel on all fours on a soft mat. Raise one leg until it is straight behind you. Don't arch your back. Do the work with your muscles.

- When you progress, lift your opposite arm in front of you at the same time you lift one leg. Hold.

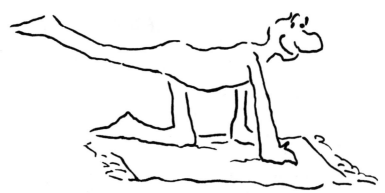

Figure 21.11. Some people with specific back disorders do better with modified back exercises.

Surprising Back Exercises. Push-ups are surprisingly good for your back. They use a lot of back and abdominal stabilization just holding the "ready" position. Even if you are not able to do push-ups, hold the ready position. Don't let your back arch—that is the same problem while standing up that drops your weight onto the low back and makes it hurt in the first place. Keep elbows slightly bent. If your arms are so weak that you lock out the elbows, strengthen them, but don't use that as an excuse to hurt your elbow joints next.

Do back exercises standing up. Just as detailed in Chapter 7 on abs, you need to exercise your back the way you need it in real life—isometrically and standing up so that you retrain how to stabilize against gravity and loads.

Secure the middle of a long rubber tube around a doorknob or other device at waist height. Hold both ends in front of you and stand far enough back that you create the desired tension on the band. Pull both arms straight down to your sides and hold. Repeat. If you consciously hold proper posture while doing this, you help all your torso-stabilizing muscles. Now, with both arms still straight, lift both arms up overhead and hold without letting your back arch or lean backward. The whole idea is to train you to use good postural mechanics during motion. Repeat. Keep breathing. Turn to the side and use the same concepts to design exercises to strengthen your back to hold strong and steady during common movements.

> The whole point and benefit of "doing" back exercises is lost when you just do back exercises without thought to using the exercise to retrain your muscles and brain how to hold good posture all the time.

Healthy Stretches

Good range of motion in all directions helps prevent back pain. Warm up before you stretch. Warm-up means just what it says. Raise your body temperature. Slow jogging, bicycling, or anything that gets you to break a light sweat will make stretching safer. See Chapter 5 on warm-ups. See your physician before attempting any back exercises and for a back exercise program that suits your own back health.

Hamstring and Lower Back Stretches. Leaning over at the waist for toe touches does stretch your back and hamstrings, but it is not the best stretch for regular use. Although it often feels good on tight muscles, it's tough on your back in the long run. A safer back stretch is to lie on your back and stretch one leg at a time by holding it straight in the air and pulling it gently toward you.

A variation of this stretch, where the bent knee is pressed to the chest, produced an injury reported in the March 1993 *New England Journal of Medicine*. A compression injury named "stretcher's scrotum" occurred when a man performing the stretch wore restrictive gym shorts, squeezing the testes between the bent leg and the body. The journal cautioned that practitioners prescribing such stretches for back pain should recommend that males wear loose, stretchable pants. Another good hamstring stretch is to stand with one heel propped up on a chair, keeping the inward curve of your lower back, standing with your foot pointed straight forward, and sticking your behind out a little. Hamstring stretches are covered in Chapter 6.

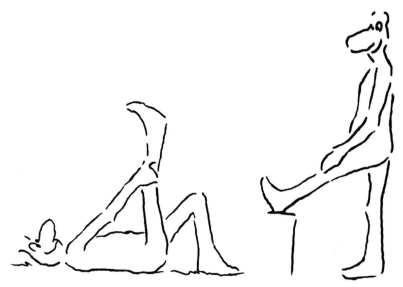

Figure 21.12. These two good stretches for your hamstrings are done without bending over from a stand. Bending over from a stand is tough on your back. When doing this stretch while standing, keep your back upright in normal alignment, rather than bent over forward.

Hip Stretches. Hip flexors, the muscles that bend your hip and raise your leg, as in walking, were covered in detail in Chapter 6 on stretching, and Chapter 7 on abdominal muscles. Tight, short hip flexors are common. Hip flexor stretches are important to back health, but unfortunately neglected.

Note: If you have a hip replacement, do not do any exercises without clearing them with your hip team. You can dislocate the prosthetic (your artificial hip).

An easy way to stretch your hip flexors is the lunge. The lunge is often done improperly so that there is little or no stretch on the hip flexors. To do it properly, stand with your feet comfortably apart, then slide one foot in back of you as far as you can do comfortably. The trick is to not lean forward, and not arch backward, but tuck your behind under you. You will feel the stretch in your forward leg where it normally creases in front, in an area about the size of a small pancake. Try lowering gently by bending your knees, keeping your body upright. This turns the stretch into a wonderful, combined dynamic stretch and leg strengthener. This is also a healthy way to pick up things. Many people bend wrong all day to get things—bending at the waist. Use the lunge instead and get free exercise all day.

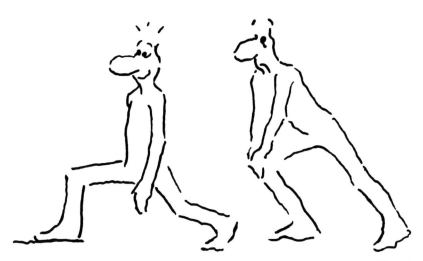

Figure 21.13. The lunge is a good hip flexor stretch for the back leg. Avoid leaning forward or you won't stretch your back leg, but may stress your forward knee. Stand upright and tuck your behind inward until you feel the stretch in the back hip. Try bending your knees to lower and raise your body for a great leg strengthener. Use this to bend for things all day for a built-in workout without ever going to a gym.

Other hip muscles that easily tighten are those that turn your leg outward, called external rotators. They are in the back of your hip. A wonderful stretch for them can be done lying down or sitting.

- Lie on your back, both knees bent, feet on the floor. Cross one ankle over the other knee. Push your crossed knee away with your hand. If you can't reach your knee, pull your foot on the floor closer to your behind (or get longer arms). Lift your foot from the floor so that both legs come toward you. Keep pushing your crossed knee away with your hand. Do both sides.

- Here is the same stretch done in a chair or on the edge of the bed: Sit upright, preserving the small inward curve of your back. Cross one ankle over the other knee. Push your crossed knee down with your hand. Keep your body upright. If you curl your back, you will not feel this stretch. Lift your chest up and arch your back. Press your lower abdomen to your leg. Don't curl your upper body or tilt your head down. Do both sides.

The inside of your hip also gets tight from sitting all day. The following stretch is a good combination hip and balance exercise:

- Stand on one leg. Bend the other knee to the side and put your foot against the inside of your standing leg. In yoga this is called the "tree pose." Bring your bent knee straight out to the side. Don't slouch, stick your behind out, or slump your hip forward. Use a mirror for positioning. To help you start out, try it with your back against the wall. Bring your bent knee as close to the wall as you can without turning your body. Raise your hands overhead, keeping them touching the wall (or close, until you can touch). To progress, bend sideways as a tree would bow in the wind. Keep arms, back, and knee against the wall.

- Try the same stretch lying down. Lie flat and straight. Bend one knee to the side with foot against the inside of the straight leg. Press the bent knee to the floor (gradually). Raise arms overhead, keeping them close to or on the floor. Repeat on the other side.

Now that you have stretched outward, stretch your hips inward.

- In the same pose on the floor, keep your foot touching your knee and rotate the bent leg over the other leg toward the floor. Keep your shoulders and back on the floor. Do both sides.

- Sit with both feet on the floor, widely separated. Bring your knees together. Or lie on your back, knees bent, feet separated. Straighten your legs and roll your leg inward. Cross your ankles with feet turned in. Experiment with comfortable stretches.

- Lie on the floor or bed, flat and straight. Cross one leg over the other leg, both knees fairly straight. Keep moving the crossed leg like the big hand of a clock. The bottom leg points at 6 on the clock face. The moving leg moves past 7, then 8, then 9. Maybe even 10 or later. Then come back down through 9, 8, 7, to 6 again. Turn your hip but keep shoulders against the surface. Work until you can go all the way around the clock to 12, then back to 6. Do both sides.

Back Stretches. Many exercise programs concentrate on bending forward, forward, and more forward. For back health, add stretches in the other direction. Try these two after bicycling, gardening, cleaning floors, prolonged sitting, or any activity where you lean forward for prolonged periods:

- Stand up with your hands on your low back. Lean back into an arch. Lift your upper back upward, not downward, squashing your low back. Don't let your low back "crease." Use your muscles to control the curve of your low back into an even curve along your whole back.

- Another variation is to lie facedown. Slowly, gently press up, keeping your hips on the floor or bed. Go only to the point where you feel stretch, not pain. As above, don't crease at one joint; use muscles to curve your whole back evenly.

If you habitually stand with your back arched, your low back may tighten to the point where you can't straighten it. All the ab exercises in the world won't help you control your posture because you're stuck in the "booty-out" posture.

- Lie on your back, with knees bent and feet on the floor. Can you flatten your back against the floor using abs? Can you bring your knees to your chest? Practice this until you have low back mobility. Try "child's pose," called that because babies and young children often sleep like this. Sit on the floor (or bed) on your hands and knees. Bend your knees and lean back on your heels to bring your head to your knees. Rest there, breathing full normal breaths. If it hurts your knees or back, stop and try it face up instead, curling knees toward chest in a comfortable range. If that hurts, don't do it at all. If you have a bulging disk, this is not a good exercise. Stay with back extension under supervision.

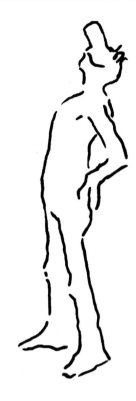

Figure 21.14. Take frequent breaks from sitting or working to stretch your back and neck in the other direction.

Neck Stretches

- For healthy neck range of motion, don't roll your head; just align your ears over your shoulders and look down, look up, look left, look right, and tip each ear to each shoulder. The bones of your neck are not made to roll around each other, a motion called circumduction. Excessive rolling is just wear and tear, and can be uncomfortable for people with neck complaints.

Forced neck stretches, like shoulder stands, push discs outward to the back, increasing risk of herniation over time. Forced head turning and rotation by practitioners has been documented to sometimes result in stroke, even death from tearing neck blood vessels.

- Commonly, neck pain from a forward-head posture is along the top of each shoulder, down from your neck, and around your shoulder blades. A good stretch to relieve this is to put one hand behind you in the opposite back pants pocket (or imaginary pocket). Keep your face straight forward, then gently tilt your head toward your hand.

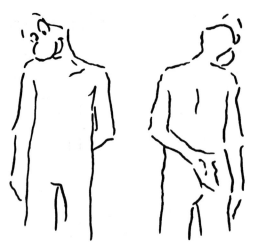

Figure 21.15. This stretch takes the tightness out of your neck and shoulders. Tip your ear toward your shoulder, keeping your face looking forward, not down. It takes only a moment to do this one. Try it often.

Tips for Avoiding Back and Neck Pain

- Stand and sit keeping the normal inward curve of your lower back. Don't let your back arch more. Don't reverse the curve by sitting round-shouldered and round-backed.

- Don't stand, lift, or reach overhead by exaggerating the arch in your low back.

- Use a lumbar roll when sitting. Get one for the car and one for work.

- Regularly stretch your hamstrings, hip flexors, back, and neck. See Chapter 6.

- Strengthen your back with exercises that include extension. Stretches are not strengtheners. You need to actively contract your back muscles to make them stronger. Ab exercises alone are only one side of the ring of support that you need.

- Do leg exercises that develop your thigh and behind muscles (quadriceps and gluteal muscles) for the shock absorption your back needs, and the leg strength needed to lift with your legs, not your back.

- Any time you bend down, bend your knees, keeping your body upright.

- Use proper lifting technique. When lifting anything, get close, face the weight, feet apart, bend your knees. Keep your torso upright. Lift slowly. Keep the weight close to you.

- Stand up after every half hour or so of sitting, and stretch your back in the other direction.

Treating Back and Neck Pain

Because most ordinary back or neck pain goes away by itself (although temporarily), much confusion results about what relieved it. If you tried a home remedy, however far-fetched, you think the remedy worked. For this reason, the market is flooded with snake-oil potions for back pain. Understandably, many back and neck pain sufferers will try anything.

Address the Cause. Many people take back pain remedies, then go right back to the standing, sitting, and lifting problems that gave them the trouble in the first place. Then they eventually get more back and neck pain. They don't understand it. They call it stress. They try chiropractors, acupuncture, prescription and over-the-counter medications, herbal remedies, psychotherapy, and prayer. They do everything except change the postural habits that got them into the mess. Some wind up in surgery, and still their pain persists. They think they are cursed. They are told they have to learn to "live with pain." Luckily, it does not have to be that way. See your physician for a good diagnosis and a referral to a solid back exercise program to speed recovery and decrease your chance of it recurring.

> People take back pain remedies, then go right back to the bad habits that gave them back pain in the first place. They don't understand when their pain returns, because they thought they were "fixed." But they didn't fix the cause.

Diagnosis. Get an accurate diagnosis from a physician specializing in orthopedics. The Greek word *gnosis* means "knowing" or "recognizing." *Dia* is a word element that, in this context, means "completely." It's crucial to know completely. Getting rid of pain and the disability that goes with it means treating the cause. Don't let any practitioner treat you without knowing what's wrong first, particularly for severe pain.

First Aid. Even though accurate diagnosis is so important, immediate treatment for most back pain is similar. Reduce inflammation that causes pain by briefly using anti-inflammatory medications and ice packs. Relax muscular spasm with muscle-relaxing medications and stretches. Medications are meant to be used only for the first day or so. Muscle relaxers are not appropriate for long-term use for most back pain. The entire purpose is to knock out the spasm right away, then let your body heal. If you have back muscles in spasm, the pain can be crippling, but it can be a simple matter to get out the spasm. A trained massage therapist, physical therapist, or osteopath can identify spasm and stretch it out with special release techniques.

The relief is quick and seems to be miraculous, but it is often a simple matter. Muscles are not supposed to be left in spasm or produce a long-term condition. For more on muscle spasm, see Chapter 30 on leg cramps.

Identify the things you do that caused the problem. Don't just injure your back, allow it to go into spasm and pain, and go to someone to "fix" it. It is not a fix. Make easy modifications in your routine to avoid the whole problem in the future. Then, as pain subsides, begin a good back-exercise program to increase your resistance to future injury. Use ice after your workouts and at the end of every long day. The old thinking of long bed rest for back pain has been found to be counterproductive. It just further weakens and deconditions you. You need activity and the right back exercises.

Pain can usually be tremendously reduced with proper exercises that relieve the muscle spasm or stop compressing and pushing on your discs. Recent studies have emphasized how important it is to get early exercise after back injury, and how damaging bed rest can be.

What About Shots? Maybe you knew someone who had terrible back or neck pain, got a shot, and was immediately fine. These shots are usually a special anti-inflammatory, delivered right into the swollen, inflamed area. This is an alternative to taking anti-inflammatories by mouth, and is often quick and effective. Anti-inflammatories reduce the space-occupying swelling and pain, and stop the pain/spasm cycle that is so important to eliminate early in the pain process. Two important cautions are that corticosteroid injections temporarily stop the healing process and make the area temporarily weak and susceptible to tearing. Be careful to take it easy after these shots, to do no further harm to the area.

Surgery Rarely Needed. Surgery for disc herniation and most other back pain is rarely necessary. This happy discovery was made when back patients were referred to physical therapy for back exercises to condition them for the physical stress of surgery. By surgery time, most of the people didn't need it. There are many problems from surgery. There is the strain of the surgery itself and deconditioning from the recovery period. Your bones need your discs for cushioning and to keep from grinding bone directly on bone. After surgery to remove all or part of a disc, you are subject to early wear and tear, possibly predisposing you to early arthritis. That is why surgeons try to leave as much of the disc as possible when doing disc surgery.

Spinal fusion is surgery to fuse one vertebra to the next. It is the extreme, last resort. The area no longer moves at all. The immobile area does not function normally and transfers compensating strain to other areas. The vertebrae and discs above and below the fused sites must move more for you to have even close to the function you had before your surgery. That means much more wear and tear on those sections than they were designed for. A problem with spinal fusion is that the person must sometimes return to have the next segments fused too, when they wear out from the trauma of working overtime next to a fused segment.

Most herniations, and their associated inflammation, will heal, shrink, and go back into place—if you let them, and that big "if" is up to you. Watch your posture while sitting and standing. When you sit, use a lumbar roll. See your physician for a prescription for back exercises that are right for you. Extension exercises usually bring good results to reduce pain, slowly allow the disc to return into place, and strengthen muscles to keep your posture healthy for your back. These exercises are easy for you to do yourself at home after a bit of instruction.

> What's the most effective treatment for back or neck pain?
> Not drugs, not surgery. Just simple exercises.

When You Wake Up. Disc pain is usually worst upon waking in the morning because your discs customarily swell a bit overnight. For injured discs, this normal swelling increases the pain. The thing you don't want to do when you wake is to sit at the edge of the bed in flexion. No one should do that, particularly not anyone with disc trouble. It puts outward pressure on discs when they are the most vulnerable. Instead, turn facedown and lie propped slightly on your elbows, in extension, for a few moments or so. Lying prone reduces pain and pressure. (But don't fall back to sleep.)

> When you first wake up, turn facedown and lie propped slightly
> on your elbows for a few moments, instead of sitting.
> In most cases, it's better for your discs.

When you get out of bed, and any time you get up from a lying-down position, roll to your side first, then push up with your arms, rather than "curling up" with a sit-up motion. Rolling to the side is a good back habit for everyone.

When making beds in the morning, don't lean over and lift. Bend your knees, keep your torso upright, and use the usual safe-lifting mechanics.

Back and Neck Pain Myths

All of the following statements are false. Each is covered in this chapter and the previous one. Understanding the mechanics of back pain is key to changing the cause, instead of just doing "remedies."

- Back and neck pain happens because evolutionarily, we began walking upright on two legs.

- Back pain is usually from lifting something the wrong way one day.

- Once you have back pain, you'll always have back pain.

- Back or neck pain is usually a serious, long-term condition.

- Women get more back pain than men.

- When you get back pain, it is important to get bed rest. The more, the better. Several days to a week is best, not getting out of bed except for bathroom activities, if that.

- For back pain rehab, abs classes are the best exercise.

- You can herniate a disc just from sneezing or getting out of bed in the morning, so it is practically unavoidable, and therefore it doesn't matter how you lift things.

- When you have back pain, it is important to take it easy, and sit down often to conserve energy.

- Back pain is a normal part of getting older.

Practice "Safe Necks"

This section detailed the mechanics of back and neck care that apply to most back pain. There is much you can do to easily prevent back and neck pain so that you don't need to treat it. Good mechanics is the key to keeping your back and neck healthy and pain free.

Back and Neck Pain Myths (cont'd)

- Eventually, you will need surgery, the most effective, true cure for back pain.

- If you have back pain, you should sleep on a board or hard mattress.

- You should be an adult and stop complaining about back pain. You must learn how to cope and live with it. You should go to a pain clinic to learn how to accept the pain.

- The back is a very different system anatomically than the rest of you, so is very difficult to fix.

- No one knows what causes back pain.

- If back pain is caused by a bad disc, you are really finished.

- "I don't need to know about back pain because I do yoga (tennis, karate, swimming...)."

- "I don't need to know about back pain because I went to the doctor and got it fixed."

- "I don't need to know about back pain—the last time I had back pain, I took vitamin xyz (or meditated, or rubbed on a potion, or did deep breathing, or _____), and that cured it after only a few days."

- The x-ray shows nothing, so that means you are a lying, complaining, wimpy, whining, attention-seeking hypochondriac.

Resources for More Information

American Physical Therapy Association   (www.apta.org)
1111 N. Fairfax Street
Alexandria, Virginia 22314-1488
(800) 999-APTA • (703) 684-2782
fax (703) 684-7343
Booklets, referrals to local physical therapists, and on-line computer resources.

American Podiatric Medical Association   (www.apma.org)
9312 Old Georgetown Road
Bethesda, MD 20814
(301) 571-9200

Calcium, Protein, Space Flight, Exercise, and Your Bones— A Detective Story

Current recommendations for the prevention of osteoporosis may actually be detrimental to health.

— J. Strain, researcher at the Biomedical Sciences Research Centre, University of Ulster, in Med. Hypotheses. 1988 Dec; 27(4): pp333-8.

Join me on an international detective story. The beginning is deceptively simple. Your bones need calcium; milk has calcium. Then questions begin creeping in. Why do some vegetarians have a lower incidence of osteoporosis than the general population? Why do some groups of Japanese, whose calcium intake is historically low, develop osteoporosis, while others don't? Why do African Bantu women, who eat relatively little calcium, have low rates of osteoporosis? Why doesn't the very high-calcium diet of Eskimos prevent their suffering the highest rate of osteoporosis in the world? Why do astronauts lose bone in space, no matter what they eat?

The detective story opens with four separate studies. Researchers at the Mayo Clinic found no correlation between calcium intake and age-related bone loss after bone finishes forming in early adulthood. Then, at Tufts University, researchers concluded that calcium had no effect on preventing bone loss in the first five years or so after menopause. From Cornell came a study in 1989 reporting: "It was not clear that increased calcium intake has a significant impact on osteoporosis or other chronic diseases that have been linked to calcium nutriture." More work published in the *Journal of the American Medical Woman's Association* concluded that calcium intake alone will "neither guarantee optimal bone growth nor protect against bone loss if other critical factors are missing."

The search for these critical factors begins with a trip back in time and the realization that calcium cannot only be excreted from your body before it has any chance of connecting with your bones, but driven from existing bone.

Your Changing Bones

Your bones are alive. They continuously break down and rebuild. Throughout your life, you make new bone cells and break down and assimilate old ones. That recycling process is your body doing its normal business of cell maintenance. You exchange about three to five percent of your bone cells every year this way. All is well as long as you replace at least as much as you lose, like money in your bank account. As you age, you do less bone making and more bone losing. That isn't bad by itself. It depends how much bone you start out with and how much you lose. The good news is that these are things you can control, to a large extent.

What Is Osteoporosis?

With osteoporosis, you lose too much bone, leaving spaces in your bones, making them porous and fragile. *Osteo-* is a Greek word element meaning "bone." *Porosis* means "porous." Osteoporosis is a serious degenerative bone disorder. Because bone loss is painless until you break a bone, you probably won't know that bone loss is happening in your body. Fractures then easily occur from little or no noticeable cause. Healing is long, sometimes never occurring.

The Toll of Osteoporosis

Osteoporosis takes a heavy toll.

- An estimated 1.5 million osteoporotic fractures occur in the United States yearly. That works out to 4,110 fractures every day or one every 21 seconds.

- Osteoporosis-induced hip and spine fractures are a major cause of illness and death among older women and, as they live longer, among men as well.

- In 2002, the number of people in the United States aged 50 and older at risk for osteoporosis and low bone mass was 44 million.

- One woman in three over the age of 65 will suffer fractures of the spine, and from 10 to 15% of all white women will fracture their hip.

- Hip fractures are fatal within one year in up to about 20% of cases.

- Half of those surviving a hip or spine fracture never walk unaided again, leaving about a quarter of the elderly female population of the United States disabled by severe osteoporosis. These risks exceed a woman's risk of developing breast, uterine, and ovarian cancer combined.

- Occurrence in women is higher than in men; but osteoporosis in men is a substantial problem in medicine and society. One in eight men over age 50 will have an osteoporosis-related fracture. This risk is greater than his risk of prostate cancer. The death rate in the year following a hip fracture is nearly twice as high for men as for women.

Why Young People Need to Know About Bone Health

Osteoporosis is not something that just happens to old people; it begins in youth. Your bone density in later years depends on what you are doing right now. Risk factors during youth can reduce the bone density of a 20- or 30-year-old to the equivalent of someone in their seventies.

Until your mid-thirties your bones are in an active growth phase that will determine your peak amount of bone. Building high peak bone mass in youth is like saving more money in the bank now for retirement later. It allows you to lose bone later in life through normal processes, without falling to dangerously low amounts as you make "withdrawals." After a variable plateau period up to around age 40, bone loss begins silently, varying greatly from your genetically determined potential, depending on your food and exercise habits.

Like heart disease, bone loss is a gradual process. The time to actively direct its course is now, to prevent it from becoming serious later. Once bone loss becomes serious, it is not easily reversible. By the time osteoporosis is usually diagnosed, from 50 to 75% of bone may be gone from your skeleton.

> Developing the most bone mass you can by the time your skeleton matures in adulthood may be the best protection against bone loss and fractures later on. It may be that low peak bone mass, not greater-than-average bone loss, causes osteoporosis.

Where Does Osteoporosis Affect You?

Three sites are most at risk for osteoporosis:

- Wrist.

- Upper back.

- Upper leg bone where it joins your hip. This upper leg bone is what usually breaks when you hear of someone "breaking their hip."

When bone thins too much in your upper back bones, they slowly begin to crush. Because of many forces on these bones, the front of each vertebra crushes more than the back, giving a wedge shape to each bone, like triangles of cheese. Wedge fractures create the classic humped-back or "Dowager's Hump," with height losses up to five inches. The Hunchback of Notre Dame probably had osteoporosis.

Falls may fracture a wrist that would not have otherwise broken. A broken wrist may be a warning sign of osteoporosis impending in the hip or back. Tooth loss is another early warning sign. So much bone is lost from the jaw that teeth loosen, then are lost.

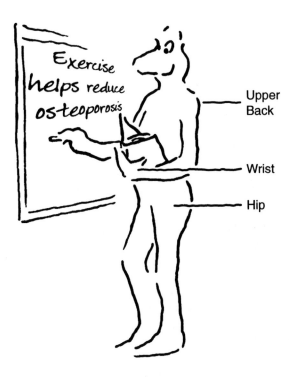

Figure 22.1. The main sites of bone loss with aging in both men and women are your upper back, wrist, and hip. The time to prevent problems later is now.

Why Are These Particular Sites at Risk?

About 1% of your skeletal calcium is readily available to supply your daily body processes. This bone pool is stored mostly in your spine bones, called vertebrae, and the ends of your long bones in a spongy, supportive mesh called trabecular bone (tra-BECK'-you-lar). When your body needs calcium, it takes it first from these stockpiles. The result is fractures of the wrist and vertebrae. These fractures occur mainly in women, because of decreased estrogen around menopause. Elderly men also may suffer from vertebral crush fractures.

In men and women over age 75, both trabecular and cortical bone are lost. The dense surface of your bones is called cortical bone. Long bones like those in your arms and legs are mostly cortical bone. Loss of too much cortical bone causes hip fractures. These fractures occur easily, even from normal stresses, because of the weakened bone structure.

Factors Affecting Risk

It is unfortunately common to believe that osteoporosis prevention is simply a matter of drinking milk. There are many factors in osteoporosis, not all of which are completely understood. There are at least four major determinants of how much bone mass you can achieve in your younger years, how much you later lose, and consequently, of fracture risk: genetics, nutrition, hormonal factors, and exercise.

Genetics. Different ethnic and racial groups differ in natural bone density. Everyone loses bone with age, but the bones of Caucasians are typically less dense than those of African-Americans, Hispanics, and Asians at all age levels. Osteoporosis most often affects Caucasians.

There also may be inherited tendencies to osteoporosis among families. Bone density in healthy mother-daughter pairs seems to match up pretty well. Daughters of women with osteoporosis often have lower bone density in similar body sites as their mothers. Peak bone mass and density may be influenced by fathers too. These tendencies can be countered with practices to protect bone density, described later in this section.

Nutrition. The role of high calcium intake in adulthood is not really clear. You not only need to get enough calcium, you need to avoid too much of things that cause you to lose calcium from your bones, and things that interfere with calcium absorption. Of the major determinants of risk of osteoporosis, nutrition is one of the easiest to take charge of in your life.

Protein. A succession of well-controlled studies published since 1920 showed increased urinary calcium loss with increased meat in the diet. In 1988, a published study by the Center for Mineral Metabolism and Clinical Research in Texas concluded that calcium loss due to the animal protein of milk raises the risk of osteoporosis. Studies find that animal protein in meat and dairy increases calcium loss, even with high calcium intake, and even when the animal versus vegetable diet is the same in sodium, potassium, calcium, phosphorus, magnesium, and total protein. The high sulfur content of animal protein raises acid production in your system. The acid increases bone calcium loss and reduces your ability to absorb it.

One study found that by age 80, 1,600 women on a lacto-ovo vegetarian diet for at least 20 years had lost only 18% bone mineral compared to closely paired meat-eating women, who lost 35%. The effect of animal protein to increase urinary calcium loss and decrease bone density is also thought to raise risk of another disease of bone loss—tooth loss from gum bone ridge resorption. The less animal protein, the less the loss.

Copper. A 1988 study from the University of Ulster linked mild dietary copper deficiency with osteoporosis in both humans and animals. Medical literature states copper is abundant in normal diets but doesn't consider common barriers to copper utilization. The lactose in dairy products can interfere with copper metabolism. High sugar intake increases urinary excretion of both calcium and copper.

Vitamin D. Availability of Vitamin D, required for calcium absorption in the small intestine, dwindles with aging. Your kidney reduces Vitamin D synthesis, you have less outdoor sun exposure, and the function or number of Vitamin D-binding receptors in your intestine declines.

Caffeine. Caffeine may make you excrete more calcium in your urine, but relation to risk is not certain.

Alcohol. Osteoporosis is more common in alcoholics than in nonalcoholics of the same age. Alcohol is directly toxic to bone cells. Alcoholism contributes to bone loss through poor nutrition, liver disease, poor calcium and Vitamin D absorption, and by interfering with parathyroid gland function. Your parathyroids are four little kidney-shaped glands near, or on, your thyroid gland. They secrete a hormone you need to metabolize calcium and phosphorus.

Smoking. Smoking, like alcohol, is directly toxic to bone cells. Cigarette smoking also interferes with calcium absorption and estrogen, and is associated with earlier menopause and bone loss than in nonsmokers.

Calcium. The issue of calcium requirement provokes all kinds of debate. Many factors affect calcium absorption and excretion, making it difficult to pin down just how much calcium you need. In the 1960s and 1970s, major textbooks of medicine did not consider calcium important in osteoporosis development or prevention, or only considered calcium malabsorption disorders. In the 1980s and 1990s, a calcium mania swept the public. Although much is still unknown, it is pretty well-established that calcium intake influences bone mass formation until adulthood. In this way, calcium reduces subsequent osteoporosis risk since someone with high bone mass at age 30 may lose bone through normal aging, yet have sufficient bone remaining at age 75.

However, studies seem to show that calcium alone does not guarantee optimal bone growth in youth. Neither will it prevent bone loss with age in men, with estrogen-withdrawal in women, or with immobilization as in a cast or with bed rest, or with amenorrhea (ay-men-or-REE'-ah), which is absence of the menstrual cycle. It is also not even a sure bet that increased dietary calcium affects bone density once you reach adulthood. There are just too many other variables. You need to remember all of them in order to have healthy bones, not just eat calcium.

> Just drinking your milk or taking calcium pills will not stop osteoporosis. Bone density depends on many things. One big factor is how much exercise you get.

Other Nutritional Factors. Obviously, many nutritional factors are involved in the health of any body system. Many other vitamins and minerals, not discussed here, play small and interacting parts in your continually changing bones. The purpose here was to identify the major players and give an overview of the processes.

Hormonal Factors. Several hormones influence bone density and risk of osteoporosis in both women and men.

Menopause and Amenorrhea. One effect of the hormone estrogen is that it increases calcium retention in your bones. Estrogen level is a strong predictor of bone mass over time. Estrogen levels drop with amenorrhea (loss of periods before menopause), and with natural and surgical menopause. Surgical menopause removes the ovaries, called oophorectomy (oo-for-EK'-tuh-mee). Menopausal women lose large amounts of bone, regardless of calcium intake. The bones relied on estrogen. During the first menopausal years, withdrawal of the body's estrogen production is a major change. It takes time to adjust to the loss. But by then, much loss has occurred.

Many things may cause menstrual irregularities, or loss of the menstrual cycle entirely (amenorrhea) in premenopausal women. It is popular to blame vigorous exercise, with some authorities going as far as stating that athletes who experience amenorrhea should be banned from further training. Exercise alone is not sufficient to cause amenorrhea. Greatly decreased body fat and poor nutrition are involved. It seems to be an obvious and natural safety feature that, in evolutionary times, if conditions were harsh with lack of food and constant, difficult travel, then conditions were unfavorable for reproductive survival. Physical resources were better reserved until easier times.

Physical exercise is important to preserving bone mass. Stopping an amenorrheic athlete from exercising is counterproductive. Investigation into other contributing factors can allow the athlete to continue vigorous training, with all its benefits of health and well-being.

> Hormone levels affect bone density in men too.

Reduced Hormone Levels in Men. Testosterone has many functions, including regulating bone mass. The stress of extended periods of extreme exercise on the body seems to send a signal to the brain to decrease levels of two hormones that stimulate the testes to produce testosterone. As hormone levels go down, risks of various reproductive and bone density problems go up, just as in women. Much attention in the literature is paid to the role of hormones, exercise, and bone density in women, but unfortunately little about the phenomenon in men.

Depo-Provera. The contraceptive Depo-Provera (medroxyprogesteroneacetate) reduces estrogen production. Women taking Depo-Provera can lose bone mass in the early years of use, and can have bone density values below normal. Bone loss in the later years of Depo-Provera use normally levels off, until it approaches the normal rate of age-related fall.

Endometriosis Treatment. Treatment with nafarelin for endometriosis increases bone loss. Adding norethisterone (NET) to nafarelin treatment seems to have a bone-sparing effect. Ask your physician if this pertains to you.

Steroid Anti-inflammatories. Long-term corticosteroid (steroid hormone) treatment is sometimes given for several conditions, including rheumatoid arthritis. Over years of use, steroid anti-inflammatories can cause bone density loss and increase risk of fracturing for both men and women. Osteoporosis prevention and bone-building medications are an important issue for anyone taking steroid anti-inflammatories for long periods of time.

Anorexia Nervosa. Anorexia nervosa is a condition of abnormal loss of appetite and refusal to eat. It results in emaciation and malnutrition. Anorexia nervosa is a major risk factor for osteoporosis in both men and women for several reasons. The diet is severely calcium deficient, and the loss of muscle and total body weight decreases resistive forces on bones. Bones need a physical stimulus for maintaining thickness.

Anorexia can lead to decreased reproductive hormones in both men and women. Estrogen and testosterone both help maintain bone density. The malnutrition of anorexia can lead to loss of regular menstrual function, which is another risk factor for osteoporosis.

Exercise. Exercise is crucial in osteoporosis prevention. The job of your bones is to support your body against the pull of gravity. Your bones develop more when there is more need for them to resist gravity. The physical stress of muscle pulling on bone during exercise stimulates bone to thicken and strengthen. By contrast, lack of mechanical stress from lack of exercise; prolonged immobility during bed rest, being in a cast, or paralysis; a sedentary lifestyle; and weightlessness during space flight leads to bone loss regardless of how much calcium you eat. Bone loss from extended immobilization may become permanent after about six months of inactivity. Bed rest so effectively reduces bone density that it is used as a model for bone loss in the microgravity of space.

Animals that hibernate go without activity for long periods. Their bodies produce chemicals that prevent bone loss. Humans are strongly susceptible to bone loss from inactivity, and need resistive exercise to keep bones dense and strong. Like muscular atrophy from lack of exercise, the bone atrophy of osteoporosis is a "use it or lose it" disease. Sedentary lifestyle is a major risk factor. Without exercise, you lose calcium from your bones no matter how much calcium you eat.

> Osteoporosis is "bone atrophy" from several causes,
> including lack of exercise.
> Sedentary lifestyle is a major risk factor for osteoporosis.

Physical activity can increase bone mass in all age groups. Movement alone is not enough; there must be active muscular resistance. Weight-bearing activity, for example, walking or jogging, increases bone density, primarily of the lower body. Weight-loading exercise, usually weightlifting, can increase bone density at all sites, including the upper body. Like nutrition and unlike genetics, physical activity is a potentially controllable risk factor.

Your body weight is another important influence on bone density. Carrying your body weight around is exercise. Obesity increases bone density. Higher-weight postmenopausal women often have higher estrogen levels, another protective factor. Very lightweight people reduce the weight load on hip and leg bones. Reduced bone density from low body weight is a problem for extremely light and anorexic people. These people benefit by weightlifting exercise to help build muscle and bone.

What About Swimming and Scuba Diving?

Swimming is not a weight-bearing activity. It is a point of great interest to swimmers and scientists whether swimming can increase bone mass. Muscles still pull on bone to move you through the water, but is it less than during weight bearing? It depends how hard you work. Studies report that tough swimming workouts give plenty of bone-building resistance. If the only exercise you get is a casual swim, it is wise to augment that with weightlifting and weight-bearing activities.

Like swimming, scuba diving is not a weight-bearing sport, except when you are lugging all your gear around. Regularly lifting scuba gear is a good weight-loading activity for healthy backs. If you are able, carry your own tanks to get weight-lifting exercise. If your back is already osteoporotic, it may not be good to carry or wear your tank before you get into the water. The weight could further compress fragile vertebrae. In this case, don your tank in the water. Buoyancy underwater helps offset the weight of a tank. Check with your physician about diving safely if you have osteoporosis.

How Much Calcium Do You Need?

With so many interacting variables, your calcium need varies. You need more calcium if you lose calcium from smoking, drinking alcohol, and eating high amounts of animal protein. High intake of animal protein may cause calcium levels to become inadequate in situations where a tendency to low dietary calcium already exists. You may do well with less calcium if you exercise and reduce factors involved in calcium loss.

Although much is unknown, it is established that calcium intake influences bone mass until adulthood. In this way calcium reduces subsequent osteoporosis risk, since someone with high bone mass at age 30 may lose bone through normal aging, yet have sufficient bone remaining at age 75. After the skeletal maturation of adulthood, you still need calcium daily, although it is not known if calcium intake over a certain minimum influences bone density.

Neal Barnard, M.D., President of the Physicians' Committee for Responsible Medicine (PCRM), reminds us that, "Excessive calcium intake does not fool hormones into building much more bone, any more than delivering an extra load of bricks will make a construction crew build a larger building." PCRM filed a complaint with the Federal Trade Commission against ads showing celebrity milk mustaches, stating that some deceptively imply that just drinking milk will prevent bone loss.

Whether or not extra calcium will help, it is important to get enough calcium. In 1997, a panel of the Institute of Medicine, National Academy of Sciences, recommended the following daily minimum amounts of calcium:

- 1,300 mg/day for adolescents

- 1,000 mg for adults 18 to 50

- 1,200 mg for adults over 50

Some authorities feel that most people do not get enough calcium. See your physician to determine your calcium needs.

Calcium Sources

What are good sources of calcium? Where do cows get theirs? You can't digest grass, but dark green vegetables like spinach, collards, and kale are good sources of calcium. It used to be often stated that certain components of these plants, called phytate and oxalic acid, would depress calcium absorption, making them far less effective than dairy sources. However, calcium absorption from both low- and high-phytate soybeans has been found to be close to that of milk, with absorption from low phytate soybeans slightly higher than that of milk. Another recent study found interference by oxalic acid to be less than previously thought.

Broccoli has more calcium per calorie than any other food. Tofu has plenty, depending on how it is processed. Seaweed is another good, yet frequently overlooked, source. Fruit has calcium. So do almonds and sunflower seeds. Better yet, fruits, vegetables, nuts, and legumes have the element boron, which may participate in preventing osteoporosis. Milk has little boron. Meat and eggs have none. Because calcium absorption goes down with increased intake, spread out your daily dose into spaced intervals to increase absorption.

Can You Get Enough Calcium Without Dairy? Although dairy products are the prevailing calcium source in many Western countries, they are not the only source, or in many cases, the best source. Dairy products contain high amounts of calcium that is well absorbed. Still, there are problems with dairy for many people:

- Dairy is one of the most potent causes of allergy.

- Dairy is a major source of fat and cholesterol, increasing risk of several chronic diseases of the heart and blood vessels.

- Capacity to break down the milk sugar galactose decreases with age, and some people just have low levels of the enzyme that breaks it down. Galactose is associated with cataracts and ovarian cancer.

- Dairy products contain lactose. Most people lose the ability to digest lactose after childhood, causing gas and pain. This makes sense evolutionarily. In most of human history, people did not consume milk after weaning. We evolved not drinking milk, and with no need to keep producing digestive enzymes.

- Lactose may interfere with copper metabolism. Mild deficiency of copper, common in Western diets, is related to the development of osteoporosis.

- Daily protein can promote a specific auto-immune reaction in susceptible people that hurts insulin-producing cells in the pancreas, raising incidence of insulin-dependent diabetes.

- Cow's milk is not chemically like human milk. It has toxic effects on human babies. Cow's milk must not be given to human infants.

- The animal protein in dairy directly increases urinary calcium loss.

> It is not difficult to get adequate calcium
> without dairy products.

Many non-Western people get more calcium than the average American, from nondairy sources. Peruvian Indians eat cereal mixed with powdered calcium carbonate rock. Contemporary hunter-gatherers have a high calcium intake, three times higher than the average middle-aged American woman, without eating any dairy.

High-Calcium Foods

Source	Milligrams of Calcium (mg)
1 cup tofu processed with calcium sulfate	868
1 cup dulse seaweed	600
1 cup navy beans and 2 corn tortillas	370
1 cup milk	291
1 cup amaranth	280
1 cup spinach	200
1 cup kale	200
1 cup broccoli	180
1 cup soybeans	175
1 tablespoon blackstrap molasses	140
1 cup fortified orange juice	120
1 cup dried apricots	100

What About Calcium Supplements?

Calcium supplements are major sales items, even though major health organizations recommend getting calcium from food, not supplements. The U.S. Food and Drug Administration recommends checking the labels of many kinds of bottled calcium pills, to avoid bone meal and dolomite sources because of their high content of lead and other toxic metals. Calcium carbonate and calcium citrate are good alternatives.

Calcium absorption among the various supplement tablets is generally good, particularly between meals, except in people who underproduce stomach acid. For these people, taking calcium tablets with a meal benefits absorption. Since three times the dose is needed for some people to absorb the same amount of calcium, absorption fraction should be assessed by a physician before beginning a supplement regimen. Most, but not all, supplements are easily absorbed. A common test is to put the calcium tablet in a glass of vinegar. If it dissolves within 30 minutes, it is more likely to be absorbed in your digestive tract than those that won't dissolve in the vinegar.

How to Reduce Your Risk of Osteoporosis

- One of the most important things you can do to reduce your risk of osteoporosis is to get regular exercise. One effective bone-building exercise is lifting weights, including packages and bags. Also important is resisting your own body weight during weight-bearing exercise like walking, dancing, running, skating, and skiing. Rest weight on your hands by doing push-ups and arm balancing, because your wrist is one of the three main sites of bone loss.

- Get adequate calcium from a variety of vegetable sources, and spread your intake throughout the day.

- Avoid meat diets.

- Quit smoking.

- Drink less alcohol.

- If you drink a lot of alcohol, get screened periodically for Vitamin D deficiency and bone loss.

- Avoid chronic use of medications that cause bone loss, like anti-inflammatory steroids (cortisone, prednisone, prednisolone), thyroid medication, some anticonvulsants, and Depo-progesterone.

- Limit consumption of sodas, since they contain phosphates.

- Talk to your health care providers about the various drug treatments to prevent and combat osteoporosis. Until recently, estrogen replacement was often considered the only way to maintain bone mass in the first five years after menopause. But there is more to bone density than just estrogen or estrogen's several forms, and estrogen replacement alone may increase risk of uterine or breast cancer in susceptible women. Estrogen replacement is also not a great idea for women at risk for stroke.

Other hormones influence bone density, including testosterone, which women naturally produce, and progesterone, which balances estrogen's effects. Some medications act like a combination of estrogen, progesterone, and testosterone. These medications are developed in hope of preventing problems like hot flashes, skin atrophy, mucus membrane drying, and risk of heart attack without the old problems of estrogen replacement. Hormone replacement (and any bone-saving program) needs to be used in a broad program of health care that includes exercise, getting out in the sunlight, reducing risk factors, and good nutrition. Since many more women die of heart attack than hip fracture or cancer, the benefits of properly conducted hormone replacement are hoped to outweigh the smaller risk of cancer for those not at risk, but problems remain.

Nonhormonal drugs are available that work to prevent and treat osteoporosis without the problems of hormone replacement. Bisphosphonate therapy slows bone deterioration. There are several kinds, including Fosamax (alendronate sodium) and risedronate (Actonel). Various calcitonin nasal sprays (like Miacalcin) use a synthetic form of calcitonin, a hormone your body produces in several forms. It allows your body to keep the bone it builds, so it is used both to prevent and treat osteoporosis. Calcitonin sprays are for women more than five years past menopause who are losing too much bone and don't take estrogen.

New "designer estrogens" like Raloxifene (Evista) are selective estrogen receptor modulators (SERM). That means they select some parts of your body to help the same way estrogen does, but not other parts of your body that don't need it or could be harmed by it. In that way they can have bone- and heart-saving benefits without the risks of breast and uterine cancers sometimes associated with estrogen replacement therapy. Ideally, a selective medication would have all the good effects of hormones, and none of the bad. Nothing is available like that yet, not even in your own body.

There are hopes for plant-based remedies as new pharmaceuticals. There are also many "herbal" products that claim to help avoid osteoporosis and menopausal symptoms. These products, sold over the counter in health food stores, are not regulated the same way as pharmaceuticals, meaning any claim can be made for them. Talk to your doctor about which might help you. Some interfere with other medications you may be on, or cause you to bleed too much if you have surgery, even dental surgery.

Anyone with risk factors for osteoporosis and a history or risk of stroke, heart disease, or any cancer should weigh the relative benefits and risks of the various medications with their physician. Develop a complete program that includes doing physical activity and changing bad nutrition habits that contribute to the whole spectrum of post-menopausal problems.

Osteoporosis Risk Reduction

Reduce	Increase	Consider
Inactivity and sedentary lifestyle	Physical activity, including weight-bearing activity	Osteoporosis prevention medications after menopause
Animal protein	Vegetable protein	Bone-density evaluation
Alcohol	Weightlifting	Nutritional assessment
Smoking	Vegetable-based calcium	Reducing caffeine, salt

Important Answers

So the detective story, while not solved, revealed crucial clues. Populations in Japan whose low protein intake comes primarily from plant sources have normal bone growth and low rates of age-related osteoporosis, even with calcium intakes half that recommended in the United States. In their genetic relatives eating a modern diet, high salt and protein intake aggravates calcium deficiency in old age. African Bantu women eat less than half the currently recommended calcium, and have low rates of osteoporosis. They eat predominantly plant protein. Their genetic relatives living in the United States eating the Western diet of high animal protein suffer rates of osteoporosis and fractures similar to those of other North Americans. Eskimos have a high-calcium diet—nearly twice the recommended amount—and are physically active, yet suffer the world's highest rate of osteoporosis, which scientists relate to their high-animal-protein diet.

> Calcium is not the whole story in bone health.
> Getting enough calcium is crucial, but without other
> critical factors, it is not a cure-all.

Osteoporosis affects both men and women. Attaining high peak bone density when younger reduces the chance of lowering bone mass to unhealthy levels in later life.

Factors affecting your risk:

- How much exercise you get.

- Your total nutritional picture.

- Your heredity.

- Your hormonal status.

Reducing calcium loss may be as important as getting enough calcium. Factors that increase your calcium loss:

- Lack of exercise.

- Smoking.

- High alcohol intake.

- High-protein diet.

To build bone and reduce bone loss:

- Increase physical activity.

- Get adequate nutrition.

- Use bone building programs after menopause (determined by your physician).

> The most important message is to not wait until later.
> Preventing osteoporosis later depends on what
> you are doing right now.

Resources for More Information

Physicians for Responsible Medicine   (www.pcrm.org)
P.O. Box 6322
Washington, DC 20015
(202) 686-2210

National Osteoporosis Foundation   (www.nof.org)
1232 22nd Street N.W.
Washington, DC 20037-1292
(202) 223-2226

23

Body Fat—It's Not All Bad

Am I fat? I've fallen down and not even known it.

– Pat McCormick

Some people worry when they don't fit into their tightest suit. Others don't worry until they can't fit into the car. A quick look around reveals that being a little plump seems to be the norm. Is that all bad?

When Does Fat Help You?

You could not live without a certain amount of body fat. Fat is a necessary part of every cell in your body. Your nerves could not conduct signals rapidly enough for you to function without their fatty wrapping.

Body fat keeps you warm in the cold. Without a certain minimum of body fat, you lose your reproductive ability.

Fat pads the discomfort of sitting and standing, carrying shoulder bags and backpacks, and suffering blows to your internal organs. High body weight, whether from fat or lean, provides the loading your bones need to stay dense and strong. Heavy people have low rates of osteoporosis.

Success in different sports depends on characteristic body sizes and compositions. Football linemen almost always have more than an average amount of fat compared to other athletes. Fat weight is an advantage to linemen for the added mass and padding for blocking ability. Increased muscle mass accompanies the extra fat weight to carry the whole package around.

Sumo wrestling is another sport where extra fat weight helps. Linemen and sumos don't have to run around much. It's not a big disadvantage to carry extra weight. Other sports where the players have more fat than average for athletes are baseball, discus throwing, ice hockey, and swimming.

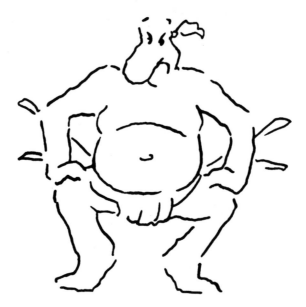

Figure 23.1. High body fat benefits some activities, like sumo wrestling.

Study after study confirms a direct relation between body fat and keeping warm in the cold—helpful in sports like swimming, ice hockey, ice fishing, skiing, and other cold-weather activities. You don't have to be obese to experience thermal benefits. Any amount of fat adds insulation.

Because of the extra work of carrying around extra fat, a heavy person generally develops extra muscle mass. Heavy people not only have more pounds of fat than lighter people, but more pounds of muscle. Extra muscle comes in handy in work like lifting things, and keeping warm in the cold. Consider the extra fat as a built-in daily weightlifting regime.

Fat increases buoyancy, adding safety and comfort to swimming. A little fat on your legs lets you float more horizontally, which is a better body position for moving efficiently through the water for scuba diving and swimming. Skinny legs tend to sink, ruining streamline.

When Does Fat Hinder You?

Extra fat weight is a burden to carry across distance or against gravity. Extra fat weight is more work to carry around. The high-calorie cost of transporting extra weight makes low body fat advantageous to gymnastics, climbing, and any sport where you have to run around. World-class distance runners almost always have extremely low body fat. Runners and gymnasts, along with boxers and wrestlers, often adopt unhealthy dietary restrictions trying to keep their weight low enough to help them in their chosen sport.

The same fat that keeps you warm in the cold makes you warm in hot weather, too. One predisposing factor to overheating is being large, round, and fat.

Having enough fat for health, comfort, and optimal performance in your sport is important. The next chapter describes the problems of too much of a good thing.

Body Fat of Athletes in Different Sports
(in no particular order)

Higher-Fat Athletes	Lower-Fat Athletes
Swimmers	Distance runners
Football linemen	Gymnasts
Sumo wrestlers	Acrobats
Baseball players	Climbers
Ice hockey players	Boxers
Water polo players	Wrestlers

24

Problems of Being Overweight

Those who think they have no time for bodily exercise
will sooner or later have to find time for illness.

– Edward Stanley

Fat has benefits, covered in the previous chapter. Too much fat has drawbacks, such as increased risk of orthopedic problems, heart attack, stroke, diabetes, certain cancers, gastrointestinal problems, even snoring.

It is estimated that over 40% of American men are overweight, compared to just under 30% of American women. Paradoxically, up to one-half of American women but only one-fourth of American men are estimated to be on a weight-reduction program at any point in time. This seems to be the case, even though women may be less active in organized exercise activities and sports. The disparity often results in a phenomenon called "The Flintstones," where couples consist of an overweight man and a slimmer woman.

More Work

It takes extra energy, work, and calories to carry extra fat around, depending on the work load. This is why a heavy man may work harder and closer to his maximum than a lighter man or woman to do physical activity that moves his body against gravity—for example, walking, running, climbing a hill, ascending stairs, and dancing. This is often the case even if the lighter person has a lesser physical capacity.

On one hand you could say that extra work is free exercise and you should be happy about it. For heavy people in good physical shape, the extra work falls within their comfort range. For those in so-so to poor shape, this work can be beyond the capacity of the out-of-shape heart to supply itself and the body with oxygen, beyond the capacity of fat-narrowed blood vessels to conduct enough blood, or past the ability of the joints to chronically support the weight.

Illness and Injury

First, there's the obvious. Backaches, sore knees, achy feet—all more common for those who are overweight. There's the old-hat stuff about heart disease, stroke, cancer, osteoarthritis, and gall bladder trouble. A large percentage of adult-onset diabetes cases in predisposed men is triggered by obesity. Adult-onset diabetes deteriorates blood vessels, sometimes ending in blindness and loss of your legs. Being overweight is one of several factors that, combined, result in diverticulitis, a painful inflammation of the large intestinal wall. Being overweight is a contributor to hernia, which eventually affects one out of eight men.

Snoring

Then there are the problems no one tells you about. High body fat is a key contributor to serious snoring and its more problematic relative, sleep apnea. Sleep apnea is a sleep disorder where the snorer stops breathing during sleep, sometimes hundreds of times per night. The large, heavy neck and throat of an overweight person leads to upper airway obstruction. Bouts of oxygen starvation occur during sleep, and the person may frequently wake up gasping and snorting. Over time, lack of oxygen to the blood vessels results in fatty deposits in the blood vessels of the heart and brain. This is thought to be one of the mechanisms for the higher incidence of stroke and cardiac irregularities in people with this sleep disorder.

Other long-term, harmful effects from snoring-related sleep disorders are more subtle but equally dangerous—the repeated awakenings from the snoring and apnea result in chronic daytime sleepiness. This sleepiness is documented to greatly increase the risk of serious automobile accidents, up to seven times the normal risk, according to some estimates.

Sleep apnea is sometimes called the Pickwickian syndrome, after the "Fat Boy" in Dicken's *Pickwick Papers,* who was obese and sluggish in the daytime. In Greek mythology, Ondine (alternately spelled Undine) was a water sprite who cursed a poorly behaving man to thereafter breathe only voluntarily, not automatically. When he fell asleep, he stopped breathing and suffocated. For modern sufferers of Ondine's curse, losing weight is often the first line of medically prescribed treatment.

Death

A man just 20% overweight is twice as likely as a normal-weight man to die before age 50 from a weight-related disease. Just 20%. That's a man who should weigh close to 170 pounds (77 kilograms) but weighs over 200 pounds (91 kilograms).

Scary Stuff

Then there's the scary stuff. "Cognitive decline" was linked to circulatory disorders resulting from obesity in a Cornell Medical College study published in the February 1992 *Clinical Geriatric Medicine*. Data reported in the September 1992 issue of *Hypertension* indicate that men with long-term high blood pressure lost more left-brain tissue than men with normal blood pressure. A high percentage of high blood pressure cases link to being overweight, even without high salt intake. The researchers suspect the specific areas of brain tissue loss affect memory, language, and "finding your way around."

25

Body Fat—
How to Tell How Much You've Got

You know you're getting fat when you can pinch an inch on your forehead.

– John Mendoza

Many people carry more than a healthy amount of body fat. How do you know if you're one of them? There are many tests, some you can do yourself at home or the gym with simple equipment. Some require only minimal training. Others need sophisticated measurement machinery run by skilled operators and interpreters.

In general, for your own use, focus on the ideas, rather than the specific numbers. Reducing your fat weight helps to lessen your chance of the diseases and problems mentioned in Chapter 24, "Problems of Being Overweight," particularly if you are at risk for them anyway. But finding out what the tests are and how they are done is an interesting story.

Apples and Pears

Where you carry your fat is as important as, or some say more important than, how much you have. The apple versus pear test requires only a mirror. Carrying fat primarily in the upper body and abdomen gives an apple shape to your figure. Lower body fat distributed on the hips and thighs makes a body more pear-shaped. Apple-shaped people seem to have a greater risk of obesity-related disease like heart disease, colon cancer, diverticulitis, diabetes, and high blood pressure than pear-shaped people. In short, beer bellies are more of a health risk than thunder thighs.

Waist-to-Hip Ratio

The waist-to-hip ratio test further defines the apple vs. pear test. It just looks to see if your waist is big compared to your hips. You find this out by taking your waist and hip measurements, and dividing the waist by the hip measurement. Answers above 0.8 for women and 1.0 for men indicate a tendency toward the more problematic apple shape. For example, waist 37 inches, hip 36 inches (94 cm and 92 cm). The answer is 1.03, not good for anyone.

Insurance Tables

One way to predict health, according to insurance companies, is to check your weight against values in their insurance company tables that tell the ideal weight for your height. According to the height and weight tables of the Metropolitan Life Insurance Company, if you are more than 20% above their supposed ideal weight, you are considered obese. Exercise scientists recommend against relying on insurance tables, as there were problems in the procedures for developing them, and like other tests limited to height and weight, they ignore that you could have any amount of body fat for your height and weight.

Body Mass Index

The Body Mass Index (BMI) compares how heavy you are relative to your height. To calculate BMI, divide your weight in kilograms by your height in meters squared. According to this test, if your BMI is over 25, you are fat. Above 30, you are considered obese. This test, like insurance tables, does not distinguish very muscular people from those overfat, and misses light, yet high-fat people.

For example, at 5'10" (1.78 meters), a weight above 174 pounds (79 kg) is fat; weight above 209 pounds (95 kg) tips your BMI over 30. At 5'4" (1.63 m), your BMI passes 25 at weights above 146 pounds (66 kg), and 30 at weights above 175 pounds (80 kg).

Feet and Meters, Pounds and Kilos?

The United States still uses units of measurement historically based on royal anatomy and pottery: the foot, gallon, pound, etc. Most of the rest of the world uses the metric system, with comparable units of the meter, liter, and kilogram. How to convert one to the other?

Kilos to Pounds: 1 kilogram is about 2.2 pounds, so multiply the number of kilos by 2.2 to get pounds.

Pounds to Kilos: 1 pound is about 0.45 kilograms, so multiply the number of pounds by 0.45 to get kilograms.

Meters to Feet: 1 meter is about 3.3 feet, so multiply the number of meters by 3.3 to get feet.

Feet to Meters: 1 foot is about 0.3 meters, so multiply the number of feet by 0.3 to get meters.

Somatotyping

Height and weight tests do not account for your musculature and body dimensions. Somatotyping is a method of classifying your body according to three characteristics—thinness, fatness, and muscularity. Thinness is called ectomorphy. Fatness is called endomorphy. Muscularity is called mesomorphy. Each type has specific characteristics of limb and body dimensions, with varying proportions of fat, bone, and muscle.

No one is only one somatotype. Everyone is a mixture of the three types in differing amounts. Some people predominate in one type, giving them the long, linear, and delicate appearance of the ectomorph; the round, soft, and short-necked look of the endomorph; or the hard, square, and rugged muscled body of the mesomorph. In football, many players score high in both mesomorphy and endomorphy. Swimmers are usually endo-mesomorphs. Gymnasts are usually ecto-mesomorphs. Sprint runners score higher in mesomorphy than distance runners. Coaches use somatotyping to identify those who would excel in different sports.

Casual somatotyping is done by the eyeball technique. Complete somatotyping requires trained analysis, photographs, or close inspection of naked subjects in three planes, caliper skinfold measurements, reference tables, and equations.

Anthropometrics

As part of somatotyping, or as a separate assessment, the size of the body's frame is determined with calculations using measurements of bone lengths and widths. Knowing frame size helps determine optimum weight. One test, the Heath-Carter, measures elbow width, knee width, biceps circumference, and calf circumference. Another anthropometric test, the Skeletal Frame Technique, measures widths of the shoulder and hip. The Tipton technique computes the minimum healthy weight for a given frame based on width and depth of the chest, and width of the ankle, wrist, and hip at two sites.

Index Tests

The Ponderal Index is your height divided by the cube root of your weight. Ponderal Index is used to determine degree of endomorphy. The Quetelet Index is another simple index of general body proportion. The Circumference test is nothing more than the familiar tape measure around the waist, hip, chest, leg, arm, or whatever.

The Jiggle Test

Jump in the air. When you land, see how long it takes for all your parts to stop jiggling. Higher times indicate higher fat amounts.

Measuring Percentage Body Fat

The different assessments talked about so far give an indirect estimation of your fat distribution. If you want to find out how much fat is actually attached to your body, you need body composition tests. These tests estimate what percentage of your total weight is just fat.

Why Measure Percentage Body Fat? A slender-looking person of normal weight can have a high amount of body fat. Another person weighing above average for their height may have heavy musculature and little body fat. The second person is above average weight, yet has low body fat. The first is normal weight and overfat, even though they don't seem to be. The difference is in their amount of body fat relative to their total weight, or percent body fat.

What's "Average" Body Fat? For comparison purposes, a healthy body fat is usually given as 10 to 15% for men and 15 to 25% for women. Percentages lower than that are considered thin. Higher figures are considered to be fat. Figures very much above those are considered to be very fat. As an interesting note, recent studies reveal the average American, male or female, is closer to 22% fat.

Are You Fat?

Apples and Pears. Is your body apple-shaped with fat primarily in the upper body and abdomen, or pear-shaped with fat mostly on the hips and thighs? Those with the apple shape tend toward obesity-linked disease.

Waist-to-Hip Ratio. Take your waist and hip measurements. Divide your waist measurement by your hip measurement. Stay below 0.8 (women) and 1.0 (men).

Insurance Tables. Compare your weight against values in tables. More than 20% over this weight range indicates that you are considered obese. Less reliable than other methods.

Body Mass Index. The Body Mass Index (BMI) measures how heavy you are compared to your height. Divide your weight in kilograms by your height in meters squared. If your BMI is above 25, you are considered fat. If over 30, you are considered obese.

Somatotyping. Somatotyping classifies your body according to three characteristics—thinness (ectomorphy), fatness (endomorphy), and muscularity (mesomorphy).

Anthropometrics. Measuring bone lengths and widths at specific joints tells the size of your body's frame—small, medium, or large, which helps determine optimum weight.

Index Tests. Several different index tests measure body proportion.

The Jiggle Test. Jump in the air. When you land, see how long it takes for all your parts to stop jiggling. Higher times indicate higher fat amounts.

Body Fat Tests

The only way to directly find out the specific amount of body fat you have would be to cut your body apart and try to scoop out all the fat stores. Even this direct method would miss fat deep inside and scattered around internal organs. All the other body fat tests are estimates.

There are several methods for estimating your percentage of body fat. These tests are called body composition analysis. Accuracy of some tests is poor, others moderate, to pretty accurate, to within a few percent. Calipers, hydrostatic weighing, and near infrared interactance are a few of the most common ones.

Calipers. Calipers measure the thickness of your folds of fat. This is also sometimes called the "pinch test." Calipers are a small, simple, and inexpensive instrument. There are several caliper tests that use up to 10 sites on your body. Simple equations translate the sums of different sites into percent fat. Caliper measurement is painless unless the tester too enthusiastically grabs and squeezes. The error of measurement of testing percent fat with calipers can be large, up to about 3 to 7%, varying greatly with the experience of the tester, making it not a true measure but a gross estimation. Caliper testing is often misused, particularly in health clubs. If a first reading shows 25% fat, then weeks later after an exercise program the second reading is 22%, it does not necessarily mean the person lost 3% fat. The large error of measurement makes it impossible to tell. Not all calipers read the same either. It is like a bathroom scale that weighs you at 160 one time, at 170 the next, and at 150 the third time.

Hydrostatic Weighing. Hydrostatic weighing, also called underwater weighing, is currently the gold standard of body composition analysis techniques. It has the lowest percentage error of all current body composition tests. There are two main methods of underwater weighing, and several different equations. One underwater weighing method uses Archimedes' principle. Density is mass divided by volume. You know your mass, and can find your volume with water displacement.

Another method obtains body volume by subtracting your weight in water from weight in air. You sit on a scale in a tank of water and exhale as fully as you can with your head under water. The air that is left in your lungs after you exhale maximally is called residual volume. Residual volume can either be directly determined before the underwater weighing, or estimated with population charts. Your body density is determined from equations of your weight under water minus your residual volume. The final reading can be off if you are unwilling to exhale completely underwater and hold the exhale for as long as it takes for the tester to get a good measurement. Being gassy can also affect your results.

Near Infrared Interactance (NIR). NIR is a technique based on the absorption of light in your fat versus your lean mass. Generally, manufacturers haven't burdened themselves with input from scientists in developing it, and there is some feeling that the technology has a long way to go. Some units claiming to use infrared interactance don't use it, rendering the unit even less accurate.

Other Tests. Sophisticated body composition analysis includes bioelectric impedance, potassium ion determination, ultrasound, CAT scans, creatine absorption, proton absorptionmetry, and nuclear magnetic resonance imagery. These tests require expensive equipment and need further validation to know just how good they are.

What to Do?

Once you know your body composition, what can you do about it if you don't like it? The next chapter explains what you can do about the shape you're in.

26

What to Do About the Shape You're In

It is a hard matter, my fellow citizens, to argue with the belly since it has no ears.

– Cato the Elder (Roman politician and general)

But argue with the belly we do. Constantly. Weight control is a multibillion-dollar industry of widgets, gimmicks, and programs, some legit, some less so.

Weight control also is usually a dismal failure. People trying to lose weight lose muscle, bone, water, electrolytes, but not an appreciable amount of fat. When they regain the weight, as most dieters do, they gain back fat. Plenty of people want to put on lean weight, but wind up putting on fat weight. The body is designed to survive. Fat helps that to a degree, so the body holds dearly to its fat. What if you don't like the idea of holding dearly to your fat? If you and your physician have determined you have more than enough of a good thing, what can you do about it? This section describes what to do to lose a little, what not to do, and why we even have body fat at all.

Why You Have Fat and Plants Don't

You don't often see a fat plant. With few exceptions, like avocados, coconuts, and other nuts, plants don't store their energy in the form of fat. We do. Why is this?

Being fat is often equated with being heavy, ponderous, weighty. Yet fat is lightweight compared to protein and carbohydrate. The same volume of fat weighs less than muscle protein. One of fat's famous traits is being light enough to float.

Fat has twice the calories as the same quantity of carbohydrate or protein by weight. In that way, fat stores more energy than carbohydrate or muscle. This lightweight, energy-dense storage form is the reason animals use fat as a storage vehicle. If you have to carry your energy around with you, it makes sense to make it a lightweight package.

Plants are mellow. Plants don't go places often. Their storage medium does not require weight control. They store most of their energy as carbohydrate. The extra weight is not a metabolic burden. Plants are heavy for their size. Ask any tree.

Why are avocados and coconuts exceptions? Because they, like other seeds and nuts, are the portion of plants that must move. They travel to new locations to germinate. They typically store fat to make their energy suitcases lighter.

Animals store little energy in the form of carbohydrate. Meat has, for all practical purposes, no carbohydrate. This is true even though your muscles stock a carbohydrate called glycogen that you use in short bouts of exercise. Your carbohydrate cache is so small that your muscle, and the muscles you eat if you are a meat eater, is partly protein, a good deal of fat (even in lean cuts), but no carbohydrate that makes any difference nutritionally.

> Plants store their energy as carbohydrate, which is heavier than the same volume of fat. The extra weight is not a burden since plants don't travel. Avocados and coconuts are exceptions because they, like other seeds and nuts, are the portion of plants that move to new locations to germinate.
>
> Animals carry their energy around with them, so it makes sense to carry it in a lightweight package—fat.

Why You Get Fat

So, humans have fat, but why so much in some cases? The difference between fatter and thinner people is mainly the amount of exercise they get and what kind of food they eat.

It's easy to be sedentary, particularly in a lifestyle geared around the automobile and television. Daily life is not active anymore. Humans evolved to move as part of all activities needed for life and fun. Modern habits take away the daily movement you need for keeping healthy. Movement has become artificial and something you have to stop your life to go do. Many people become so unaccustomed to movement that they get too tight-jointed to cut their own toenails, and don't use their muscles even to bend and walk normally. Weekend warriors rarely exercise enough for it to count as regular exercise. It's easy to pack on pounds if you don't routinely move as part of your normal daily activities.

> Being fat usually results from too little exercise.
> Active movement should be part of normal life, but has
> become artificially segregated into stopping your real life
> and "doing exercises."

How to Lose Fat: What Not to Do

Don't Believe Gimmicks. People flock to outrageous weight-loss regimes, programs, gizmos, and outright hoaxes. Why are starvation, dehydration, stomach stapling, unhealthy fad diets, vibrating machines, and amphetamines considered acceptable, while normal daily movement and exercise are avoided as extreme? Avoid unhealthy gimmicks in favor of a healthy lifestyle. Healthy exercising is detailed in Part I of this book.

Don't Fad Diet. Fad diets restrict your nutrition, are usually not healthy, and don't keep the weight off in the long run. Severe calorie restriction by itself is rarely successful and hard to sustain. Remember that many so-called diets are just gimmicks. Just because something is called a diet doesn't mean it is a weight-loss diet. After all, anything you eat is your diet—it could be all ice cream and cardboard boxes.

Don't Restrict Water. Water is not fat. Losing water weight has no effect on fat loss. You need water to be healthy. Don't restrict water in hopes of losing water weight. Dehydration is unhealthy in general for your body, and it lowers your exercise capacity and ability to thermoregulate. For those who eat when they're not hungry, a glass of water is a good substitute.

Don't Lose Weight Quickly. Weight lost quickly usually returns just as quickly. It's also tough on your heart. Avoid rapid weight loss unless your physician has determined that the benefits outweigh the risks. The more slowly you lose weight, the more likely it is to stay off.

Don't Believe Claims of Spot Reducing. Spot reducing is a myth. The idea of spot reducing is to lose fat from a specified area by repetitive movement of that area. If that were true, then the people selling spot-reducing devices would have thin mouths from all their talking, typists would have skinny hands, and bicycle riders would have skinny legs. If you want to lose fat, then do aerobic exercise like walking, running, biking, cross-country skiing, rowing, or swimming.

Remember Error of Measurement. Don't believe health club personnel who measure your body fat with calipers at intervals and state that you have lost 2% fat, or 5% fat, or whatever percent since starting their program. The error of body fat measurement inherent in caliper testing is too high to compare specific percents over time. Trust the fit of your clothing. See Chapter 25, "Body Fat—How to Tell How Much You've Got," for more about fat measurement.

Don't Hate Yourself. Accept yourself if you have a little more to adore. If you are meant to be big, appreciate the advantages. Be sure to exercise and trim food fat for health. Anorexia and starvation are passé. Being big isn't for everyone, but neither is being too thin. There's no reason you can't be big-boned, large, healthy, and happy, too.

Summary—

How to Lose Fat: What Not to Do

- Don't believe gimmicks.

- Don't fad diet.

- Don't eat high-sugar, high-calorie foods just because they are "fat-free."

- Don't restrict water.

- Don't lose weight quickly.

- Don't believe claims of spot reducing.

- Remember error of measurement.

- Don't hate yourself.

How to Lose Fat: What to Do

There are many easy, fun, and healthy ways to lose fat. Here are a few.

Give Peas a Chance. Remember, animals have fat and plants generally don't. Eat more plants. Meat, even lean cuts, often has more than the maximum amount of fat recommended by the American Heart Association. Vegetables and grains are a good source of carbohydrate that fuels your body. Plants are a good source of protein, but, unlike meat, have no cholesterol and little fat. It used to be thought that plant protein was not as good as meat protein. In the modern diet there is little chance of not getting enough of the different kinds of protein you need from vegetable sources. There is no need to carefully combine plant proteins, as once thought. Your body does that for you automatically, as you eat over time. Vegetable meals are also cheaper than meat meals.

Eat Low-Fat. Sensible eating means not starving yourself. Just exchange a few bad food preferences for healthier ones. Find low-fat substitutes for habitual high-fat snacks. Chapter 15, "Calculating Food Fat," explains how to tell how much fat is in the foods you eat, and lists fat contents of common foods. Develop some fun, healthful, new food preferences.

> Not all calories are the same. When you eat 100 calories of complex carbohydrate, your body burns 25 calories just to digest the carbohydrate. When you eat 100 calories of fat, your body burns just three calories to process it.

Eat More Filling Food. Your stomach will stop bothering you for more food when it thinks it has plenty. Studies at Tufts University found that low-calorie but physically "heavy" food like cantaloupe can make you feel fuller than an airy donut. Why eat a few high-calorie crackers, when a glass of water or a cup of spinach can make you feel stuffed? A slice of whole grain bread can fill you more than a couple of slices of fluffy white bread. These foods used to be called "stick to your ribs"—the hearty, heavier foods.

See Your Physician. See your physician to determine your general state of health and percent body fat. Choose a physician skilled in this area.

Exercise. Exercise is the key to losing excess body fat. Exercise doesn't only mean going to the gym. Find a few regular activities that you enjoy, that fit your lifestyle, and that you can build into your ordinary day without it being a chore.

Reclaim Built-In Exercise. Many activities of daily living are built-in exercise. Devices like garage door openers benefit those with health problems that would be aggravated by opening the heavy door. For others, opening the door twice a day by bending and lifting properly, so many days per week, would give you extra muscle and lose you a few pounds of fat per year. You can find many other examples throughout your day, like swapping walking and biking for driving, steps for elevators, push mowers for power mowers, carrying your own packages and golf clubs for using a cart—you get the idea. Exercising in a gym is really a substitute for having an active lifestyle. Some people prefer to drive to a health club and take the elevator to their exercise class. Others hate the gym, and are thrilled to find they can avoid it by having a fun, active life.

Very important—lift properly all day. Most people bend right over at the waist many dozens of times daily. You know you shouldn't lift like this, but you do. Keep your torso upright, your behind under you, and use your legs. Lifting right is a built-in calorie burner, saves your back, and strengthens your knees and legs when done properly. Stand up properly all day. It burns more calories and is good for your joints.

Have young children and think there's no time to exercise? They *are* your exercise. Lift babies overhead up and down, three sets of 10. They love that. Lift properly as taught in Chapter 7 on abs and Chapters 20 and 21 on back pain. Is the baby getting bigger and heavier? Perfect. The increasing weight will increase your strength. Do squats and lunges holding your baby. Up and down and up and down. They love the ride. Babies have a natural grasping reflex equal to the grip of world-class climbers. Don't squander that gift. Plop them on your leg and do leg lifts front, back, and side. Do push-ups with them on your back. Do "monster" push-ups—put baby on the floor, face up, and straddle him with your arms. Do push-ups so that your face comes down to his. Blow raspberries each time you lower. Do "peek-a-boo" back extensions—lie facedown, face to face. Lift your upper body off the floor using your back muscles. Hold your arms out to the side. When you lower back to the floor, cover your eyes with your hands. Lift back up and open your hands to reveal who it is. Bend properly for the hundreds of times a day you need to bend with young children around the house and all the times they play "the gravity trick" with their things and food. Teach them to be active as they grow. Take them skating, biking (helmets and sensible safety), and to all kinds of fun activities. When you go out, carry them in arms or on your back, not in a push-carriage. Interact with them.

Check Things Out. Read about fitness and nutrition from schooled sources, so you can identify the hype and sales pitches.

Lift Weights. Weightlifting is important to fitness. Lifting weights alters your body composition toward the lean, burns calories, and helps you get fit and have more fun through an active life. Remember that lifting your body weight is lifting weights. Bend properly. Get up from the chair often. Get up and down from the floor. See Chapter 3, "Improving Your Fitness," for specifics on what kind of lifting gives what kind of results.

Have Fun. Find an active pastime you enjoy and count it as exercise. Like to go dancing? Live it up once a week and count it as one exercise class. Walk to the grocery store and carry home packages. That's two. Like to window-shop? Sightsee? Bicycle? Roller-skate? Garden? Play catch with children? Carry piggy-back? Be creative.

Be Happy. Be happy. Why not?

Summary—

How to Lose Fat: What to Do

- Eat low-fat. Try more vegetables and grains. Fruits make good desserts.

- Try heavier, low-calorie foods. They fill you more than physically lighter, higher calorie foods.

- See a physician skilled in nutrition and exercise.

- Get more exercise.

- Find all the things that you can do in a day to be more active without going to a gym.

- Educate yourself. Read about fitness and nutrition. Carefully choose sources with real medical information, not hype and sales.

- Lift weights. Aerobics are not enough. Weightlifting increases your lean mass, which burns more calories than your fat weight. Lift children. Use your body weight for weightlifting by bending properly.

- Stand up straight. It burns more calories than slouching. Think how much that could add up to every day.

- Get lots of fun activity. Do things you used to love. Enjoy being active.

- Be happy. It's healthy.

27

Cardiovascular Disease

The trouble with heart disease is that the first symptom is often hard to deal with: sudden death.

– Michael Phelps, M.D.

What condition kills more people than any other? Cardiovascular disease. It's the number one noninjury cause of death, beginning at age 30 for men and 40 for women. Nearly half of all deaths in the United States each year are from cardiovascular disease, which includes heart attack and stroke. It kills twice as many men and women as cancer. Most men dying a sudden death during physical activity have been found to have underlying heart disease. The good news is that cardiovascular disease is largely preventable, by things you can do yourself at home.

How Does Cardiovascular Disease Affect You?

Cardiovascular disease keeps you from enjoying your life in several ways:

- It can end your life at a young age.
- It reduces your physical capacity to deal with exertion.
- It limits your ability to go out and enjoy life.

- Environmental stresses on your body from weather extremes of heat and cold are hard enough on your cardiovascular system. Cardiovascular disease greatly limits your ability to cope with these extremes safely. Even men with no underlying heart disease usually show greater blood pressure and other cardiovascular responses, such as irregular heartbeats, than women during activities in the cold.

- For men who have cardiovascular problems, the combination of work and cold in activities like shoveling snow or just having fun in the snow can be lethal.

Cardiovascular Disease Affects More Than Just Your Heart

Your blood vessels can clog up all over your body, not just in your heart. One common place is your brain. Reduced blood flow to your brain can hurt your mental processes. "Hardening of the arteries" may explain an older person's senile behavior. An often-missed warning of heart attack and stroke is confusion and change in reasoning powers.

Blood vessels clogged with cholesterol plaques in your lower leg cause pain and problems when walking. Oxygen can't reach the muscles, and they cry in pain. Sometimes, they just stop working, causing a limp, a condition called claudication, which comes from a Latin word meaning "to limp."

Another interesting place is your Achilles tendon, the large "string" that attaches your calf muscle to your heel. High cholesterol levels can stiffen the area and predispose it to injury, increasingly common in middle-aged men.

Another body site also concerns men. An often ignored warning signal of dangerously narrowed arteries is decrease in erectile function. High blood pressure, high cholesterol, and smoking are major risk factors. Men with this warning sign should check the possibility of cardiovascular disease with their physicians.

All these injuries are more common in industrialized nations because of the link to vascular problems from Western diet and sedentary lifestyle. Seventeenth century English physician Thomas Sydenham summarized it, "A man is as old as his arteries."

How Your Blood Vessels Are Involved

Your blood vessels aren't just inert pipes. They are living and responsive. The lining of your blood vessels is a layer of flat cells called endothelium. Your endothelium regulates how your blood vessels dilate and constrict. Normally, the endothelium makes a chemical called nitric oxide, which relaxes vessels and prevents spasms. When fat, diabetes, smoking, and other stresses upset your endothelium, it stops making nitric oxide. Constricted vessels make your blood less able to flow smoothly and more likely to cause heart attacks or blood clots.

Your endothelium knows when cholesterol enters your bloodstream. Cholesterol slows your lining's ability to regulate cell growth, which builds up plaque. Lowering your cholesterol lets the endothelium function well enough again that heart disease symptoms subside even with the plaque.

Removing the plaque that blocks arteries is a common medical treatment. But in many patients the blockage comes back. Besides the fact many of them didn't change their diet and they still didn't exercise so that plaques built back up, something else was going on. The procedure to remove plaque seems to make the body think there is an injury to the endothelial wall. White blood cells come to the rescue at the site of the removed plaque as if it were a wound. This is like relatives barging into help you when you don't want them. Inflammatory proteins build up tissue that blocks the artery again. Healthy diet and exercise can reduce plaques without this injury process so that your blood vessels stay clean and open.

Risk Factors for Cardiovascular Disease

There are major and minor indicators of your chance of developing cardiovascular disease. Although some factors are more serious than others, all are cumulative, meaning the more you have, the greater your risk.

Four Top Risk Factors. Until recently, there were three top risk factors:

- Cigarette smoking.

- High blood pressure.

- High blood cholesterol.

Now a fourth major risk factor has been identified—no real surprise.

- Lack of exercise.

These four are the most predictive factors of your risk.

Other Common Risk Factors. Your risk usually increases with:

- Age.

- Family history of cardiovascular problems.

- Diabetes.

- High body fat.

- How much fat you eat, particularly animal fat.

- Being male—men develop cardiovascular disease, on average, about 10 years younger than women.

- Cocaine use. Even with no other risk factors present, you may have a sudden heart attack if you use cocaine.

Too Much Iron. An intriguing risk factor is high blood iron level. Iron in the body is usually found in a form tightly bound with a protein, as in hemoglobin. Iron is an oxidant, and when it becomes available in unbound form, it turns on several harmful reactions with oxygen that damage your cells. People with high iron levels have been found to develop high rates of heart disease. Conversely, premenopausal women who lose small monthly amounts of iron, and vegetarians and athletes who often run a bit low, have lower incidence of heart disease than the rest of the population. High iron levels may also be linked to unusual fatigue, and possibly cancer. It's another good reason to cut back on red meat, which has a high iron content.

About 2% of Americans have a genetic disorder that prevents them from processing iron, a condition called hemochromatosis. The high iron levels that they build sometimes cause heart failure. Recent news is that even slightly high iron levels may raise risk even in those without the faulty gene, particularly men who don't have the benefit of monthly blood loss. This seems to be more common than previously thought. James Cook, M.D., an iron specialist at the University of Kansas Medical Center, states, "No one, unless he or she has been diagnosed with an iron deficiency, or belongs to a high risk group, should routinely take iron supplements." How common is hemachromatosis? Dr. Victor Herbert, chief of Mount Sinai's hematology and nutrition lab in the Bronx, states, "Only 6% of Americans have iron deficiency anemia. Twelve percent have a hemochromatosis-related iron overload."

Not Enough Fruit and Vegetable Vitamins. Besides the well-known association between cardiovascular health and healthy eating in general, many vegetables have folic acid. Folic acid, a B-vitamin, has several functions in your body. One is to lower your levels of a substance called homocysteine. Homocysteine occurs naturally in your body and has many roles. But in high amounts, it is associated with heart attack and stroke. The average meat-centered Western diet can result in deficiencies of common vitamins, including folic acid.

Folic acid deficiencies might be responsible for 15 to 40% of heart attacks and strokes, depending on the study cited, a large number in either case. Eating more folic acid won't make up for a sedentary lifestyle and unhealthy eating habits, but getting enough folic acid (about 400 micrograms per day) seems to be important to cardiovascular health. Find folic acid in green leafy vegetables like spinach, brussels sprouts, lettuce, and many fruits, including oranges and apples.

Sleep Apnea. Sleep apnea was detailed earlier in the chapter on the problems of being overweight. "Apnea" means to stop breathing temporarily. In sleep apnea, the sleeper stops breathing, sometimes hundreds of times per night. They may make loud, labored snores and efforts to breathe. The episodes of apnea starve their bodies of oxygen. Low oxygen seems to make fatty plaques deposit in their blood vessels. Sleep apnea is a risk factor for stroke and heart attack. The many nighttime awakenings also cause chronic daytime sleepiness. This sleepiness greatly raises the risk of serious automobile accidents. Sleep apnea is a serious sleep disorder. An effective treatment for sleep apnea is losing weight.

The Four Top Risk Factors for Cardiovascular Disease

Cigarette smoking
High blood pressure
High blood cholesterol
Lack of exercise

Other Risk Factors

High dietary fat
Diabetes
High body fat
Cocaine use
Increasing age
High iron
Sleep apnea
Being male

What Is Your Risk?

There are several pen-and-paper assessment tools to help you determine your own risk. The following page shows one from the Michigan Heart Association. It is one of the older assessments, but a good and easy one to start with. Circle the number in each category that best describes you. Then total your score.

Cardiac Risk Index

	10 to 20	21 to 30	31 to 40	41 to 50	51 to 60	61 to 70
Age	10 to 20	21 to 30	31 to 40	41 to 50	51 to 60	61 to 70
Score	1	2	3	4	6	8
Heredity	No known history	One relative over 60 with cardio-vascular disease	Two relatives over 60 with cardio-vascular disease	One relative under 60 with cardio-vascular disease	Two relatives under 60 with cardio-vascular disease	Three relatives under 60 with cardio-vascular disease
Score	1	2	3	4	6	8
Weight	More than 5 lbs below standard weight	-5 to +5 lbs standard weight	6-20 lbs overweight	21-35 lbs overweight	36-50 lbs overweight	51-65 lbs overweight
Score	0	1	2	3	5	7
Tobacco Smoking	Nonuser	Cigar and/or pipe	10 cigarettes or less a day	20 cigarettes a day	30 cigarettes a day	40 cigarettes or more a day
Score	0	1	2	4	6	10
Exercise	Intensive occupational and recreational exertion	Moderate occupational and recreational exertion	Sedentary work and intense recreational exertion	Sedentary work and moderate recreational exertion	Sedentary work and light recreational exertion	Complete lack of all exercise
Score	1	2	3	5	6	8
Cholesterol or, % fat in the diet	below 180 mg / No animal or solid fat in diet	181-205 mg / 10% animal or solid fat in diet	206-230 mg / 20% animal or solid fat in diet	231-255 mg / 30% animal or solid fat in diet	256-280 mg / 40% animal or solid fat in diet	281-330 mg / 50% animal or solid fat in diet
Score	1	2	3	4	5	7
Blood Pressure	100 upper reading	120 upper reading	140 upper reading	160 upper reading	180 upper reading	200 or over upper reading
Score	1	2	3	4	6	8
Gender	Female under 40	Female 40-50	Female over 50	Male	Stocky male	Bald, stocky male
Score	1	2	3	5	6	7

RISKO with permission and courtesy of Michigan Heart Association © Michigan Heart Association

Results of Cardiac Risk Index _____

If your total score is:

6 – 11 – Your risk is well below average.
12 – 17 – Risk below average.
18 – 24 – Risk generally average.
25 – 31 – Risk moderate.
32 – 40 – Risk at a dangerous level.
41 – 62 – Danger, urgent. See your physician now.

Reducing Your Risk of Heart Disease

You can't do much about your age, gender, or family history. Happily, there are plenty of things you can do. Of the four major risk factors, you can directly control how much you exercise and smoke, and indirectly control high blood pressure and cholesterol with exercise, supervised medication, and healthy nutrition. Most cardiovascular disease has a large nutrition and fitness component. You can reduce your risk through healthy eating and exercise habits.

Adopt Healthy Habits. You've heard it before. Exercise more, quit smoking, and eat less sugar and fat. It gets easier the more you do it. Many fatty foods are an acquired taste. After switching to low-fat foods for a while, you'll be surprised to find how greasy the fatty foods taste when you try them again. When you eat fewer sweets, you crave them less. You'll also notice your weight and blood pressure drop if they were previously high, further reducing your risk. If you have diabetes, you can usually reduce its severity with better nutrition and more exercise. You win all around.

Start Healthy Habits Young. It's not just older people that get heart disease. Autopsies on American soldiers killed in Vietnam and Korea showed that the majority already had moderately advanced atherosclerosis. Autopsies of children who die of causes other than cardiovascular disease reveal that artery clogging can begin as early as childhood, the product of a sedentary lifestyle and the modern diet of chips, fries, burgers, and ice cream. Habits developed early, both good and bad, are more likely to be kept throughout your life.

Clogged arteries begin in youth. Heart disease is not just something that happens suddenly to older people.

Eat More Fruits and Vegetables. Make vegetables the main part of your meals, instead of being just side dishes. Fruit can make easy and good-tasting snacks and desserts. See your physician, registered dietitian, or exercise physiologist for a program to cut dietary fat and learn how to eat more healthfully.

Lower Your Blood Cholesterol. Two thirds of heart attacks happen to people with cholesterol readings over 200. The average cholesterol reading in the United States is around 220. Cholesterol poses a double hazard. It slowly deposits on blood vessel walls and makes blood vessels more likely to suddenly squeeze shut, contributing to ministrokes that warn of serious illness to come. Your blood cholesterol can rise when you eat high amounts of cholesterol and lots of saturated fats.

Cholesterol is found only in animal products, such as eggs, dairy, and meat. Your liver makes all the cholesterol you need. You don't have to eat any at all. For more on cholesterol, see the next chapter. The amount of saturated fat you eat relates to your blood cholesterol levels. Cutting back on saturated fat helps reduce your risk of high cholesterol. Saturated fats are mostly found in meat, dairy, and hydrogenated vegetable oils.

Consider Estrogen After Menopause. After surgical or natural menopause, a woman's risk of cardiovascular disease rises until it just about matches that of a man. Estrogen replacement reduces a woman's chance of heart attack by about half. Speak with your physician about the benefits and risks of the different replacement options that apply to your current state of health.

Pick Up the Phone. An easy thing to do. Call your physician to ask how to reduce your risk. If you don't have a personal physician, call a physician referral service to find a physician that fits your needs and likes.

Donate Blood. Some experts recommend regular blood donations to avoid high blood iron levels that may relate to disease risk. This usually is only for certain people with abnormally high iron levels. *The British Medical Journal* reports on a study from Finland of 2,600 men. Nearly 10% of the men who had not donated blood in the two previous years suffered a heart attack. Only one of the 153 who had donated blood had a heart attack in the same period of time. Although it is possible that the men who had donated blood were more health conscious in general, the connection in the study seemed to be strong. Call your local Red Cross for information on donating blood—to help someone who needs blood, and possibly yourself.

Get in Better Physical Shape. Being out of shape is a vicious cycle. You are not able to do enough exercise to improve your health. So you become more out of shape, and more unhealthy. Your risk of a problem brought on by exertion rises. Being in better shape lowers your risk of cardiovascular disease while exercising, and improves your ability to do the amount of exercise you need to become healthier.

Have a Social Support Network. Behavioral researchers report that having a social structure of friends is heart-healthy. Speculated reasons include that friends share health information, and that the support of friendship reduces physical and emotional stress. Many people socially isolate themselves. How can they develop a better network of friends? Writer and philosopher Ralph Waldo Emerson observed, "If you would have a friend, you must first be one." Make time for friends, accept people as they are, and respect their secrets. That will go a long way to developing and keeping friendships.

Know the Symptoms of a Heart Attack. If you get chest pain, chest tightness, shortness of breath, or pain down one arm, go immediately to a hospital emergency department. Don't dismiss these warnings as indigestion. Don't ignore these symptoms in a woman. Cardiovascular disease is the number one disease of both women and men.

Get Medical Care Right Away. Even if the pain goes away, it doesn't necessarily mean you didn't have a heart attack. How well the hospital can care for you if you are having a heart attack depends on how quickly you get there. Delay reduces the effectiveness of the many treatment options available. Quick treatment (within six hours) prevents more extensive, irreversible damage to your heart. Call for help instead of trying to get to an emergency room yourself. Some people have a full-out attack while driving to the hospital, and never make it there. Call ahead to ask your doctor to meet you there.

Be Proactive, Not Reactive

The reactive approach is to sit around, get clogged blood vessels, wait for the physician to prescribe drugs, worry, have surgery, have a stroke, have a heart attack. Your heredity is not your destiny. If your father had heart disease, you're not doomed. On the other hand, the more common approach is, "My father (or mother) didn't have heart disease, so I have nothing to worry about." Neither is completely true. Be proactive with preventive care. Cardiovascular disease develops largely through unhealthy habits, making it, fortunately, largely preventable.

How to Reduce Your Risk of Heart Disease

- Adopt healthy habits. Exercise more, quit smoking, and eat less sugar and fat.

- Start healthy habits young. Habits developed early, both good and bad, are more likely to be kept throughout your life.

- Eat more fruits and vegetables.

- Lower your blood cholesterol by exercising more and eating less saturated fat.

- Consider estrogen replacement. Heart attack risk rises sharply after menopause. Estrogen replacement reduces a woman's chance of heart attack by about half.

- Call your physician or physician referral service to find a physician. Find out how to reduce your risk through healthy exercise, health, and nutrition plans.

- Donate blood. It's not certain, but possible, that regular blood donations help to avoid high blood iron levels that may increase disease risk.

- Get in better physical shape. Being in better shape lowers your risk of cardiovascular disease while exercising and improves your ability to do the amount of exercise you need to become healthier.

- Have a support network of real friends.

- Know the symptoms of heart attack.

- Get medical care right away. If you get chest pain, chest tightness, shortness of breath, or pain down one arm, go immediately to a hospital emergency department.

Resources for More Information

American Heart Association   (www.americanheart.org)
National Center • 7272 Greenville Ave. • Dallas, TX 75231-4596
1-800-AHA-USA-1 or (800) 242-8721

American Red Cross   (www.redcross.org)
For referral to a CPR class or blood donation near you, call (800) 42-CROSS

Iron Overload Diseases Association   (www.ironoverload.org)
433 Westwind Drive • North Palm Beach, FL 33408-5123
(888) 678-4766 • iod@ironoverload.org

28

Good and Bad Cholesterol Explained

Avoid fried meats, which angry up the blood.

– Rule 1 of the 6 Rules of Staying Young by Satchel Paige

You're going out for the day. Got your keys? Yes. Jacket? Yes. Wallet? Yes. Favorable lipoprotein ratio? Huh?

What Is a Lipoprotein?

You've probably heard of the different kinds of lipoproteins as "good cholesterol" and "bad cholesterol." Lipoproteins aren't just cholesterol. Lipoproteins are large molecules that your body makes out of cholesterol, fat (lipid), and protein. Lipids won't dissolve in your blood or travel through your blood on their own, so they have to be carried around by helpful proteins.

There are five kinds of lipoproteins. This chapter covers two: high-density lipoprotein, or HDL (good cholesterol), and low-density lipoprotein, or LDL (bad cholesterol).

Lipoproteins and Cholesterol

Cholesterol is one of three lipids ushered around your blood by lipoproteins. Cholesterol is a necessary ingredient in your body. Why? It is a precursor of your steroid hormones, including all your sex hormones, and a precursor of your bile acids, which handle fat digestion. Your body uses it to make Vitamin D, and it is a necessary part of every cell membrane in your body.

In excess, cholesterol deserves its bad reputation. Too much cholesterol in cells lining your arteries builds up deposits called atherosclerotic plaques (*athero* means "gruel-like," and *sclerosis* means "hardening"). About a third of all American adults have cholesterol readings high enough to indicate a high risk of heart disease. According to physician Dr. Dean Ornish, the "average" American has a cholesterol reading around 220, and the average American develops heart disease. Dr. Ornish is known for his work with reducing heart disease through a program that includes very low dietary fat.

"Bad" Lipoproteins and Heart Disease

Low-density lipoprotein is called "bad cholesterol" for a good reason. Fatty plaques that narrow blood vessels are made of LDL and VLDL (very low-density lipoproteins).

LDL picks up 60 to 75% of the cholesterol from the fats you eat and from your liver, which makes cholesterol, and takes it to the cells of your blood vessels and muscles. Because LDL carries most of the cholesterol, a high amount of LDL in your blood translates to higher risk of heart attack and angina pectoris (*angina* means "pain," and *pectoris* means "chest").

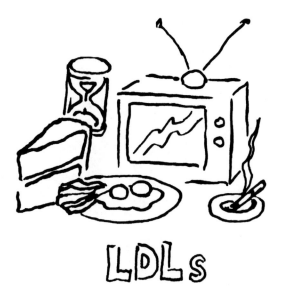

Figure 28.1. You don't eat bad cholesterol or low density lipoproteins (LDLs); your body makes them. Your body can wind up with too much LDL when you eat too much animal fat or saturated vegetable fat, smoke, take drugs such as anabolic steroids, and don't exercise.

What "Good" Lipoproteins Do

High-density lipoprotein (HDL), popularly called good cholesterol, removes cholesterol from your bloodstream and does not collect or stick to the inner linings of your arteries. HDL contains an enzyme that helps break down deposits and takes "used" cholesterol away from the cells back to your liver for recycling and excretion. The higher your HDL level, the lower your risk of heart disease.

Dr. David Hsu of Stanford University Hospital describes the four main functions of HDL:

• It is an airport baggage handler that tags and de-tags chylomicrons, VLDLs, and IDLs (the very low and intermediate density guys) with protein tags that identify them and allow them to be picked up out of your blood (the conveyor belt) by the correct recipient at the correct destination. The tags are called apoproteins.

• It is a maintenance person, picking up garbage (free cholesterol) from peripheral tissue (e.g., from cell membranes of dead or live cells) and storing it, using an enzyme that makes the cholesterol even more willing to stay inside the HDL maintenance person.

• It is a porter that carries cholesterol back to the liver, where the HDL is broken down and the cholesterol released into liver cells to be used as needed.

• It is a trader, and trades cholesterol stores with VLDLs and LDLs for fats.

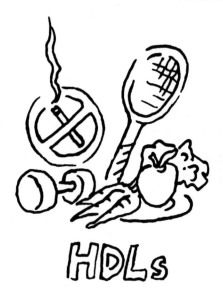

Figure 28.2. You can increase your good cholesterol, or high density lipoprotein (HDL) level, by avoiding smoking, avoiding drugs such as anabolic steroids, eating less animal fat and more vegetables, and exercising more.

What Distinguishes High From Low Density?

The names "high" and "low density" come from two characteristics of lipoproteins. The first is lipid content. LDL has more lipid than HDL. Normally, when you call something "low," you think of a smaller amount. But the higher lipid content of LDL decreases the density because fat is less dense than other body constituents. Think of cream floating on milk. Heavy cream has more fat than light cream, making it less dense. Although it weighs less than light cream, it's called heavy for its higher fat content. In the same way, LDL has more fat but lower density.

The names "high" and "low" also come from the way they're packaged. Loosely packed LDL cholesterol floats through the bloodstream to your cells. Cholesterol released from the cells tightly crams into HDL for the voyage back to your liver.

One way to remember which is which:

HDL = Healthy
LDL = Lousy

How to Get Less LDL and More HDL

Improving your ratio of good to bad cholesterol is not so difficult. Lipoproteins ferry LDL and HDL to and from each cell in amounts determined by your food choices and activity level. Although blood vessel diseases like heart attack and stroke are the number one killers in the United States and Great Britain, they are practically strangers in half the world. In those areas, intake of animal products and fat is low, activity level is high, and smoking is almost unknown.

Eat Less Saturated Fat and Cholesterol. LDL levels may be directly related to eating saturated fat, although the question of how much dietary fat intake affects the pattern of HDL and LDL cholesterol levels has not been answered for certain. It is agreed that saturated fat increases the rate of cholesterol formation, and that people, especially those at risk of heart disease, who already have a heart condition, or are overweight, should limit cholesterol, and, more importantly, saturated fat in their food.

You get saturated fat from all animal sources like meat, fowl, dairy, and eggs. In contrast, vegetable oils are not saturated except tropical palm and coconut oils. Beware of ingredients in packaged foods like hydrogenated vegetable oils. Hydrogenation artificially saturates vegetable oil.

Cholesterol is part of every cell membrane in animals, giving the outer cell area part of the structure it needs. Plants don't need cholesterol around their cells because they have rigid cell walls. That's why only animal products have cholesterol. There's no need for you to eat cholesterol to get the amount your body needs to do its job. Your liver manufactures all you need—even if you eat no cholesterol at all.

Quit Smoking. If there weren't already enough reasons for you to quit smoking, here's another: Smoking lowers HDL.

Avoid Anabolic Steroids. The male hormone testosterone depresses HDL levels, one reason men's risk of heart disease is higher than women's risk. Taking extra male hormones called anabolic steroids plummets HDL levels.

Exercise. Exercise more effectively changes HDL/LDL ratio than dietary change and weight loss. Endurance exercise increases HDL and its important enzyme, and decreases total blood cholesterol and LDL in both men and women. Altered blood lipid profile may be one of the principal mechanisms of reduced risk of heart disease through exercise.

Several studies published in well-accepted medical journals report that more exercise and less dietary cholesterol and fat may not only stop coronary artery disease from progressing, but reverse it.

How to Lower Your "Bad Cholesterol"

- Eat less saturated fat and cholesterol.

- Quit smoking.

- Avoid anabolic steroids.

- Exercise.

Your Cholesterol Ratio

Your total cholesterol reading is determined by your LDL and HDL levels. You raise your risk of heart disease if you have too much total cholesterol and if you have too little good cholesterol (HDL). High levels of circulating HDL in relation to LDL are usually more important than your total amount of blood cholesterol.

Your total, and the ratio of good to total, is a number easily determined by blood testing. In general, the lower your cholesterol ratio, the lower your risk of heart disease. The optimal ratio is 3.5 or lower.

Cholesterol Ratio Before an Exercise and Low-Fat Diet Program:

$$\frac{\text{Total cholesterol 200}}{\text{Good (HDL) cholesterol 50}} \quad = \quad 4.0 \quad \text{This is a high ratio.}$$

Cholesterol Ratio After a Program to Raise Good Cholesterol:

$$\frac{\text{Total cholesterol 180}}{\text{Good (HDL) cholesterol 60}} \quad = \quad 3.0 \quad \text{This is a good ratio.}$$

Occasionally, people who eat very low-fat diets, particularly vegetarian diets, lower their LDL level so much that their cholesterol ratio becomes high. This should not be mistaken for an unfavorable ratio. These people have a lower-than-average risk of heart disease. The big picture of blood fats is what is important.

A Priority

Much attention is paid to the few yearly deaths by sensational events such as plane crashes. At the same time, hundreds of thousands of people die every year by the frying pan. Heart disease is still the number one killer of both men and women. What will change that, more than any drug or fad health food, are healthy food choices and regular exercise. So get rid of the cigarettes, get more vegetables on your plate, and get exercising.

Resources for More Information

National Cholesterol Education Program   (www.nhlbi.nih.gov/about/ncep/)
National Heart, Lung, and Blood Institute, NIH
Public Health Service; U.S. Department of Health and Human Services
(800) 575-WELL

American Heart Association   (www.americanheart.org)
National Center
7272 Greenville Ave.
Dallas, TX 75231-4596
1-800-AHA-USA-1 or (800) 242-8721

29

Headaches

One man's food is another man's poison.

– Socrates

Foods or actions that cause no pain to some people can trigger a terrible headache in others. Two thousand years ago, physicians required their patients to fast as part of their medical exams. Often, the patients' symptoms would stop.

Many headaches are caused by things you can change, meaning that many headaches are preventable. This section is not intended for use as a medical diagnosis, and is by no means complete, but is a look at possible mechanisms and things to do for relief.

Types of Headaches

There seems to be a continuum between the various kinds of headaches, particularly tension-type and migraine. These types of headaches may represent ends of a single continuum rather than being distinct from one another. Modern headache centers take an integrated approach to understanding the types of headaches, leading to better diagnosis and treatment. The types of headaches are described here separately to introduce them in an organized fashion.

Tension-Type Headache. Previously called muscle-contraction headaches, or tension headaches, these can occur when you tense the muscles of your face, brow, scalp, and neck for lengthy periods. For example, frowning and brow furrowing over taxes or other stressful paperwork; tensing over a desk, computer, or workbench; shouldering the phone to your ear; or clenching your teeth. The pain is steady, felt on one or both sides of the head, or can often feel like a tight band around the head. Since tension headaches are often triggered by stressing the head and neck muscles for long periods of time, tension headaches typically start late in the day and resolve with sleep. Tension headaches usually disappear after the stress is over, but if you habitually tense your muscles day after day, you can have pain from it day after day.

Migraines. The pain of migraine headaches is thought to result from inflammation of the blood vessels surrounding the brain. Nausea, vomiting, and sensitivity to light and sound may occur. The pain can be so terrible that even a word meaning "depression or unhappiness" (*megrems*) comes from a Middle English variant of migraine.

Migraine can occur with or without an "aura"—neurological symptoms appearing 10 to 30 minutes before a classic migraine. An aura may include flashing or zigzag lights, lines, and dots; dimmed vision; tingling in the face or hands; weakness of an arm or leg; speech difficulties; or confusion. Migraine usually starts on one side of the head and may spread to the other side. Left untreated, attacks can last up to three intensely painful days.

Migraine without aura used to be called common migraine, because it is more common than migraine with aura. When warnings occur, they might include fatigue, mental fuzziness, mood changes, or unusual fluid retention. These symptoms, as well as those of the aura, indicate that the generator of migraine is in the brain, not the blood vessels. Untreated, common migraine pain can last up to three days. If it lasts longer, it is called migraine status.

There are several other kinds of migraine. Hemiplegic migraine produces temporary paralysis on one side of the body (hemiplegia). Basilar artery migraine (named for a problem in a major brain artery called the basilar artery) is often seen in young women. In ophthalmoplegic migraine, the pain is around the eye and causes droopy eyelids and double vision.

Dr. William B. Young of the Jefferson Headache Center in Philadelphia explains migraine origins. "Ten to fifteen years ago, it was state of the art to say that migraine began with changes in brain blood vessels. Today, we have evidence that migraine sufferers have a lowered threshold of the 'migraine generator' within the brain. One theory is that this generator is in the brainstem, involving serotonin cells. Another theory is that an aura, or an aura-like phenomenon in the cortex of the brain, starts a cascade of events that leads to migraine pain including inflammation of the blood vessels surrounding the brain."

Cluster Headaches. These headaches are rare, but they are so painful and have such a characteristic pattern that they deserve mention. They occur mostly in men.

Cluster-headache sufferers experience severe bouts of pain on one side of the head for about an hour, one to three times per day. Often, cluster headaches occur at the same time every day, "clustered" into a period of weeks or months, then disappear for months to years, only to recur. Eye tearing, lid drooping, and nasal stuffiness are characteristic. Sufferers may pace, bang their heads, rock, and become irritable during the attack. The pain can be so intense, it has been called the "suicide headache."

> Neurologist Jim Burke, M.D. at Albert Einstein Medical Center in Philadelphia explains cluster headaches. "These headaches are different than migraine headaches. People who are experiencing a cluster headache will be pacing the floor holding their head, while a person experiencing a migraine will look for a dark, quiet room."

Traction and Inflammatory Headaches. These come from a variety of other problems, from stroke to sinus infection. Traction headaches can result from pulling, stretching, or pushing pain-sensitive parts of the head, for example, with tight hats, collars, and hair barrettes. Inflammatory headaches may come from elsewhere in the body, signaling problems like meningitis, trigeminal neuralgia, glaucoma, tooth infections, or problems of the sinuses.

Common Headache Triggers

Many things common in your everyday life can trigger headaches. Responses to triggers are individual. Here are a few.

Head and Neck Posture. A very common and very overlooked cause of tension headache is poor back and neck posture. Holding your head forward of the midline of your body is called a "forward head." The weight of your head held in front of your neck rather than over it fatigues and strains neck muscles, overstretches the ligament down the back of your neck, and puts pressure on your cervical discs. Pain from a forward head is usually felt down the back of the head and neck, along the top of the shoulders, between the shoulders, and under and along the shoulder blade.

Many people have a forward head without knowing it. A forward head is accentuated if you crane your neck while driving, using computers, or watching TV. Many exercises common in gyms make a forward head worse: pulling your neck forward for abdominal work, craning and tensing your neck while lifting weights, and tipping your neck forward while lifting or pulling a bar in back of your neck. (Healthier substitutes for these exercises are in Chapter 9, "Good and Bad Exercises.") A forward head is easily prevented with proper posture. Bring your head into healthy alignment by holding your ears above your shoulders, rather than letting your head crane forward of the midline of your body. Stand with your back and behind and heels against a wall and see if the back of your head touches the wall. It should touch without lifting your chin or arching your back. Similarly, you should be able to lie flat on the floor comfortably without a pillow. If these don't feel natural, you are too tight to hold your head in healthy posture and need to stretch your shoulders and chest more to the back so that they don't curl you forward. Chapters 20 and 21 provide more information on how to correct a forward head.

Food. For migraines, it is unusual for food to be the only trigger, but food is often part of the cause. Classic food triggers are chocolate, red wine, beer, walnuts, peanuts, liver pâté, yogurt, lima beans, salted and cured meats (ham, corned beef, sausage, bacon, lunch meats), dried meats, pickled herring, chicken livers, and aged cheeses like blue cheese. These foods contain the chemical tyramine, which constricts arteries, the first step to getting a migraine. The difficulty in finding out which foods are problems is that migraines often take a day or two to "bloom" after eating trigger foods. By then, the connection is long forgotten.

Other headaches come from processed meats, like hot dogs. Processed meats contain nitrite compounds, which can dilate blood vessels in susceptible people, causing pounding head pain. Other times, specific foods can set off an allergic reaction, resulting in headache. If avoiding certain foods does not reduce the number of headaches you get, resume your regular diet. Don't become a "migraine hermit."

Alcohol. Nonmigraine headache is common after too much wine, whisky, brandy, or rum, because these drinks (unlike vodkas) are high in headache-causing substances called congeners. Migraine and cluster headaches are different from alcohol hangovers but may occur with a hangover because they can both result from drinking alcohol. Cluster headaches may start shortly after a drink is taken.

Caffeine. Sometimes, too much caffeine can cause a headache. But for people who habitually drink caffeine drinks, caffeine withdrawal can bring on a headache, which is a vicious cycle among some coffee and soda drinkers. Some coffee drinkers find that they will have a headache until their morning coffee, making it difficult to cut back or quit drinking coffee.

Sleep. A classic nonfood trigger for migraine is altered sleep schedules, such as sleeping later than usual. Napping with your head propped on the arm of the couch can trigger some back-of-the head headaches.

Sleep apnea, a sleep disorder where the sleeper stops breathing, sometimes hundreds of times per night, drops oxygen levels. Many physical problems result. People suffering sleep apnea have daytime sleepiness, and often wake up headachy from the many periods of oxygen starvation. Loud snoring and gasping are clues to sleep apnea, which occurs most often among very overweight people. See Chapter 27, "Cardiovascular Disease," for more on sleep apnea.

Eyestrain. Close work, an eyeglass prescription that is not just right, and glare are often factors in starting a headache from eyestrain. To reduce chance of eyestrain, remember to look up and at a distance away from your work regularly, to let your eyes focus on different distances. If you wear glasses, have your glasses prescription checked. Make sure it is the right strength for you, and that all the other considerations of grinding the glass for your prescription have been faithfully met. Make sure that the distance between the pupils of your eyes was measured correctly, then ground correctly into your lenses. Ask your optometrist or optician to check the base curve and axis of your lenses. Make sure your glasses fit properly and are the right distance from your eyes. If you don't wear glasses, have a good eye exam to see if you need correction, and to check the health of your visual system.

Less Common But Still Important Contributors

Tight Hats. Wearing a tight hat can cause a headache, producing a type of tension headache sometimes known as "hatus-too-tightis."

Carbon Monoxide Poisoning. Headache is a common flag of an uncommon problem —carbon monoxide poisoning. This can come from a faulty heating system at home, exhaust system in your car, blocked chimneys, or using kerosene lanterns, heaters, or stoves indoors, in tents, and in campers. People have been poisoned by riding in the back of trailered boats or recreational vehicles when exhausts are drawn inside. You can't smell, taste, or see carbon monoxide. Carbon monoxide poisoning can be serious, even fatal. Small, inexpensive home carbon monoxide detectors are available in stores, usually next to the smoke detectors. Make sure your home has good ventilation.

Drugs. Regular, long-term use of pain-suppressing drugs, both prescription and nonprescription, lowers your own body's natural pain-suppressing ability. Sudden withdrawal from these drugs can rebound you into a headache.

Hyperventilation. Sometimes, people begin to breathe too deeply and quickly for any number of reasons, including fear and excitement. Such breathing quickly lowers body carbon dioxide levels, sometimes enough to cause limb tingling, dizziness, lightheadedness, headache, or other odd sensations.

Teeth and Jaw. Toothaches start some headaches. Biting, grinding, and clenching teeth at night during sleep can cause jaw fatigue and sometimes head and neck pain. Poorly fitting dentures can cause jaw misalignment and pain. Someone with a dysfunction of the jaw joint, called the temporomandibular joint (TMJ), may become headachy from chronic clenching at night, or even chewing food day after day.

Sinusitis. Sinusitis occurs when one or more of your sinus cavities fills with bacterial or viral fluid and becomes inflamed. The infection may start in your upper respiratory tract and spread to your sinuses. Sinusitis may involve allergies to irritants, such as cigarette smoke, dust, ragweed, and animal hair. According to the NIH, "Research scientists disagree about whether chronic sinusitis triggers headache."

Nitroglycerin. People who get angina pectoris (meaning "chest pain" in Latin) are often prescribed nitroglycerin pills or patches to wear. Nitroglycerin dilates blood vessels, which improves blood flow and oxygenation, relieving chest pain. The nitroglycerin is important to relieving chest pain, but users often get headaches because brain blood vessels dilate, too.

Other Contributors

Headaches can come from allergies, air pollution, bright sunshine, hunger, thirst, cigarette smoke, dust, and fumes from chemicals and paint. "Benign exertional headaches" can occur when starting physical activity, such as running, lifting, and even coughing, sneezing, or bending. These headaches are more common in men and rarely last more than a few minutes. Fatigue, glaring or flickering lights, even changes in the weather, can set off headaches.

Combinations of Things

Determining what triggers your headaches can be tricky. Often, it is a combination of things that singly would do little to cause pain. For example, you may endure a tough day, a high smog count, and an uncomfortable office chair or car seat, and drink too much coffee because you didn't sleep well the previous night. Then you go out for dinner that night and have red wine and a chocolate dessert. That might be the final straw, producing a killer migraine the next day.

Treating Headaches

During the Stone Age, medical shamans treated headaches by cutting holes in the patient's skull with flints to let the demons out. The term for this practice is trephination. Not only did patients survive trephination, it seemed to be popular. Some skulls recovered from that period show more than one healed trephine hole. Trephining was practiced until the Middle Ages. By the ninth century, a headache remedy from the British Isles was to drink "the juice of elderseed, cow's brain, and goat's dung dissolved in vinegar."

Understandably, headache sufferers often will do almost anything to relieve the terrible pain. Fortunately, today there are better remedies.

A Dynamite Headache Story

Nitroglycerin is an explosive used to make dynamite and blasting gelatin. It is also used in medicine to reduce chest pain. Now who made such a connection, and what does that have to do with headaches?

The story goes that World War II dynamite factory workers endured throbbing headaches as an occupational hazard. When they left their positions after the war, their headaches stopped, but some of them began dying of heart attacks. Why was this?

People whose blood vessels are narrowed by fatty deposits can't get enough blood to their heart, reducing their oxygen supply. Their heart must pump harder against narrowed areas, increasing oxygen demand. When oxygen supply doesn't meet oxygen demand, their heart cries out in pain, called angina pectoris. A physician may prescribe nitroglycerin, which dilates the blood vessels of the heart, restoring blood flow and relieving pain. It also dilates the blood vessels of the head. Headaches are a characteristic symptom of too much nitro.

Nitrates are the active ingredient in nitroglycerin. Munitions workers had been inhaling airborne nitrates on the job, sometimes causing headaches, but also dilating their coronary blood vessels. After discontinuing exposure, the vasodilatory effect was rapidly lost. Their blood vessels constricted to their previous size. Headaches vanished. But those workers with coronary vessels already diseased from the usual causes—high-fat diet and lack of exercise, fell victim to blocked blood flow to their hearts. By leaving the ordnance plants, they lost the protective vasodilatory effect of their workplace air.

Nitroglycerin is very explosive. Dynamite is close to 75% nitroglycerin. Because it is mixed with inert materials like sawdust, wood pulp, or diatomaceous earth, it will detonate only with a fuse or the kick of a blasting cap. But medicinal nitroglycerin will not blow up because it is only about 1% nitroglycerin and is packed in an absorbent, inert material that reduces its volatility. Just watch out for headaches.

Tension-Type Headaches. Ordinary muscle-triggered headaches go away when you stop tensing your face, head, and neck. Acute muscle-contraction headaches can be relieved with a hot shower or moist heat, and over-the-counter pain relievers like Tylenol®. Training for better head and neck posture can reduce much of the pain that is common down the back of the neck, into the shoulder blades, and along the tops of the shoulders (see Chapters 20 and 21 on back and neck pain). Physical therapy and gentle exercise of the neck may be helpful. Pushing your fingers against your forehead, from brows to hairline, slowly, repeatedly, and firmly, seems to be a helpful massage for tension headache.

Some people have fierce tensing habits, triggering chronic headaches. They need to retrain their postural habits and learn not to tense their muscles. They can do this through good physical therapy and exercises, and the various kinds of biofeedback, relaxation training, and counseling.

Migraines. According to neurologist and headache specialist Dr. William Young, the most commonly prescribed drugs used to relieve migraines are ergotamine tartrate, DHE, and sumatriptan. They can be taken at the beginning of a migraine to stop it cold. Combination medicines containing Excedrin® or Midrin® can be effective. Dr. Young stresses the importance of not overusing pain medications (more than two to three days a week), or a daily rebound headache may result. Rebound headaches can be severe enough to require hospitalization.

During a migraine, it helps to seek a dark, quiet room, and use cold packs. Sometimes it helps to press on the bulging artery in front of the ear on the painful side.

Cluster Headaches. Medications commonly prescribed for cluster headaches include drugs like caferget, DHE, and sumatriptan. Since one of the mechanisms proposed for at least one stage of cluster headache is enlarged and inflamed brain blood vessels, various treatments aim to reduce the size of the enlarged blood vessels using ice hats or oxygen. When you breathe pure oxygen, your body constricts brain blood vessels to protect your brain from the ill effects of too high levels of oxygen. Breathing 100% oxygen has been known to help relieve some cases of headache, but there are very little good data on this. Breathing oxygen at higher than usual pressures in a hyperbaric chamber is also under study. Most people with cluster headaches require medication. Pain medications rarely work, but more specific treatments are successful in the vast majority of cases.

Trigeminal Neuralgia. Also called Tic douloureux (painful tic). This condition can cause brief "lightning bolts" of facial pain, set off by the smallest touch or movement of the face or mouth. It comes from a problem of a facial nerve called the trigeminal nerve. This nerve supplies your face, teeth, mouth, and nose with sensation, and also lets you chew. People with trigeminal neuralgia may fear chewing or brushing their teeth because those actions can set off the pain.

Treatment for trigeminal neuralgia involves various medications, taken regularly for prevention. In other cases, surgery directly on the trigeminal nerve can stop the episodes.

Acute and Chronic Sinusitis. Home treatments include hot facial compresses, sniffing salt water mixtures to reduce irritation and swelling, pain relievers, decongestants, and keeping your home free of allergens (shag rugs, cats, whatever the trigger irritant). In addition to over-the-counter decongestants, some people get rapid results with spicy foods and hot peppers. Others take steam baths. Medical treatment may involve allergy shots, vasoconstrictors, and inhaled steroids to shrink swollen, inflamed membranes and allow better drainage; other compounds that reduce the amount of inflammation-causing histamine released; and, occasionally, antibiotics if the problem is bacterial.

When to See a Physician

Many headaches don't require medical care. Headaches from the occasional missed meal, muscle tension, or poor posture are easily remedied. But some headaches signal serious problems, such as head injury, stroke, or disease. According to the National Institutes of Health, you need prompt medical care for the following:

- Sudden, severe headache (reaching a maximum in less than one minute).
- Headache associated with convulsions.
- Headache accompanied by confusion or loss of consciousness.
- Headache following a blow to the head.
- Headache associated with pain in the eye or ear.
- Persistent headache in a person who was previously headache-free.
- Recurring headache in children.
- Headache associated with fever.
- Headache that interferes with normal life.

Preventing Headaches

To avoid tension-type headaches, good posture is important. Check to see if you hold your head in a forward posture (see Chapters 20 and 21 on back and neck pain). Avoid teeth clenching and grinding. Look in the mirror to see if you habitually purse your lips, furrow your brow, squint, or look surprised. Relax and enjoy your day. Some people keep a mirror at their desk to catch candid reflections when they are not "posing" for a mirror.

Common methods to prevent migraine headaches include medications, biofeedback training, stress reduction, regular exercise, and eliminating trigger foods and activities. To find food triggers, keep a food diary. For one week, write down every food you eat, and the time of day. In the same space, note how you feel. Also log the weather, what work and exercise you did that day, and anything else you think may relate. Review your food/headache journal after one week (or longer if you did not have a headache during that time). Look for what happened in the 24 to 48 hours before your headache.

Some migraine patients need preventive medications, taken daily, which can begin to control headaches in three to six weeks. Vitamin B2 (riboflavin) has been shown effective for some migraine sufferers. The dose is 400 milligrams a day, a very high dose, although with few reported side effects. Your physician can determine which migraine treatment, or combination of treatments, is right for you.

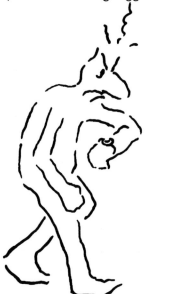

Figure 29.1. A tension-type headache in the making.

Finding the cause is important to ending inflammatory and other headaches. For example, headaches from temporomandibular joint (TMJ) problems can be corrected with devices for the mouth, and retraining chewing habits.

See your physician for assessment to identify what kinds of headache you get and what usually triggers them. Take a good look at your posture, nutrition, exercise, physical condition, and surroundings. Have your teeth and eyes checked. Have your furnace and chimneys checked. Find out if you tense your face and neck. Find out if you have allergies. Keep a list of what you eat to see if you have any trigger foods. Then, as obvious as it sounds, work to avoid things that give you headaches.

Resources for More Information

National Headache Foundation   (www.headaches.org)
(888) NHF-5552 • info@headaches.org

American Council for Headache Education (ACHE)   (www.achenet.org)
19 Mantua Road • Mt. Royal, NJ 08061 • (856) 423-0258

30

Leg Cramps
and What to Do About Them

For this, be sure, to-night thou shalt have cramps,
Side-stitches that shall pen thy breath up; urchins
Shall, for that vast of night that they may work,
All exercise on thee; thou shalt be pinch'd
As thick as honeycomb, each pinch more stinging
Than bees that made 'em.

— Prospero, in The Tempest, Act I, Scene II

What Are Leg Cramps?

Muscles contract to move your bones. That's their job. The muscles that move your bones around are voluntary muscles. You tell them when to contract. After you stop telling them, they relax. When a muscle contracts too much, too suddenly, and does not relax again, that is a cramp. It is a spasm. It hurts. Leg cramps usually occur in your calf, foot, or hamstring muscles, but occasionally affect the quadriceps muscles in the front of your thigh, or other muscles.

Calf Cramps. Your gastrocnemius, or calf muscle, is the prominent, fleshy muscle at the back of your lower leg, below your knee. It attaches from your knee to your heel. Its main job is to pull on your heel to point your foot down, an action called plantarflexion. Plantarflexion flexes your ankle toward the sole, or plantar surface, of your foot. You can (usually) easily see the "string" that your calf muscle attaches to your heel to pull with. The string is a tendon called the Achilles tendon. When your calf muscle cramps, it pulls your Achilles tendon more strongly than usual and won't let go, which pulls your foot downward into a pointed (plantar-flexed) position, and holds it there painfully.

Foot Cramps. Your foot muscles that curl your toes down extend along the bottom of your foot from your heel to your toes. When these muscles cramp, they pull your toes, usually your two middle ones, downward toward the sole of your foot—painfully—and hold them there in spasm.

Hamstring and Quadriceps Cramps. A hamstring cramp will hurt in the back of your upper leg, and contract your hamstring muscles enough to make your knee bend. A quadriceps cramp will tighten the front of your thigh, causing your leg to straighten out painfully.

Why?

There is one very common reason why people get cramps in their calves and feet, and several uncommon reasons for cramps in general. First, the less common reasons:

People like to say that not eating enough salt, or bananas, or any particular food causes leg cramps, but that is an unlikely reason. In Western societies, a deficiency of salt or potassium is hard to get. The average Westerner eats many times the amount needed. The body helpfully "pees" it all out until levels are normalized again. Biochemical reasons why an overstressed muscle may cramp are not pinned down. Scientists would love to know the chemistry, too. Some people may get cramps from too much salt or potassium loss because of disease, diuretics, or large fluid losses from prolonged vomiting and diarrhea. But it seems that in the general population muscle cramps during exercise are not from large electrolyte disturbances.

An uncommon cause of constant, severe calf cramps is cirrhosis of the liver. A rare possibility is certain inherited disorders that specifically cause leg cramps. Sometimes, the pain is not muscle cramps at all, but from other conditions confused for cramps. Arteries of the leg can plug up for the same reasons blood vessels anywhere in the body plug up—vascular disease is not just of the heart. When a person with narrowed leg arteries starts activity, the legs need more blood than can fit through those vessels, and the leg cries in pain for oxygen. That is called claudication, from a Latin word meaning "lameness." Those at highest risk are sedentary people, smokers, or people fond of high-fat diets. Another issue is pregnancy, which often presses on vessels exiting to the legs, causing leg pain and cramping.

Those are some uncommon reasons for leg cramps. Now what is the usual reason?

The Most Common Reason

Foot and leg cramps are most often caused by holding your leg, ankle, and foot muscles tightly, rather than letting them swing fluidly when you walk around all day. Tight shoes that restrict your toes or the natural range of motion of your foot when walking change the way your legs need to move, and can shorten the muscles into being more cramp-ready. The extra work of tensing the muscle makes it overexert, another factor in cramping.

> You can get leg cramps from holding your leg, ankle, and foot muscles tightly, rather than letting them swing fluidly during walking.

Calf cramps during swimming are most usually caused by kicking with tight ankles, and holding the foot at a rigid angle. The rigid, unyielding way the foot and leg are held overstresses the muscles trying to do the work of moving you. Cramps at the bottom of the foot are usually from kicking with toes curled or hooked. Tightly hooked toes, either by habit or finning in fins too large or too small, tightly contracts the muscles at the bottom of the foot, which easily go into spasm. Sometimes, a swimmer will bend the knees too much, too hard while finning, overstressing the hamstrings, the muscles at the back of the thigh, causing them to cramp as well. In a pool, pushing too hard off the wall to do a start or turn can contract the calf muscle too tightly, making it cramp.

> The most common reason swimmers get leg cramps is kicking with tight ankles and hooked toes.

What to Do

Relieving a cramp can be easy and quick. A cramp is a contraction of a muscle. To release it, pull the muscle to lengthen it. You pull in the opposite direction that the cramp is pulling. The following cramp releases work whether you are running, swimming, or lying in bed.

For Calf Cramps: Calf cramps pull your foot down. To stretch the cramp out, pull your toes up toward the front of your leg and hold. Don't point your foot or start activity again too soon, or the muscle will likely cramp again.

For calf cramps while swimming in shallow water, stop and stand on the non-cramping leg and stretch the cramping leg. In deep water, take a big breath and hold it. Float facedown, grasp the offending foot, and do a cramp release while floating. This position makes you resemble a jellyfish with a surface floating body, and arms and legs trailing underwater like tentacles. Remember not to point your foot, or resume the bad kicking that cramped you in the first place. The muscle needs time to settle down.

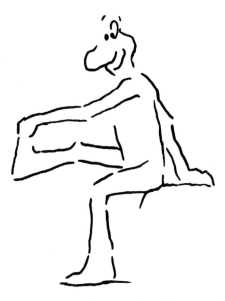

Figure 30.1. To stop a cramp, stretch the muscle in the opposite direction. To stretch out a calf cramp, pull your foot back and straighten your leg.

For Foot Cramps: Foot cramps pull your toes down. Grab your toes, pull them back, and hold. While wearing fins, grab the fin tip and pull up and back just as you would for a calf cramp, described above, paying attention to pulling your toes back.

For Hamstring Cramps: Hamstrings are the triple set of muscles in back of your upper leg. When they contract, whether by choice or by cramp, they bend your knee. To uncramp the hamstrings, straighten your knee and hold.

For Quadriceps Cramps: Your quadriceps are a set of four muscles (thus the name "quad") in front of your upper leg. When they contract, they straighten your knee. To uncramp the hamstrings, bend your knee and hold.

For Other Cramps: The principles are the same for any spasm your muscles may experience. A common nonleg cramp is a "stitch" in your side, which is a cramp of the diaphragm, your breathing muscle. A "stitch" may occur during a run or other active sport. One way to stretch out a "stitch" is to take a big breath, and hold it while attempting to breath out against the held breath. The pressure stretches things a bit and often releases the cramp. Other people find relief by raising their arms and straightening up, changing from the bent-over position which contracts the muscles.

Back spasms are also common. They can be ruinously painful, frightening, and hindersome to your range of motion and activities. But they are just cramps like all the others and can often be quickly stretched out and relaxed with the proper exercises. They should not be left in spasm for any period of time. Like any other cramp, this makes the muscle more ready to continue the cramp cycle. See Chapters 20 and 21 on back and neck pain for more on this.

What About Walking and Pounding?

You may have heard about walking around to stop a leg cramp, or pounding the muscle. These are not very effective, but can work coincidentally. Sometimes, people with a calf cramp jump up and walk, which bends back the foot, lengthening the muscle enough to stretch out the spasm. Sometimes, the pounding can push a muscle enough to lengthen it, but pounding is likely to make it contract more in sheer defense. Just stretch a cramp, and release the stretch slowly.

Should You Work Through Leg Cramps?

Should you allow a cramp to continue cramping and just ignore it, or keep swimming or whatever you're doing? No. Allowing a muscle to remain in spasm starts a vicious cycle. Spasm itself makes the muscle more "irritable," and ready to cramp again. Just after releasing a cramp, it usually feels like it wants to cramp again. If you point your foot, for example, after a calf cramp and contract the calf muscle again, chances are the calf will cramp again. Besides that, why stay in pain when cramps are so easy to reverse?

How to Prevent Leg Cramps

Daily Habits. Don't walk around all day holding your leg, ankle, and foot muscles tightly. Don't wear tight, uncomfortable shoes, or shoes that you may think are comfortable but that restrict your toes or the natural range of motion of your foot when walking. Take time to exercise, relax, and regularly stretch your legs and feet.

Proper Kick When Swimmng. The most effective prevention for leg cramps from kicking while swimming is not to kick with rigid ankles or curled toes. Kicking this way is a bad habit. Many people who kick this way do not know how to kick with loose ankles and floppy feet. The hallmark of people who hold their ankles tightly while kicking in a pool is that they barely make forward progress when using a kickboard without fins on, no matter how hard they kick. Their legs often sink, and kicking is tiring. Don't hold your foot in any one position, and don't deliberately bend it up and down with your kick. Allow it to flop loosely, independent of your leg. This is one of the most important aspects to kicking properly.

Special Exercises. Perhaps you're expecting a list of push-ups, exercises with weights, or running. Here is a surprise. The most important exercise to do if you get leg cramps is a drill to retrain your foot to be completely separate from muscular control while using the rest of your leg.

- Sit on a chair with your lower legs dangling. At a pool, sit at the rim of the pool, with your lower legs dangling free underwater.

- Grasp your lower leg near your ankle with both hands. Shake your leg up and down, paying attention to how your foot moves. It should flop freely as you shake it. Don't hold it rigidly angled at the ankle. Don't hook or curl your toes. This may take some work and practice. Let it be as loose and floppy as a rag doll.

- Carefully observe that as you shake your leg downward, your foot should flop upward, and as you quickly pull your leg up again, your foot flops downward loosely. It should not yank upward as a unit. If you shake side to side, your foot should also swing freely.

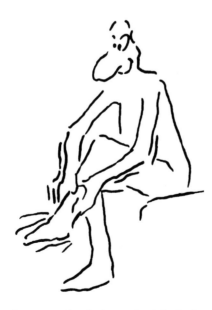

Figure 30.2. The floppy foot exercise is important to train your ankle to be loose. Shake your foot, allowing it to flop loosely in whatever direction you shake it.

Doing this exercise until you are successful is crucial for anyone who gets leg cramps while swimming. You can practice this anytime you are sitting comfortably. Someone else can shake your leg, too. Do this until you have retrained your legs' neuro-muscular patterns so well that you can flop your feet by quick, small knee movements without using your hands (or someone else's).

The test of a good, loose kick is when you can go into a pool without fins, take a kickboard, and kick with easy forward progress. Most people who have tight ankles make little, sometimes no, headway. Those with tight, hooked ankles, who also use a large deep swinging kick, can find themselves traveling backwards. Think of tight ankles, held rigidly at an angle from your leg, as airplane flaps. Trying to move forward with tight ankles is like trying to accelerate with your flaps down. With practice, you can loosen your ankles, develop an easy, powerful kick, and eliminate the majority of your leg cramps while swimming.

Leg Stretches. Another useful exercise (although not to be substituted for the floppy-foot drill) is stretching the back of your legs. It's been noted by some muscle-dynamics scientists that in societies without sit-down toilets, the habitual squatting stretches the appropriate muscles, making calf and foot cramps rare.

No More Leg Cramps

Do regular, easy stretches for your legs and feet, and build up the muscles of your feet and legs so they can handle exertion better. Leg cramps are not something you have to put up with.

31

Funny Physical Facts and Foibles

*Laughter is a form of internal jogging. It moves your internal organs around. It enhances respiration.
It is an igniter of great expectations.*

– Norman Cousins

Why Does It Hurt and Tingle When You Hit Your Funny Bone?

Why do they call it the funny bone? Why isn't it funny at all when you hit it? It's called the funny bone because it's the humerus.

The humerus is the long bone in your upper arm, extending from shoulder to elbow. A nerve called the ulnar nerve runs from your spine through your shoulder and elbow to your hand. Your ulnar nerve passes closest to your skin's surface just under the knob of bone at the elbow end of your humerus. When you ding your elbow there, you abruptly compress your ulnar nerve against the bone, causing acute, temporary pain and numbness.

Your ulnar nerve runs through your elbow in a passageway called the cubital tunnel. In medicine, the word *cubital* refers to the elbow. A person taking your blood pressure will position their stethoscope in the "antecubital space," in front of your elbow. *Cubital* comes from an ancient word that you've probably heard before. If you know the story of Noah's Ark, you remember "cubits," a unit of measure that Noah used to build the Ark. A cubit is the distance from fingertips to elbow. A dinged funny bone is called *transient cubital tunnel syndrome*.

How Much Blood Do You Have to Cut Off Before Your Foot Falls Asleep?

None. The phenomenon of "falling asleep" is not related to blood, but to nerve. When you compress a nerve enough, you can temporarily cause the numbing and pins-and-needles tingling that is popularly called "falling asleep" and medically called neuropraxia (nur-uh-PRAKS'-ee-ya). One common, short duration example is banging your funny bone. Sudden compression of the ulnar nerve in your elbow is responsible for the tingling funny bone, explained previously.

Another well-known, longer duration example is the phenomenon occurring in one or both legs after sitting too long at the edge of a bench, particularly in the bathroom. This phenomenon is called "toilet seat neuropathy" in medical parlance. In this occasion, after sitting too long, you try to stand up but fall over or hop around on tingling feet. It usually reverses quickly.

Where Did the Expression "Knee-Jerk Reaction" Come From, and What Does It Really Mean?

You've probably had a physician or someone else tap you just below your kneecap. Your lower leg jumped without you thinking about it. A knee-jerk reaction is one you don't think about. In other words, it doesn't use your brain. Here's why:

Just below your kneecap is the tendon connecting your four thigh muscles (quadriceps) to your lower leg. When the tendon is hit, it stretches slightly, but suddenly. The stretched tendon sends a sensory signal, which is a signal about what you felt, up your leg to the part of your spinal cord just above your behind. The signal says, "We're being stretched too fast, and it may mean trouble; send help to contract us!" The signal is reflected (that's why it's called a reflex) to a motor nerve. Motor nerves control movement. The motor nerve in your spinal cord sends a signal to your thigh muscles, the quadriceps. The signal says, "Contract!" Your quads contract to counter the stretch. Your leg jumps without any input at all from your brain. By the time a separate sensory signal gets all the way up to your brain to tell you that your tendon was stretched, your quads already contracted quickly, making your leg jump. The simple sensory-to-motor loop that needs no more than your spinal cord to function is called a stretch reflex. You can elicit other stretch reflexes by tapping behind your ankle on your Achilles tendon, or near the crease of your elbow on your biceps tendon.

There are other kinds of reflexes. They vary in complexity, but none needs your brain to operate. Sneezing is a reflex reaction to upper-respiratory irritation. Coughing is a reflex reaction to lower-respiratory irritation. The "wink" reflex closes your eye when something tries to fly in. The "hot stove" reflex yanks your hand away from high heat in the same "sensory-in, motor-out" reaction that, like other reflexes, does not involve conscious thought to initiate action.

The simplest reaction in your body is the reflex, and the "knee jerk" is the simplest of reflexes—only two nerves and no brain.

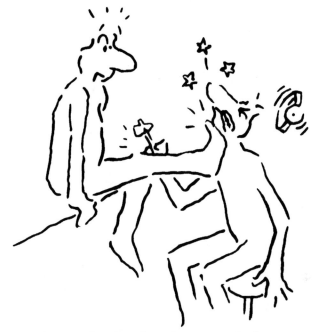

Figure 31.1. A knee jerk is a reflex that doesn't use your brain.

What Makes You Feel Pumped Up After Lifting Weights? How Does the Muscle Grow That Fast?

Your muscles don't immediately grow in the sense of adding lean weight or splitting muscle fibers. The size increase that occurs right after lifting and inflates muscles and egos is only fluid, and temporary fluid at that.

When you lift heavy weights, your working muscles contract, compressing the blood vessels in them. Circulation is temporarily reduced, or even stopped, with extreme muscular contraction.

After you finish lifting weights, a larger volume of blood and fluid than normal rushes back into your muscle, in reaction to the previous deficit. The extra blood puffs up the muscle. There's a fancy technical term for this phenomenon of extra blood puffing up muscles when they react to being contracted. The prefix for an amount greater than normal is *hyper*. The suffix *emia*, for blood, comes from the Greek *haima* (from which we get the words *hemorrhage, hemophilia, hemoglobin,* even *hemorrhoid*.) Speaking technically, pumping up is called *reactive hyperemia*.

Is It True That if You Put Sleeping People's Hands in a Glass of Water They Will Wet Themselves?

No. It is not true, but it is always worth a try for the sake of science.

Merely dipping the hand or fingers is ineffective. When you fully immerse your body in water, a real physiologic need to "go" occurs. However, even then, if you are potty-trained, the signals will not override your training. If you were immersed fully during sleep, this would still be so, as long-duration immersion experiments show.

Due to the effects of making you want to go, the increased output occurring with immersion may be called the "P Phenomenon," or PP for short. The P Phenomenon happens because immersing your body in water shifts blood away from your arms and legs to the area of your chest called the thorax. Because of buoyancy, fluids just float into the thorax. Being in a cold environment also shifts blood volumes to the thorax. That's why you often notice the P Phenomenon when stepping into a cold shower. Volume detectors in the heart notice the increase in fluid and, to normalize thoracic volume, helpfully signal your body to voluntarily show some fluid the way out.

In warm or hot water, however, the phenomenon is reduced. Blood vessels expand in your arms and legs in response to the heat. This peripheral vasodilation shifts blood to your limbs and reduces thoracic blood volume, reducing the physiologic cascade responsible for the P Phenomenon. The fact that warm water reduces the response offers even more evidence against the glass of water story, when the claim is that the water has to be warm.

The P Phenomenon even occurs in the microgravity environment of space travel. Fluids float away from the legs and into the upper body, just as during immersion in water. Astronauts have a technical term for this. They call it "The Fat-Face, Chicken-Legs Effect."

What Is the Popping Noise
When Your Joints Crack?

Joints pop in several ways. The interesting story starts with bubbles.

A certain amount of nitrogen from the air around you dissolves in your body fluids, including joint fluids called synovial fluids. When pressure is decreased, the gas can come out of its dissolved form. If that happens quickly, bubbles form. There are easy ways for this to happen, for example, popping your knuckles or squatting down and cracking your knees. More on why in a bit. Even scuba divers can do this by coming up from a dive too fast. That does not make noise, but can cause decompression sickness, where bubbles come out of solution in their bodies, get stuck, and cause pain and other problems in all the various places that they get stuck. Then the diver may make a lot of noise. Cracking your knuckles doesn't cause or relate to decompression sickness, although the bubble formation can be similar. Exactly how and why is extraordinarily complex. A summary of a few of the basics follows.

Gases like carbon dioxide and nitrogen are present in dissolved form in your body fluids. They are held in solution by the pressure of air around us and by gas pressures in your body. If you pull your finger joint so that it enlarges briefly, the slight vacuum formed creates a temporary low-pressure cavity. The low pressure pulls gas molecules out of solution, forming bubbles in a process called vacuum cavitation. The bubbles quickly collapse. Pop. It takes time for the gas to redissolve before the joint can crack again.

Another way bubbles can form besides enlarging the joint space is crushing the muscle against bone, as during some kinds of knuckle and knee cracking. Pop.

Studies have also looked at body tissues (in a laboratory) that are full of dissolved gas (the tissues, not the laboratory). These tissues had no bubbles, even after experimentally subjecting them to large pressure reductions. However, when energy was added by moving the tissue (as happens with muscle contraction), bubbles readily formed. Pop. Pop.

Not all joint cracking is due to bubbles. Often, it involves tendons moving quickly over adjacent bony knobs, making a distinctive noise. Pop. Tendons are tough, inelastic fibers that connect a muscle to a bone. Snapping tendons occurs routinely in many people's shoulder, elbow, hip, back, and ankle joints. Occasionally, tendon snapping occurs in the knee. This kind of snapping, unlike knuckle popping, can be repeated within short intervals, sometimes during every step when walking. Pop. Pop. Pop. Tight muscles can cause that, and specific stretching exercises can relieve it. On rare occasions it is so painful, constant, and detrimental to sports activity that surgery is performed to move the tendon to a slightly different position to avoid the snapping.

Another reason for joint popping can come from using bad sitting, standing, and lifting postures all day. As muscles tighten and contract unevenly, tendons or ligaments can get pulled slightly away from their accustomed track. People often learn that they can "crack" their back to restore a more comfortable position. Pop. Although it often feels good, it is not a miracle cure. It is better to learn to identify and minimize the muscle stress that caused the need in the first place.

How detrimental knuckle and other joint cracking may be to your joints depends on degree. It's probably safest to avoid any vigorous trauma to your joints. Joints are important parts of your body. Joint deterioration is related to the extent of abuse, genetics, and other not-well-identified factors. Although not a certainty, chronic, traumatic joint stress may be a contributor to early wear and tear that may lead to arthritic degeneration.

Not All "Knuckle" Popping Is in Your Body

Marine propellers cavitate bubbles by similar mechanical forces as knuckle popping. The rotating propeller blade rapidly forms low-pressure areas. Dissolved gas cavitates out of the water near the blades. When these many tiny bubbles suddenly form then collapse with great vigor against the blade, they make noise and eventually pit the blade. Pop. Pop. Pop. Anticavitation devices are important tools to extend the life of propellers and minimize military submarine noise.

Why Does Hair Grow Back Thicker and/or Darker When You Shave It?

It doesn't. This old tale is hard to kill. There is a reason hair seems to change, when it really doesn't. All body hair is thicker, and usually darker, at the base than the tip. When you shave, you cut off the thinner, lighter tips. When the rest of the hair shaft starts growing past the skin line again, you see only the thicker, darker part of the hair you cut. When that decapitated hair finally reaches the end of its cycle and falls out, the hair growing to replace it is not altered from its original shape or genetically determined color. If you shave again before this happens, you will feel the stubby growth again soon enough.

As far as boys shaving for the first time, the beard typically becomes coarser with the passing years of manhood, shaved or not. Hair change with maturation should not be confused with effects of shaving.

Why Are the Areas on the Side of the Head Called Temples?

The word "temple" comes from the Greek word for "time." The sides of the face near the ears are usually the first to go gray, evidencing the inevitable passage of time.

Does Oxygen Make You Feel Good?

Breathing oxygen is popularly thought to help football players, make you feel good, cure headaches, and work wildly as an aphrodisiac. All these claims have been firmly disproven—except one.

Chapter 4, "What Does 'Aerobic' Really Mean?" explained that breathing oxygen will not help football players. The sprints and tackles in football are so short that the body fuel that is used is quick and ready stored fuel, not oxygen. Football may be a hard sport, but it is not an aerobic one.

Studies by the Department of Internal Medicine at Baylor University, reported in the *Journal of the American Medical Association,* found no advantage to breathing 100% oxygen on recovery from exhaustive bouts of exercise, no difference in performance during a second bout after breathing 100% oxygen, and that the professional athletes who served as subjects could not identify whether they were breathing 100% oxygen or room air. In other studies, a percentage of subjects who were told they were breathing oxygen but received room air reported elevated mood.

Breathing supplemental oxygen benefits exercise if breathed *during* long duration, heavy exercise. Heart rate and blood levels of lactic acid decrease, and time to exhaustion increases. Still, carrying oxygen tanks while jogging or biking presents interesting practical problems. If you want to get more oxygen to your cells for greater long-distance ability, there is another way to do it yourself. Regular aerobic training enhances your body's entire oxygen-carrying and -using system.

As for effect on libido, there is no evidence of any physical aphrodisiac capability of oxygen. The placebo effect is potent in this area.

It is in relieving cluster headaches that oxygen seems to work. Breathing 100% oxygen constricts brain blood vessels. One of the mechanisms proposed for at least one stage of cluster headache is enlarged brain blood vessels that inflame and hurt. Oxygen is under study as a treatment for cluster headache (more on this in Chapter 29, "Headaches").

Oxygen is a good invention, no doubt. Many purported properties are fiction. But some are real. You can feel good about that.

GLOSSARY

A

Acetabulum   [From Latin *acetum*, "vinegar," from which we get acetic acid. Acetabulum is a shallow vinegar vessel or cup.]   Cup-shaped hollow in your hipbones, where the head of your upper leg bone (femur) fits. The socket of the ball and socket joint. Your acetabulum is located at the junction of the three hipbones, the ilium, ischium, and pubis bone. See Femur, Ilium, Ischium, and Pubis.

Acromion   [From Greek *akros*, "extreme," or "tip" + *omion*, diminutive of *omos*, "shoulder."] The bone of the outer end of your shoulder, formed by your shoulder blade (scapula) winging around to the front of your shoulder. Your collarbone attaches in front.

Adenosine Triphosphate (ATP)   (uh-DEN'-oh-sin try-FOS'-fate) [Named for its adenosine base plus three phosphates.]   The molecule made in your body that supplies energy to your cells for all your biochemical processes. It has two phosphates held on by low-energy bonds, and a third with a high-energy bond. ATP releases energy by breaking off the phosphate with the high-energy bond, becoming adenosine diphosphate (ADP). In extreme situations, ADP loses another phosphate to become adenosine monophosphate (AMP), but little more energy is gained, as that is a low-energy bond. You have three systems that make ATP—one is aerobic and two are anaerobic. See Aerobic Metabolism, Anaerobic Metabolism, and Creatine Phosphate (CP).

ADH   See Antidiuretic Hormone.

Aerobic Capacity   See Endurance, Cardiovascular.

Aerobic Exercise   Activities that are long and intense enough to benefit your cardiovascular system, but not so intense that your *an*aerobic energy-making systems have to do much work. Just sitting in a chair uses your aerobic metabolism for about 100% of your energy needs, but it is not an aerobic exercise. Sprinting down the street at top speed is exercise, but is so high intensity that your anaerobic systems predominate; your aerobic system can't supply energy fast enough. Jogging, swimming, or bicycling for 20 minutes or longer at a pace where you are not greatly out of breath is aerobic exercise.

Aerobic Metabolism   System of making ATP (an energy molecule) using oxygen with stored carbohydrate, fat, and protein. Aerobic metabolism goes on all day and night, even when you're sitting around or sleeping, making a distinction between aerobic metabolism and aerobic exercise. In animals, it takes place in the cells' organelles, called mitochondria. Your aerobic system has two pathways, the Krebs cycle and the electron transport chain. You make most of your ATP in the electron transport chain. When you exercise aerobically, oxygen carries off hydrogen ions, transforming lactic acid back to pyruvate, which can be used to make ATP. It also means that lactic acid does not get a chance to build up as it does when you are anaerobic. Your aerobic system allows you to generate energy for long, low- to moderate-intensity activities. Your aerobic metabolism can supply much energy, but can't do it very fast. Your *anaerobic* systems allow you to do quick, high-intensity activities. The combination of systems makes your exercise capacity versatile. See Adenosine Triphosphate (ATP), Anaerobic Metabolism, Electron Transport Chain, and Krebs Cycle.

Aldosterone (al-DOHS'-tur-own) [Named for its chemical structure containing an aldehyde and a sterol.] Steroid hormone secreted by your adrenal gland and regulated by your kidney. Helps you retain salt and water, and excrete potassium, to maintain their healthy balance in your body.

Allergy [From Greek *allos*, "other" + *ergon*, "action."] Condition where a person may react with sneezing, itching, and skin rashes to things like pollen, foods, or microorganisms, which cause no reaction in other people. Term coined by Austrian physician Pirquet, around the early 1900s.

Amenorrhea (ay-men-or-REE'-ah) [*a-*, "without" + Greek *men*, "month."] Long-term cessation of menstruation due to several causes, most notably low estrogen. A risk factor for osteoporosis.

Amphetamines [Composite word from A(lpha) + M(ethyl) + PH(enyl) + ET(hyl) + amine.] A group of stimulant drugs, sometimes used to increase athletic performance, to reduce fatigue, or to reduce hunger as an ingredient in diet pills. They are sympathomimetic, as they mimic the activation of your sympathetic nervous system, primarily by releasing nerve transmission chemicals called catecholamines, especially epinephrine (adrenaline) and norepinephrine (noradrenaline) from nerve endings. See Catecholamine, Ergogenic Aid, Sympathetic Nervous System, and Sympathomimetic.

Anabolic Steroids Drugs capable of increasing muscle growth. Not all steroids are anabolic, for example, the anti-inflammatories prednisone and cortisone, and Vitamin D. Since anabolic steroids have many dangerous effects along with their muscle building ones, they are prescription substances. Bodybuilders sometimes try to find nonregulated sources. There are no true anabolic steroids sold in health food stores, although many products that are just regular food have labels suggesting that they have anabolic effects. This is not illegal. Become educated to watch out for such misleading claims. See Ergogenic Aid.

Anaerobic Capacity Ability of your body to use special stored fuel, not oxygen, for rapid-onset, short-duration, intense activity. Because it is not an oxygen-using (aerobic) system, it is called anaerobic. You use your anaerobic system for sprinting, swimming against hard currents, lifting heavy weights, and any short, intense activity. You can improve your anaerobic capacity by exercising anaerobically, that is, practicing short, intense exercises. See Anaerobic Metabolism, and compare to Aerobic Exercise and Aerobic Metabolism.

Anaerobic Metabolism Two systems of making ATP, a special energy molecule, without using any oxygen. The first system is your ATP-CP system of stored ATP. Your second anaerobic system is glycolysis. It is important for you to have systems of making energy without using oxygen for the many activities that begin so quickly, and are so high intensity, that your oxygen system is not able to supply your needs. Your anaerobic systems allow you to do quick, high-intensity activities. Anaerobic metabolism can't make much ATP, but can do it very quickly. Your aerobic system allows you to generate energy for long, low- to moderate-intensity activities. The combination of systems makes your exercise capacity very versatile. See Adenosine Triposphate (ATP), Aerobic Metabolism, and Glycolysis.

Anorexia Nervosa [From Greek *an*, "without" + *orexis*, "appetite," from *oregein*, to reach out for.] An abnormal loss of appetite and refusal to eat, resulting in emaciation and malnutrition. A risk factor for osteoporosis.

Anthropometrics (an-throw-poh-MET'-tricks) [From Greek *anthrapos*, "human being" + *metrikos*, from *metron*, "measure."] Science of identifying and comparing human body measurements, such as lengths and widths of segments, to those of other segments, and to those of other people. One use of anthropometrics is to measure bone lengths and widths at specific joints to tell the size of your body's frame—small, medium, or large—which helps determine optimum weight. Another use of anthropometrics is to predict the sport you might excel in, based on your specific body size and other anthropometric measurements.

Antidiuretic Hormone. [From Greek *anti*, "opposite or against" + *diourein* "to pass urine" (*ourein*, to urinate).] Abbreviated ADH. A hormone made in the back (posterior lobe) of your pituitary gland that makes smooth muscle contract, particularly in all your blood vessels. ADH raises blood pressure and reduces excretion of urine. Also called vasopressin (from Latin words meaning an agent that presses down blood vessels).

Antihistamine [From Greek *anti*, "opposite" + histamine.] An agent that reduces effects of an inflammatory chemical called histamine. Both histamines and antihistamines are naturally produced in your body, but you occasionally need a "boost" of an oral or injectable antihistamine. Antihistamines work by blocking or displacing histamine at its sites of action. See Histamine.

Apnea (AP'-nee-uh) [From Greek *a-*, "without" + *pnoia*, "breathing."] Temporary halt to breathing. Examples are voluntary breath holding while swimming underwater, and involuntary lapses from sleep disorders involving snoring. See Sleep Apnea.

Apples and Pears Body classification system to predict, in a very general way, a tendency toward cardiovascular risk and obesity-linked disease. People who store fat primarily in their upper body and abdomen have bodies that resemble an apple shape, while pear-shaped people store fat mostly around the hips and thighs. Apple shape is associated with higher disease risk than pear shape.

Arrhythmia [From Greek *a*, "without" + *ruthmia*, "rhythm."] Irregular heartbeat. Arrhythmias occur normally now and then among normal heartbeats, without ill effect or you being aware of them. Too many arrhythmias, occurring too often, can be harmful.

Arteries Muscular, elastic, branching system of thick-walled tubes carrying blood away from your heart to your body. See Veins.

Arthritis   [From Greek *arthron*, "joint," + *itis*, "inflammation."] Inflammation of a joint, or joints, with pain, swelling, loss of function, and sometimes deformity of the joint. There are different kinds of arthritis. Degenerative, or osteoarthritis, involves wearing away the smooth cartilage on bone ends (articular cartilage). Osteoarthritis can be because of, or along with, trauma to the joint or other conditions. Other kinds of arthritis, like rheumatoid arthritis, are due to an autoimmune attack by the body against itself. Arthritis is treated with anti-inflammatory medications and exercise.

Atherosclerotic Plaques   [From Greek *athero*, "gruel-like," + *sclerosis*, "hardening."] Irregular deposits of lipid in the lining of medium and large arteries. Associated with cardiovascular disease.

B

Ball and Socket Joint   Type of joint, found in your shoulder and hip, allowing rotary motion in every direction. The ball part is a roundish knob of one bone that fits into a cavity or socket of the other. Also called enarthrosis. See Acetabulum and Femoral Neck.

Body Mass Index (BMI)   Pen and paper test for obesity, obtained by taking your weight in kilograms divided by height in meters squared. If BMI is above 25, you are considered by this test to be fat. If over 30, you are considered obese.

Bone   Semistiff connective tissue that holds up all your other soft, squishy parts. Bones in different parts of your body have varying amounts of a dense, compact, outer layer, called cortical bone, and an inner, loose, spongy trabecular bone. The central part of your long bones is filled with marrow. Bones are covered by the periosteum. Your bones are not all hard, inorganic mineral. Bone is about 75% inorganic material and 25% organic material. The protein, or collagen, portion of bones gives them flexibility and resiliency. If you remove the calcium from a bone by soaking it in vinegar, the bone would become as flexible as a dog's rubber plaything. See Cortical Bone, Periosteum, and Trabecular Bone.

Bradycardia   [From Greek *brady*, "slow" + *kardia*, "heart."] Slow heart rate in an adult human, usually fewer than 60 beats per minute.

Bronchi   (BRON'-kai) [From Greek *bronkhos*, "windpipe."] Plural of bronchus. The two branches of your windpipe leading to your lungs.

Bursa   [From Greek, "wineskin," "purse."] A little sac containing viscous lubricating fluid, located where a tendon passes over a bone, or at points of friction between moving body structures. You have over 70 bursas in various places in your body. Chronically irritating a bursa can result in inflammation, called bursitis. Shoulder bursitis can result from bad shoulder exercises. Knee bursitis can result from too much kneeling, what used to be called "housemaid's knee."

C

Cadaver Analysis   Body fat determination technique of cutting a body open to directly measure fat stores.

Calcium Balance   Amount of body calcium gain versus loss. Positive calcium balance occurs when more calcium is absorbed from your diet than excreted. Excess calcium deposits in your skeleton. When loss exceeds absorption, calcium will mobilize (be taken) from your bone, a process called negative calcium balance.

Calipers   [Alteration of caliber.] Small instrument used for measuring diameters. Calipers used for body composition analysis measure the thickness of your folds of fat. Caliper measurement is painless, except by overenthusiastic testers. The error of measurement can often be large, varying greatly with tester experience. Calipers are often misused in health clubs. If, for example, you are measured at 25% the first time, and 22% the second time, it is incorrect to state that you lost 3% fat. Because of error of measurement, that is impossible to tell.

Carbohydrate   [From Latin *carbon* + Greek *hudro,* "water," because they are made of carbon, hydrogen, and oxygen.] Organic compounds including sugar, starch, and cellulose. Found in nutritional quantities only in plants, they are a major energy source for many animals, including humans. Animals store a carbohydrate called glycogen in their muscles and liver, but not enough to supply any appreciable amount if the animal is eaten. For that reason, meat is not considered to have any carbohydrate. See Glycogen.

Carbohydrate-Loader Drink   Beverage containing carbohydrate, used to replace fluids and delay fatigue in long endurance events. See Carbohydrate, Carbohydrate-Replacer Drink, and Electrolyte.

Carbohydrate-Replacer Drink   High-carbohydrate drink, used both to replace fluids and restock your body's carbohydrate supply after long endurance events. See Carbohydrate, Carbohydrate-Loader Drink, and Electrolyte.

Catecholamine   (cat-eh-COAL'-uh-meen) [Named for its chemical structure derived from a catechol and an amine, and so, catechol-amine.] Important family of nervous system chemicals that work as both neurotransmitters and hormones to transmit signals in your body. Some of your important catecholamines are dopamine, norepinephrine, and epinephrine. Your body makes them in sequential steps, starting with the amino acid tyrosine. Each step turns each catecholamine into the next. First, you make tyrosine into DOPA. From DOPA, you make dopamine. From dopamine, you make norepinephrine. From norepinephrine, you make epinephrine (same as adrenaline).

Cervical Vertebrae   [From Latin *cervic,* "neck."] The seven bones of your neck. They are named sequentially down from your head as C1–C7. If you tip your head forward and feel the back of your neck, your most prominent bump is your C7 vertebra. Your other six cervical vertebrae are above it. Below C7 begin your 12 thoracic vertebrae, which are the bones of your upper back. See Lumbar Vertebrae, Thoracic Vertebrae, and Vertebra.

Cholesterol [From Greek *khole,* "bile" (because it was first found in gallstones) and from which we get words like gall and gold, + Greek *stereos,* "solid."] Made in your liver, cholesterol is an important constituent of all your cell membranes, and a precursor to steroid hormones. Also influences development of cardiovascular disease. Cholesterol circulates in your blood plasma, carried around by proteins of various densities (lipoproteins). Cholesterol is the most abundant steroid in animal tissues, but not found at all in plants. See High-Density Lipoprotein Cholesterol, and Low-Density Lipoprotein Cholesterol.

Claudication [From Latin *claudico,* "to limp."] Leg pain from clogged blood vessels in your legs.

Coca Leaves [Coca is Spanish, from the Quechua *kúka.*] Dried leaves of certain small shrubs or trees, genus Erythroxylum, especially E. coca. The leaves contain cocaine and other alkaloids, and are chewed for a stimulating effect by people of the Andes to help tolerate hunger, fatigue, and altitude, or harvested and purified for making cocaine. See Ergogenic Aid.

Coccyx (KOKS'-icks) [G. *kokkyx,* "cuckoo," from its resemblance to a cuckoo's beak.] Tail bone. Small, triangular bone at the end of the spine in human beings and tailless apes. Made of four fused rudimentary vertebrae. See Cervical Vertebrae, Lumbar Vertebrae, Thoracic Vertebrae,and Vertebra.

Coenzyme A body chemical that you need to enhance or promote action of an enzyme. Coenzymes are smaller than the enzymes they work with. Usually contains a vitamin or mineral combined with a specific protein. Sometimes, coenzymes are misrepresented as able to improve physical ability if taken orally, which is not the case. Like all proteins, they are broken down into component parts to digest and pass through your intestinal wall. They will not automatically reassemble into the original coenzyme on the other side. See Enzyme and Ergogenic Aid.

Cortical Bone [From Latin *cortex,* bark.] Also called compact bone. Dense, strong bone forming the outside shell or wall of your long bones. When bone loss occurs with normal (and accelerated) aging processes, cortical bone loss occurs later than trabecular bone loss. See Bone, Periosteum, and Trabecular Bone.

Cramp [Possibly from Middle Dutch *crampe,* hook, to restrict or prevent from free action or expression.] Sudden, involuntary, painful muscle spasm, or shortening. Stretching your muscle to lengthen it releases the cramp. Cramp releases on leg, foot, and side cramps can be easily done yourself, and on back spasms, done yourself or by orthopedists, osteopaths, and trained massage therapists and physical therapists.

Creatine Phosphate (CP) [Named for its composition of creatine with phosphoric acid.] Organic compound in your muscles that stores and provides energy for muscular contraction. Breaking down creatine phosphate provides the phosphate you need to make ATP, the bottom-line energy molecule for all your body processes. Also called phosphocreatine. See Adenosine Triphosphate (ATP).

D

Disc [From Greek *diskos,* "to throw."] Round, flat, fibrocartilage cushion between certain bones. You have tiny little discs between your jawbone (mandible) and your head bone (temporal bone). Sometimes, these discs wear out, causing pain at the joint between those two bones called the temporomandibular joint (TMJ), causing TMJ pain. Your vertebral discs lie between the bones of your spine (vertebrae). Vertebral discs are commonly injured over time by bad sitting, standing, and lifting postures, particularly discs of your lower back (lumbar vertebrae). That is where you usually impose the greatest stresses when lifting, sitting, and standing improperly. See Disc Herniation and Lumbar Vertebrae.

Disc Herniation (slipped discs) Protrusion of a vertebral disc beyond its normal place. Can cause pain by itself, and also by pressing on nerves and other structures, which causes pain away from the site of herniation. Discs are pushed out of place over time by bad sitting, standing, and lifting habits, and usually easily treated without surgery, by good back habits and exercises.

Dorsiflex [From Latin *dorsum,* "back" + flex, "to bend."] Turning your hand or foot toward the upper side. To bend the ankle so your toes point backward toward the top of your foot. See Plantarflex.

Dowager's Hump Curved, hunched appearance of the upper back in both men and women, caused by osteoporotic crush fractures of the thoracic vertebrae (bones of the upper back). See Osteoporosis.

E

Electrolyte [From Greek *electro* + *lytos* and *lysis,* "soluble" or "loosening," from which we get such words as *dialysis, electrolysis,* and *analysis.*] Any substance that, when dissolved in a liquid, becomes electrically conductive because it breaks up into ions. Ions are atoms or molecules with at least one electron more or less than normal for it, giving it a negative or positive charge. For example, table salt (sodium chloride) breaks down in water into the positive sodium ion and the negative chloride ion. In physiology, the term *electrolyte* usually refers to the ions, rather than the original substance. Your cells use electrolytes to regulate processes, such as flow of water across your cell membranes. Ions propagate signals along nerves for all the thousands of functions that nerves control to keep you alive, moving, and thinking. Two of your principal positively charged ions (electrolytes) are sodium and potassium. Magnesium and calcium are also positive ions. Two important negatively charged ions are chloride and bicarbonate.

Electrolyte Drink Beverage containing electrolytes and, usually, carbohydrates to supply water, electrolytes, and carbohydrate before, during, or after exercise.

Electron Transport Chain A sequence of reactions that are part of how you make ATP energy aerobically. Electrons from the Krebs cycle get transported to oxygen by little electron carriers. The electrons pass through a series of iron-containing proteins called cytochromes (close relatives of hemoglobin). Each player in the series is increasingly fond of electrons, so that the entire series runs "downhill," and energy is produced. Energy not used for chemical work dissipates as heat. The electron transport chain is also called the respiratory chain and the cytochrome system. See Adenosine Triphosphate (ATP) and Krebs Cycle.

Endorphin   [Composite word from *endogenous* ("made from within") + "morphine-like substance."] A class of hormones produced by a number of processes, including extended, hard exercise. Not confirmed, but, along with other opioid chemicals produced in your body, possibly associated with positive mood after good workouts.

Endurance, Cardiovascular   [From Latin *indurare*, "to harden."] Ability of your heart and lungs to get oxygen and nutrients to your body for fuel during exercise. Determines how long you can go at a given pace. Needed for continuous, mid- and low-intensity walking, running, skiing, swimming, cycling, etc. Also called cardiorespiratory endurance, aerobic capacity, or functional capacity. See Aerobic Metabolism, Anaerobic Capacity, and Anaerobic Metabolism.

Endurance, Muscular   [From Latin *indurare*, to harden.] Ability of muscles to move a relatively light weight repeatedly. Walking, swimming, finning, cycling, running, and even sitting and standing up straight all day require muscular endurance.

Enzyme   [From Greek *en-*, "in" + *zume*, "yeast," from which we get the word *zymurgy*, the branch of chemistry dealing with fermenting and brewing alcohol. From the Greek word *zein*, "to boil."] A protein which speeds up chemical reactions. Enzymes function by holding other molecules in just the right way so that they can put the molecules together or break them apart. Examples of enzymes that help break apart other molecules are lactase, which breaks down lactose in milk; amylase in your saliva, which starts breaking down carbohydrates you eat; papain, a plant enzyme used in meat tenderizer that breaks down meat protein; and zymase, the enzyme in yeast that breaks down sugar into alcohol and carbon dioxide. The various synthetase enzymes help put molecules together. With notable exceptions, names of most enzymes end in the suffix *-ase*. All enzymes are proteins. Enzymes that you eat are destroyed by digestion before they can pass into your blood stream and reach your body tissues. Digesting means breaking down to components small enough to pass through your intestinal wall. It will not automatically reassemble into the original enzyme on the other side of your intestinal wall. Eating enzymes, promoted as health foods (except digestive aids), will not raise body enzyme levels. See Coenzyme.

Ergogenic Aid   [From Greek *ergon*, "work" + *gen*, "producing" or "*gen*erating"]. Products that enhance physical ability. Ergogenic aids may be nutritional, psychological, or physical. Not everything claimed to be ergogenic is ergogenic. There are many sham products on the market. Some ergogenic aids work, such as caffeine and amphetamines. Not all dietary products sold as ergogenic aids are completely healthful or non-habit-forming, such as the several stimulant herbs on the market, or products containing caffeine. See Amphetamines, Anabolic Steroids, Coenzyme, Ginseng, Ma Huang, Minerals, and Vitamins.

Extension   Increasing the angle of a joint. Elbow extension is when you straighten a bent arm. Knee extension is straightening your knee. Neck and back extension involve moving your head or torso, respectively, away from a bent-forward position. Hyperextension is extending your joint past a straight line, or 180 degrees. See Flexion.

F

Facets, Vertebral   [From Old French *facette*, "little face."] Small, smooth areas on your spine bones (vertebrae), where one vertebra fits together with the next. If injured over time with bad back posture, can be a cause of back pain. Usually associated with chronic, excessive, arching postures.

Fat   A greasy substance found in adipose tissue of animals, and in seeds and nuts. In animals, fat is the principle storage form for energy. As a food, fat gives you 9 calories per gram. Carbohydrate and protein, by comparison, give you 4 calories per gram. See Carbohydrate and Protein.

Femoral Neck   Slender part of your upper thigh bone (femur) near your hip between the long bone of your femur with the "ball" part of your femur (the femoral head). Your femoral head fits into the "socket" of your hip, called the acetabulum. The femoral neck is a common site of osteoporotic fracture. See Acetabulum, Ball and Socket Joint, Femur.

Femur   [From Latin for "thigh."]   Your thighbone (upper leg bone) between your hip and knee. It is the largest and strongest bone in your body.

Flexibility   [From Latin *flexibilis*, "to bend."] Ability to move safely and comfortably through a range of motion to do the things you want to do.

Flexion   [From Latin *flectere*, "to bend."] Decreasing the angle of a joint. Elbow flexion, for example, is bending your arm. Knee flexion involves bending your knee. (*Genu* is the Latin word for "knee," giving us the word *genuflection*.) Neck and back flexion involve curling your head or torso, respectively, toward a bent-forward position. Too much flexion in your lower back, usually from poor posture when sitting, contributes to back pain. See Extension.

Folic Acid   [From Latin *folium*, "leaf," for its common occurrence in leafy vegetables.] Substance from the Vitamin B complex group, occurring in green plants, fresh fruit, and yeast. Also called folacin, folate, and Vitamin Bc. Deficiency of folic acid is known to be associated with birth defects, and more recently with heart disease and stroke. Eating more green, leafy vegetables adds folic acid to your diet.

Food Pyramid   A schematic of seven food groups for nutritional health. The food pyramid replaces old "four food groups." Large helpings of fruits, grains, and vegetables form the large, solid base of the pyramid. Middle groups of protein include beans and nuts. Has a small sugar and fat group at the top point, indicating to eat only a small amount of them. Food pyramid recommendations stress vegetables as main dishes, with meat as side dishes if you eat meat, not the other way around.

Four Food Groups   An obsolete system of grouping foods into four categories to be eaten at every meal. It was found that diets based on the four categories were high fat, stressed too much meat and dairy, and had only about half of the minimum daily required amounts of needed nutrients.

Free Radical   An atom, molecule, or macromolecule existing temporarily with at least one unpaired electron. Electrons usually prefer to be paired. Being unpaired makes them reactive and eager either to acquire another electron or to lose the unpaired one. Some free radicals are beneficial, such as those involved in muscle contraction and in your immune response, while others are involved in disease processes. Free radicals occur normally as a by-product of breathing, and in increased numbers during exercise, in smog, from cigarette smoke, and in high-pressure oxygen environments. In 1954, Rebecca Gershman and her colleagues, in a theory now widely accepted, proposed that the damaging effects of oxygen toxicity are caused by oxygen free radicals. Because it has one unpaired electron, oxygen free radicals strongly want to take an electron from other molecules, particularly from your fatty acids and proteins. When oxygen free radicals grab electrons from your hemoglobin, cell membranes, or protein enzymes, they can't do their jobs, and become free radicals themselves, going on to grab electrons from others, in a destructive game of tag. Your body produces various antioxidant substances to neutralize many free radicals.

G

Gastrocnemius   [From Greek *gastro,* "belly," referring to the largest part of a muscle + *kneme,* "leg."] Large, prominent muscle of the calf of your leg. Attaches to your Achilles tendon and pulls on the tendon to pull your foot downward (plantarflex).

Ginseng   [From Mandarin Chinese *ren,* "person" + *shen,* collective name of a variety of herbs with fat, fleshy roots sometimes resembling the human body.] Any of several plants, or roots of plants, of genus *Panax,* particularly *P. pseudoginseng,* of eastern Asia, or *P. quinquefolius* of North America. Stimulates your nervous system, raising your heart rate and blood pressure. See Ergogenic Aid.

Glycogen   [From Greek *glukos,* "sweet" + *gen,* "making" or "producing."] The form in which glucose (sugar) is stored in your body, mostly in your liver and muscles. Glycogen is converted to glucose through a series of enzymatic steps to meet your body's rapid energy needs. See Glycolysis.

Glycogen Loading   An exercise and diet procedure to increase the amount of glycogen you can store. Greater stores of glycogen extend your exercise capacity.

Glycogen Sparing   Body process of using more fat as an exercise fuel, and less glycogen, and so "sparing" your glycogen. Glycogen sparing allows more time until your glycogen stores are exhausted, allowing you to exercise longer. Being in better shape "teaches" your body better glycogen sparing.

Glycolysis   [From Greek *glukos*, "sweet" + *lysis*, "breaking down" or "loosening," seen in such words as *dialysis, electrolysis,* and *analysis*.] Metabolic process of breaking down carbohydrates and sugars, typically glucose, to generate ATP, your "bottom-line" energy molecule. Occurs in almost all living cells. In humans, the last product generated by glycolysis while making ATP aerobically is pyruvic acid (aerobic glycolysis). When you are anaerobic, the process goes one more step to lactic acid (anaerobic glycolysis). When you have enough oxygen, lactic acid can be changed back to pyruvic acid. This series of reactions was described by Gustav Embden and Otto Meyerhof in the 1930s, and so is sometimes called the Embden-Meyerhof cycle. Glycolysis can make only two molecules of ATP from a molecule of glucose, while your aerobic metabolism can make 36. Being aerobic makes more energy, which is why your aerobic system lets you exercise longer than your anaerobic system. See Adenosine Triphosphate (ATP), Glycogen, Lactic Acid, and Pyruvic Acid.

H

Hamstring Muscles   Triple set of muscles on the back of your upper leg. Your hamstring muscles work to bend your knee and straighten your hip. Your two innermost hamstrings, or medial hamstrings, are the semimembranosus and semitendinosus muscles. Your outside, or lateral, hamstring is the biceps femoris muscle. The term *hamstrings* is also used to refer to the tendons of the three muscles, readily felt as stringy cords on either side of the hollow of the back of your knee.

Hemochromatosis   [Greek *haima*, "blood" + *khroma*, "color" + *osis*, "condition."] A hereditary disorder of iron metabolism, where you absorb and keep too much of the iron you eat. Iron deposits in the tissues, particularly the liver, pancreas, and skin, where it causes a bronze coloration and constant fatigue. Eventually, heart and liver failure may occur.

High-Density Lipoprotein Cholesterol   Popularly called "good cholesterol." Compound containing lipid (fat) and protein. HDL removes cholesterol from your blood stream, and does not collect on or stick to the inner linings of your arteries. You can increase your levels of HDL with exercise and low-fat meals. See Cholesterol and Low-Density Lipoprotein Cholesterol.

Hip Flexors   Muscles that bend (flex) your hip into a sitting position. Many people confuse hip flexor exercises that bend the hip, like sit-ups and leg lifts, for abdominal exercises that, properly done, would involve only your abdominal muscles that curl your trunk. The three major hip flexors are the iliacus, psoas (SEW'-as), and rectus femoris. The iliacus and psoas, often lumped together as the iliopsoas, are your "filet mignon" muscles. Beef animals are prevented from exercising their hip flexors to make the muscle soft and fatty for humans to eat. Tight hip flexor muscles contribute to poor posture, back pain, and surprisingly, shoulder injuries, when your shoulder has to overrotate to reach overhead because tight hip flexors do not allow full range of motion of your torso.

Histamine   [Named because it is an amine derived from histidine, and so hist (idine) + amine.] An amine released from cells of your immune system as part of an allergic reaction. Histamine powerfully stimulates gastric secretions, constricts bronchial smooth muscle that restricts breathing, and dilates small blood vessels. Sometimes, this dilation is extensive enough to cause a drop in blood pressure. See Antihistamine.

Homeostasis [From Greek *homos*, "same" + *stasis*, "standstill."] Continuous regulation of all your body's goings-on, using physiologic checks and balances to maintain your system at its set equilibrium. Body temperature, oxygen levels, pH, water balance, plasma ion regulation, calorie utilization, and many other processes are all tightly regulated. The principle was first described by French physiologist Claude Bernard, and later given its name by Walter Cannon, a Harvard physiologist.

Homeotherm (HOME'-ee-oh-thurm) [From Greek *homos*, "same" + *therme*, "heat."] Animals who generate and regulate heat internally to maintain a largely constant body temperature that is independent of, and typically above, surrounding temperature. Birds and mammals are homeotherms. Sometimes called endotherms. See Poikilotherm.

Hormone [From Greek *horman*, "to urge on."] Chemical messengers, usually peptides or steroids, produced in one body tissue and traveling through your blood to stimulate or suppress activity in another tissue. Examples, among many, are insulin, adrenaline (epinephrine), and antidiuretic hormone (ADH). Hormones regulate body processes as diverse as growth, metabolism, and reproduction, and can modify behavior.

Hydrostatic Weighing Also called underwater weighing. Body composition analysis technique to determine body fat, called the "gold standard" because it has a low error of measurement, and other tests of body composition are often compared in percentage error to hydrostatic weighing. To be weighed hydrostatically, you sit on a scale in a vat of water, then exhale all you can while keeping your entire body underwater.

Hypertonic [Prefix *hyper*, "more" or "above" + Greek *tonos*, "tension."] In chemistry, a solution containing a higher concentration of dissolved particles compared to a reference solution, usually blood or body tissues. For example, seawater is hypertonic to your blood (about three times more concentrated, contrary to popular belief that they are similar). See Hypotonic and Isotonic.

Hypotonic [*hypo*, "less," or "under" + Greek *tonos*, "tension."] In chemistry, a solution containing a smaller concentration of dissolved particles compared to a reference solution, usually blood or body tissues. For example, fresh water is hypotonic to your blood. See Hypertonic and Isotonic.

Hypovolemic Thirst One of your two thirst mechanisms. Stimulated by low body water stores. See Osmotic Thirst.

Hypoxia [Prefix *hypo* + *oxa*, "oxygen."] Condition in which insufficient oxygen reaches body tissues. Distinct from (but usually related to) hypoxemia, which is insufficient oxygenation of blood.

I

Ilium   [From Latin *ilium*, "groin" or "flank."] Widest and uppermost of three bones that make up each side of your pelvis. The ilium on each side of your hips can be felt as the "shelf" that you can rest a bundle on. See Ischium and Pubis (your other two pelvic bones).

Inflammation   [From Latin, *in* + *flammare*, "to set on fire."] Response of body tissues to an injury, bite, sting, or infection. Characterized by warmth (calor), redness (rubor), swelling (tumor), and pain (dolor). Inflammation attracts immune cells, which secrete free radicals to kill bacteria and other invaders. See Free Radical.

Insensible Perspiration   Sweat that evaporates before you are aware of it. The term sometimes includes evaporation from your respiratory tract.

Insulinogenic   [Insulin + Greek *gen*, "producing."] Substance that encourages insulin production. Sometimes, carbohydrate products are misrepresented in health food stores as special foods that stimulate insulin. Because one function of insulin is to encourage protein storage, advertisers lead people to believe that eating such food will build muscle. But just about any food is insulinogenic, and another function of insulin is to aid fat storage. Conversely, a popular high-protein diet promotes the idea that you must avoid nonprotein foods because they stimulate insulin, leading to more fat storage, and eat only high-protein foods. That also seems to be misleading (and potentially unhealthy). High-protein diets "work" because they are low-calorie, not for any insulin-stimulating or suppressing quality.

Insurance Tables   Predetermined values in insurance company tables of ranges of "acceptable" weights for various heights and frame sizes. Usually, if you are more than 20% over this weight range, you are considered by the particular tables to be obese. Sometimes used to determine approximate risk of some cardiovascular diseases, and thus eligibility for certain kinds of insurance.

Ischemia   (is-KEE'-me-uh) [From Greek *iskhein*, "to hold back" + *haima*, "blood." From *haima*, we get words like *hemoglobin, hemorrhage,* and *hemorrhoid*.] Decrease in blood supply to your cells due to constriction or obstruction of your blood vessels, for example, during heart attack or muscle spasm. Pain and loss of function follows ischemia.

Ischial Tuberosity   [From Greek *iskhion*, "hip."]   Butt bones or sit bones. Protuberance at the base of your lower hip (ischial) bones, where muscles, notably your hamstrings, attach. You can feel your ischial tuberosities as the bumps of bone that you sit on. The ischium is the lowest of the three bones that, together, make up each half of your pelvis. The other bones are the pubic bones, which fuse in front to become your anterior hip bone, and the ilium, whose crests on either side of your hip you can feel as the two "shelves" that you can rest a package upon.

Ischium   [From Greek *iskhion*, "hip joint."] The lowest of the three bones that make up each half of your pelvis. At the bottom of each ischium is a bump, called the ischial tuberosity. These are the bony bumps you sit on. See Hamstring Muscles, Ilium, Ischial Tuberosity, and Pubis.

Isotonic [From Greek *isos*, "equal" + *tonos*, "tension."] In chemistry, a solution containing the same total concentration of dissolved particles as a reference solution, usually your blood or body tissues. For example, many commercial sport electrolyte drinks are isotonic to your blood. A popular myth is that your blood is isotonic to seawater. However, it is much less concentrated, or hypotonic. Even many sea creatures have different tonicities than the sea, some higher, some lower.

J

Jiggle Test An informal test of body composition. Jump in the air. When you land, see how long it takes for all your parts to stop jiggling. Higher times indicate higher fat amounts. See Apples and Pears, Body Mass Index, Calipers, and Hydrostatic Weighing.

K

Krebs Cycle [Named for Sir Hans Adolf Krebs, who won the Nobel Prize in 1953 for this important discovery.] A cyclic series of reactions that are part of how you use oxygen to make the energy-yielding molecule ATP. It is a cycle, as the last step in the chain of reactions is making the chemical you started with (citric acid). Each of the steps in the cycle needs a specific enzyme. Electrons removed during the Krebs cycle enter your second major aerobic pathway to make ATP energy, called the electron transport chain. The Krebs cycle is also called the citric acid cycle or tricarboxylic acid cycle (TCA). See Adenosine Triphosphate (ATP), Aerobic Metabolism, and Electron Transport Chain.

L

Lactic Acid or **Lactate** [From Latin *lact*, "milk," named because bacteria in milk produce it from the milk sugar lactose in the process of making their energy. They excrete the lactic acid into the milk, which sours it.] Molecule formed by metabolizing glucose for energy, when there is not enough oxygen present (anaerobic metabolism). Lactic acid is associated with the burning feeling of muscles that occurs during anaerobic metabolism. When enough oxygen is present, lactic acid changes back to pyruvic acid, which can be used in aerobic metabolism. See Adenosine Triphosphate (ATP), Anaerobic Capacity, Anaerobic Metabolism, Glycolysis, and Pyruvic Acid.

Ligament [From Latin *ligare*, "to bind."] Tough, fibrous bands connecting bones to each other, connecting cartilage at a joint, or supporting an organ.

Low-Density Lipoprotein Cholesterol Popularly called "bad cholesterol." Compound containing lipid (fat) and protein. Dietary cholesterol and cholesterol made in your liver are transported to your blood vessels and muscles by LDL. Too much LDL can be a risk factor for cardiovascular disease. See Cholesterol and High-Density Lipoprotein Cholesterol.

Lumbar Vertebrae or **Lumbar Spine**   [From Latin *lumbus*, "loin."] Five spinal bones of your lower back. They are named, from top to bottom, L1–L5. The intervertebral discs most often involved in low-back pain are between L4 and L5 and, particularly, between L5 and S1. S1 is your first sacral vertebra. See Cervical Vertebrae, Disc, Sacrum, and Thoracic Vertebrae.

M

Ma Huang   [From Mandarin Chinese *ma*, "hemp" + *huang*, "yellow."] Asian plants of the genus Ephedra, particularly *E. sinica*, which contains the stimulant ephedrine. Ma huang is often sold in health food and oriental medicine stores in various drinks and pills for its stimulant effects on your nervous system, heart, and blood vessels, giving a "peppy" feeling. It can be dangerous in high amounts. See Ergogenic Aid and Sympathomimetic.

Meniscus   [From Greek *meniskos*, diminutive of *mene*, "moon," for its shape.] In anatomy, menisci are flat cartilaginous discs that act as cushions between the ends of your knee bones. In each knee you have two menisci, side-by-side between your upper leg bone (femur) and lower leg bone (tibia). The meniscus on the inner side of each knee is your medial meniscus. The one on the outer side is your lateral meniscus. Menisci can be torn by twisting your knee, and worn out by poor leg postures when walking. See Disc.

Menopause [From Greek *meno*, "month" + Greek *pausis*, "cessation."] Phase of life after menstrual and reproductive functions. Twenty-five percent of American women reach menopause by age 47, half by 50, three quarters by 52, and 95% by age 55. Menopause is a risk factor for osteoporosis. There seems to be a physical corollary in men, where hormonal functions taper and bone loss accelerates, among other effects.

Metabolism   [From Greek *metaballein*, "to change."] The total of all physical and chemical processes in cells and living systems as a whole, necessary for energy synthesis to maintain life.

Minerals   [From Latin *mineralis*, pertaining to mines and mining.] Dietary minerals are inorganic elements essential to the health of humans, animals, and plants. Examples are iron, calcium, potassium, sodium, and zinc.

Mole [From German *mol*, short for *Molekulargewicht*, "molecular weight."] A unit of measure to manage large numbers of atoms, molecules, ions, etc. One mole is 6.0225×10^{23}, or Avogadro's number. Also called gram molecule.

Muscle Spindles   [Named for their thin, spindle-like shape.] Small, thin, sensory organs in your muscles (and the muscles of all vertebrates). Muscle spindles are sensitive to the stretch of the muscle they are in. Also called neuromuscular spindle, stretch receptor, and Kühne's spindle. Named for Wilhelm (Willy) F. Kühne, German physiologist and histologist (1837–1900) who first identified them. See Myotatic Reflex and Proprioceptors.

Myotatic Reflex   [From Greek *myo*, "muscle" + *tasis*, "a stretching."]   Quick muscle contraction in response to a sudden stretching force on your muscle. Initiated by stimulation of muscle proprioceptors called spindles—stretch receptors in your muscles. Also called the Liddell-Sherrington reflex, the muscular reflex, and the stretch reflex. See Muscle Spindles and Proprioceptors.

N

Neurotransmitter   [Neuro is from the Greek *sinew*, meaning "string" or "nerve" + "transmitter."] Group of chemicals your body produces to send nerve impulses from one nerve ending to the next, across a tiny space called a synapse. Examples of neurotransmitters, among many, are acetylcholine, serotonin, and catecholamines, such as dopamine, norepinephrine, and epinephrine.

O

Ondine's Curse (or Undine's Curse)   Literary term from Greek mythology for sleep apnea. Ondine (or Undine) was a water sprite who cursed a deserving villain with being able to breathe only voluntarily. When he fell asleep, he stopped breathing, and suffocated. See Sleep Apnea.

Oophorectomy (oo-for-EK'-tuh-mee)   [From Greek *oon*, "egg," + *phoros*, "bearing," + *ectom*, "excising" or "removing."] Surgical removal of the female gonads, the ovaries. Sometimes done in conjunction with hysterectomy—removal of the uterus. Equivalent in hormonal effect to male castration. A risk factor for osteoporosis.

Osmotic Thirst   One of your two thirst mechanisms. Stimulated by high blood electrolyte content, regardless of your body's total water volume. That is why salty things make you thirsty, even when you are drinking (and why bars serve you salty finger food). Drinking ethanol-containing fluids also makes you thirsty because ethanol increases urination and water loss by suppressing the hormone ADH. See Antidiuretic Hormone and Hypovolemic Thirst.

Osteomalacia [From Greek *osteon*, "bone" + *malakia*, "softness."] Gradual softening and bending of bone, usually from Vitamin D deficiency. Associated with varying amounts of pain.

Osteopenia   [From Greek, *osteon*, "bone" + *penia*, "poverty."] Any decrease in bone mass below normal. Among the causes are osteomalacia and osteoporosis.

Osteoporosis (ah-stee-oh-pore-OH'-sis) [From Greek *osteon*, "bone" + *poros*, "passage," "pore" + *osis*, "a condition," from the Greek word for "suffering."] Decreased bone mass leading to porous and fragile bones that fracture easily. At-risk sites are your upper back, hip, and wrist. Healing is difficult and slow. Occurs mainly in post-menopausal women and elderly men. Important to prevention is resistive exercise, like weightlifting, and resisting your own body weight during weight-bearing exercise like walking, dancing, running, skating, and skiing.

Overload Principle   Term to describe the need for greater-than-accustomed loads to improve exercise capacity. The type of overload required is specific to the system; for example, to increase strength, you need to lift heavier weights (your muscles must contract at tensions close to their maximum). To increase endurance, you need to cover longer distances. To increase your flexibility, you need to regularly take your joints through greater ranges of motion.

Oxygen Debt   A term used as if synonymous with oxygen deficit. Refers to the extra oxygen you use during recovery from exercise to "repay" the oxygen needed but not available at the time of high intensity exercise. When energy stores decrease and lactic acid builds during your "debt" phase, you have to slow or stop exercise, and gasp for more oxygen while your limbs burn with lactic acid. The oxygen you take in during your "debt-paying" phase is used to make energy and remove lactic acid. See Anaerobic Capacity and Lactic Acid.

P

Parasympathetic Nervous System   Part of your autonomic nervous system. Works to decrease heart rate, decrease blood pressure, dilate blood vessels, and stimulate digestive secretions. Inhibits or opposes your sympathetic nervous system. Your parasympathetic nervous system nerves originate in your brain stem and the lower part of your spinal cord. See Sympathetic Nervous System.

Perfusion   [From Latin *perfundere*, "to pour."] Blood flow.

Periosteum   (per-ee-OSS'-tee-um)   [From Greek *peri*, "around" + *osteon*, "bone."] Membrane that covers your bones except at your bone ends. At bone ends, you have cartilage called articular cartilage. The periosteum is an attachment for your muscles and tendons. In young bones, the periosteum has two layers—the inner one makes new bone tissue, and the outer one is the tough, fibrous connective tissue layer that conveys blood vessels and nerves supplying your bones. As you get older, your inner, bone-producing (osteogenic) layer gets thinner. See Bone, Cortical Bone, and Trabecular Bone.

Physiology   [From Greek *phusis*, "nature" + *ology*, "study."] Study of the functions of living beings and their parts.

Pickwickian Syndrome   Informal, literary name for sleep apnea in obese people, named after the "fat boy" in Dickens' *Pickwick Papers*, who was obese with daytime sluggishness. See Sleep Apnea.

Plantarflex   [From Latin *plantaris*, from *planta*, "sole of your foot."] To bend your ankle so that your foot points toward your sole, or bottom. See Dorsiflex.

Plasma   [From Greek *plassein*, "to mold."] Clear, yellowish, noncellular, fluid part of blood. Makes up about 55% of blood volume. Plasma without the clotting protein fibrinogen is called serum.

Poikilotherm   (POY'-kill-oh-thurm)   [From Greek *poikilos*, "various" + *therme*, "heat."] Animals, such as fish and reptiles, whose body temperature varies depending on surrounding temperature. Sometimes called ectotherms. See Homeotherm.

Postmenopausal   After menopause. A woman is considered postmenopausal when she has had no menses for one year. See Menopause.

Power   [From Latin *potere*, "to be able."] In exercise physiology, power is a measure of how fast you can be strong. Exercise power is the combination of speed and strength. Someone who can lift a weight in two seconds has twice the power of someone who needs four seconds to move that same weight.

Premenopausal   Before menopause. See Menopause.

Prime Mover   Muscle or muscles mainly responsible for a particular movement.

Proprioceptors   [From Latin *proprius*, "one's own" or "self," + *ceptors*, "receiving information."] Sensory receptors in muscles, tendons, joints, and your inner ear. Proprioceptors detect changes in your position or movement. Your most abundant proprioceptors are your muscle spindles, which notice stretch in your muscles. When suddenly stretched, or stretched too far, your spindles send a signal that stimulates another signal that comes back to tell your muscle to contract. Proprioceptors help you keep your balance, and prevent muscle tears from too much stretch. Also called mechanoreceptors. See Myotatic Reflex.

Protein   [From Greek *pratos*, "first."] Large, complex, organic molecules of one or more chains of amino acids. Proteins are fundamental components of all living cells, and necessary for proper functioning. Proteins contain carbon, hydrogen, oxygen, nitrogen, and usually sulfur. Many important body components are proteins, such as enzymes, hormones, and antibodies.

Pubis or **Pubic Bone**   [From Latin *pubes*, "groin."] The front, lower part of your hipbones that form the front arch of your pelvis. Your left and right pubic bones come together in front at your pubic symphysis. The pubic bone is distinct at birth and later fuses together with your other two hipbones, the ilium and ischium. See Ilium and Ischium.

Pyruvic Acid or **Pyruvate**   [From Greek *pyr(o)*, for "fire," "heat," or "derived from acid" + Latin *uva*, "grape" (from being produced by the dry distillation of racemic acid, originally derived from grapes).] Molecule produced from breaking down glucose to make energy (glycolysis). When there is enough oxygen present for the intensity of exercise (aerobic glycolysis), pyruvate can change into another substance called acetyl CoA, which feeds into your aerobic metabolism where you can make much more energy. When there isn't enough oxygen (during anaerobic glycolysis), pyruvate turns to lactate (or lactic acid). In this case, energy is limited, and the lactate building in your working muscles causes a burning feeling. See Aerobic Metabolism, Glycolysis, and Lactic Acid.

Q

Q_{10} **Effect**   The enzyme reactions in your cells that produce energy and control body functions speed up as your body temperature rises. A 10° C rise would double the rate of enzyme reactions. This is called the Q_{10} Effect. Your internal temperature could never change 10° without severe health consequences, but the two to four degrees that a warm-up raises your temperature uses the Q_{10} Effect to boost athletic performance, make stretching safer, and soothe arthritic joints.

S

Sacrum   [From Latin *sacrum*, "sacred" (bone).] Broad, slightly curved, triangular bone forming the back wall of your pelvis. Made of five fused vertebrae. It joins your lowest lumbar vertebra from above, your coccyx below, and your hip bones on either side.

Scoliosis   [Greek *skolios*, "crooked" + the suffix *osis*, "a condition."]   Sideways curving or twisting of the spine. There may be one or more curves, and may be due to muscle and/or bone deformity, or chronic unequal muscle contractions. Associated pain can often be reduced with good back exercises.

Sleep Apnea   Sleep disorder involving snoring, where the snorer stops breathing during sleep because of upper airway obstruction, causing repeated shortage of oxygen to the brain. Sleep apnea sufferers are often overweight, heavy-necked males, but heavy females are also affected. Sleep apnea raises the incidence of stroke and cardiac irregularities. The repeated awakenings from the apnea, sometimes hundreds per night, result in chronic daytime sleepiness. This sleepiness is documented to greatly raise the risk of serious automobile accidents. Sleep apnea can be stopped, but not cured, using high-pressure air that opens airways, delivered by face mask worn during sleep. The machine is called a Continuous Positive Air Pressure (CPAP) machine. For long-term treatment, losing weight is often effective.

Somatotyping   Body classification system according to three characteristics—thinness (ectomorphy), fatness (endomorphy), and muscularity (mesomorphy). Nobody is only one type, but a combination of them, usually with one or two predominating.

Spondylolisthesis (spon-di-lo-lis-THEE'-sis) [From Greek *spondylo* + *olisthsis*,   "slipping and falling."] Slipping, resulting in abnormal forward movement, of one of the vertebrae on the vertebra below it. Sometimes associated with low back pain. Although the bones may not move back into place, the pain is often easily relieved with regular back exercises.

Spot Reducing   Any method thought to remove fat only from specific body areas. Although there are many products and potions on the market promising spot reduction of body fat, only liposuction works.

Sprain   Partial or complete tear of a ligament, from stretching past its limit of range. Usually painful.

Strain   [From Latin *stringere*, "to extend" (and from which we may get the word *perestroika*.] To injure a muscle, sometimes from overuse, sometimes from stretching past its limits.

Strength   [From Old English *strang*, "strong."] Ability to move a heavy weight one or few times.

Stroke Volume   Amount of blood ejected from your heart with each beat. Stroke volume (SV) times heart rate is cardiac output, or SV x HR = Q. If stroke volume increases with increased venous return, as with immersion or lying down, heart rate decreases to keep cardiac output constant.

Swimmer's Ear   Painful infection or inflammation of your outer ear, which is the part you can see (the auricle) and stick your finger into (the canal). Cotton swabs and scratching your canal contribute to swimmer's ear by removing protective cerumen (ear wax). Earplugs rarely keep water out, and often create conditions good for swimmer's ear by rubbing away wax and holding water in your canal. Swimmer's ear usually is easily prevented and treated with white vinegar or Otic Domeboro drops. Swimmer's ear is not related to middle-ear or inner-ear injuries caused by pressure, or to congestion of your middle ear, so decongestants do not help. Swimmer's ear does not automatically require stopping swimming or diving, just drying your ears afterward. Serious and recurring cases need medical intervention.

Sympathetic Nervous System   [From Greek *sympatheo*, "to feel with."] Part of your autonomic nervous system. Works to increase heart rate and blood vessel constriction, and reduce digestive secretions. Opposes and balances your parasympathetic nervous system. Your sympathetic nervous system nerves originate in the thoracic and lumbar regions of your spinal cord. See Parasympathetic Nervous System and Sympathomimetic.

Sympathomimetic (sim-path-oh-my-MET'-ik) [From *sympatho*, for the sympathetic nervous system + *mimikos*, "imitating."] A substance that mimics the action of your sympathetic nervous system by releasing nerve transmitter chemicals called catecholamines (especially epinephrine and norepinephrine) from nerve endings. Commonly known sympathomimetic substances are amphetamines, ephedrine (found in "health food" stimulants and certain allergy medicines), phenylephrine (powerful vasoconstrictor used in preparations to relieve nasal congestion and maintain blood pressure during anesthesia), and phenylpropanolamine (used as a nasal decongestant, a bronchodilator, and appetite suppressant). The term *adrenomimetic* has been proposed to replace the term *sympathomimetic*, which some feel to be less accurate. Adrenomimetic (add-REE'-no-my-MET'-ik) means having an action similar to that of your body chemicals epinephrine and norepinephrine. In general, the term sympathomimetic is used rather loosely, but should be used only when discussing drugs that actually produce effects that mimic activation of your entire sympathetic system, not just central nervous system stimulation. Not everything that is a central nervous system stimulant is sympathomimetic, for example, caffeine, nicotine, strychnine, and picrotoxin. Strychnine and picrotoxin are such strong central nervous system stimulants that they are considered convulsants. See Amphetamines, Ergogenic Aid, Ma Huang, and Sympathetic Nervous System.

T

Tendon   [From Latin *tendere*, "to stretch." This derivation is interesting, as tendons don't stretch greatly except with injury.] Tough, fibrous, inelastic modification of the ends of muscle, which connect your muscles to your bones.

Thoracic Vertebrae   [From Latin *thorax*, "breastplate" or "chest."] Twelve upper back bones, named T1–T12, from upper to lower. A pair of ribs attaches to each thoracic vertebra, 12 pairs of ribs in all. Both men and women have 12 paired ribs, 24 total. Men do not have one less rib.

Trabecular Bone (tra-BECK'-you-lar)   [From Latin, diminutive of *trabs*, "beam."] Spongy, branching, supporting meshwork of bone found mostly in your vertebrae and the ends of long bones. Decreased density first occurs in trabecular bone.

U

Undine's Curse   Alternate spelling for Ondine's Curse. See Ondine's Curse and Sleep Apnea.

V

Vasoconstriction   [From Latin *vas*, "vessel" + Latin *constrict*, "to compress."] Decrease in diameter of blood vessels, usually arterioles.

Vasodilation   [From Latin *vas*, "vessel" + Latin *dilatare*, "to enlarge."] Increase in diameter of blood vessels, usually arterioles.

Veins   Membranous, branching system of thin-walled tubes that carry blood from all areas of your body back to your heart for transport to your lungs. See Arteries.

Vertebra (plural vertebrae) [From Latin *verto*, "to turn."] Spine bone. Humans usually have 33 vertebrae—seven cervical (C1–C7), 12 thoracic (T1–T12), five lumbar (L1–L5), five sacral (fused into one bone, your sacrum), and four coccygeal (fused into one bone, your coccyx). Each vertebra bears the weight of all your body above it.

Vitamins [From Latin *vita*, "life" + amine, so called because they were originally thought to be amines.] Any of various organic substances essential for normal growth and activity. Deficiencies may cause various diseases and problems, but taking above a needed amount has not been shown to have beneficial effects. It is often difficult to determine a "needed amount," making the topic difficult to study.

Vo_{2max} (pronounced vee-oh-tu-max) Vo_2 is how much oxygen you consume. Max Vo_2 is the maximum amount of oxygen your system can extract and use to do exercise.

W

Waist-to-Hip Ratio A simple, general test of physical status. Take your waist and hip measurements. Divide your waist by your hip measurement. For health, stay below 0.8 for women and 1.0 for men.

Warm-up Raising your body temperature until it is more energy efficient, and safer for your joints and cardiovascular health to exercise. Best accomplished with slow, gradual increase in physical activity of your large limbs, as with walking, cycling, and slow jogging. Can also be assisted by passive heating with hot baths and local heat packs.

Weight-Bearing Activity Exercise where body weight provides the resistance, as in walking, running, dancing, skiing, skating, and hiking. Regular weight-bearing exercise is known to increase bone density and reduce risk of osteoporosis in your hip and back. You need to add weightlifting (or push-ups) to increase bone density at the third site that is most at risk for osteoporosis, your wrist.

Weight-Loading Activity Exercise where external weight provides the resistance, as in weightlifting and carrying packages. Regular weight loading is known to increase bone density and reduce risk of osteoporosis.

About the Author

Dr. Jolie Bookspan is a sports medicine specialist and physiologist who studies how the human body works during exercise in extremes of heat, cold, altitude, high and low oxygen, G-force, weightlessness, decompression, immersion, and injury states.

She has worked as a scientist at an underwater laboratory, taught anatomy at a college in the mountains of Mexico (where the entrance exam was getting up there without a nosebleed), was advisor to The Discovery Channel, and studied and researched in India, North Africa, and Asia.

She is the author of "Diving Physiology in Plain English" and three hyperbaric medical textbooks, numerous articles for technical and popular health magazines, and nine medical textbook chapters.

Left paralyzed in an accident, she rehabbed with her own methods while doctors insisted that she accept she would never walk again. Two months after walking again, a second accident left her paralyzed, even more seriously than before. She walked again years later, against all expectations.

Formerly a career military researcher and national class athlete, Dr. Bookspan has a black belt in karate, is happily married to Paul, also a black belt, and has a successful neck and back pain sports medicine practice in Philadelphia.

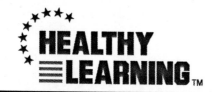